Medical Conditions Affecting
Pregnancy and Childbirth

Medical Conditions Affecting Pregnancy and Childbirth

Judy Bothamley
Senior Lecturer in Midwifery
Thames Valley University

and

Maureen Boyle
Senior Lecturer in Midwifery
Thames Valley University

Radcliffe Publishing
Oxford • New York

Radcliffe Publishing Ltd
18 Marcham Road
Abingdon
Oxon OX14 1AA
United Kingdom

www.radcliffe-oxford.com
Electronic catalogue and worldwide online ordering facility.

Every effort has been made to ensure the accuracy of these guidelines, and that the best information available has been used. This does not diminish the requirement to exercise clinical judgement, and neither the publishers nor the authors can accept any responsibility for their use in practice.

British Library Cataloguing in Publication Data

A catalogue record for this book is available from the British Library.

ISBN-13: 978 184619 240 1

Typeset by Pindar NZ, Auckland, New Zealand
Printed and bound by Hobbs the Printers, Southampton, UK

Contents

Preface

The Confidential Enquiry into Maternal and Child Health (CEMACH) report *Saving Mothers' Lives* (Lewis, 2007) highlighted a number of reasons why health professionals are encountering more women whose pregnancies are complicated by medical conditions. The number of women with cardiac disease becoming pregnant is growing each year, although this is unfortunately the most common cause of maternal deaths. Obesity, older age and the complex health problems of women born outside the UK have also been identified as key factors. Women with serious medical conditions who would have previously been unable to contemplate pregnancy are now able to access specialist care and become mothers.

This changing face of maternity care presents a challenge to midwives and midwifery education. Every woman having a baby should have access to midwifery care and this book aims to help midwives gain knowledge of medical conditions so they are confident in the support and care they provide. There are three aspects to that midwifery care.

Firstly, the midwife offers a connection with the reality of this normal life event. For the woman who has a medical condition, the experience of expecting a baby, giving birth and being a parent is the main event in her life, albeit with possible concerns for her own and her baby's health. This is a life-changing experience for her, as for any other parent, and the midwife's involvement can do much to promote an element of normality.

Secondly, the midwife can be a key person on the multidisciplinary team as her scope of practice encompasses pregnancy, labour and the puerperium, including support in adaptation to motherhood, and therefore she is in an ideal position to co-ordinate care and to provide some continuity. The woman may have an extensive medical input, an array of tests and medication as well as needing to comprehend the new aspects of her condition now she is pregnant. The midwife, in addition to her usual responsibilities, can offer explanations of diagnostic tests, liaise with other members of the team, care for the woman in a high-dependency care setting, give advice and information and listen to and respond to the woman's concerns associated with her pregnancy and her medical condition.

Thirdly, the midwife, when assessing the woman, needs to identify signs and symptoms not usual for pregnancy and recognise a medical condition or its deterioration, as well as being able to make a timely and appropriate referral.

This book aims to equip the midwife to perform these roles. Each chapter includes physiological information, explanations of the condition and principles of care for preconception, pregnancy, labour, delivery and the postnatal period. The content was determined by current areas of concern, with substantial material in the areas of diabetes, cardiac diseases and obesity as well as including more common medical conditions like asthma and anaemia. The text aims to bring together basic human physiology, knowledge of changes in pregnancy and an understanding of the condition in an integrated and accessible way. This will be valuable for midwives and of particular benefit to student midwives new to these subjects.

Although each chapter can stand alone, nevertheless reference will often need to be made across the book – for example, many conditions predispose to pre-eclampsia and thromboembolism, and therefore these sections will need to be accessed. Explanations of laboratory tests, diagnostic tests and common drugs are included in the relevant chapters. Where there is relevant literature regarding psychosocial elements of specific conditions, this is included.

The midwife has a key role in the pregnancy of a woman with complications. All women – not just those considered normal – should have access to midwifery care that will offer support throughout the childbirth process.

Judy Bothamley
Maureen Boyle
January 2009

About the authors

Judy Bothamley (RN, RM, ADM PGCEA, MA) is a senior lecturer in midwifery at Thames Valley University in London. Following nurse training in her native country of Australia she qualified as a midwife in the UK in 1983. Her varied career has included working with high-risk women in the delivery suite of a tertiary referral unit; providing continuity of care for teenagers and doing research with the partners of teenage mothers; studying the experiences of Somali woman in the NHS; and being the lead midwife in the antenatal clinic and ward. She has published material on the experience of fathers and on tuberculosis in pregnancy and has contributed a chapter on thromboembolism in *Emergencies Around Childbirth: a handbook for midwives* (Radcliffe Publishing, 2002). She is the lead for physiology teaching at Thames Valley University and has written workbook material for both postgraduate and undergraduate modules, including distance learning materials. She likes to see physiology applied to practice in a way that is easy to understand.

Maureen Boyle (RN, RM, ADM PGCEA, MSc) is a senior lecturer in midwifery at Thames Valley University in London. After working as a nurse in Canada, she qualified as a midwife in the UK in 1985 and has practiced since then at St Mary's Hospital in Paddington, London. She has specialised in the support of women experiencing complications in pregnancy and delivery, using this to underpin the development of a CPPD module for experienced midwives, *High Dependency Care for Midwives*. She has published widely, including editing *Emergencies Around Childbirth: a handbook for midwives* (Radcliffe Publishing, 2002) and *Wound Healing in Midwifery* (Radcliffe Publishing, 2006).

CHAPTER 1
Diabetes mellitus

CONTENTS
- → Definitions
- → Introduction
- → Physiology and pathophysiology
- → Blood tests
- → Pregnancy complications of diabetes
- → Type 1 diabetes: care issues
- → Type 2 diabetes: care issues
- → Gestational diabetes: care issues
- → Role of the midwife
- → Psychosocial issues
- → Commonly used drugs

DEFINITIONS

Type 1 Diabetes mellitus: established (pre-pregnancy) insulin-dependent diabetes (this may very rarely be diagnosed in pregnancy).

Type 2 Diabetes mellitus: established (pre-pregnancy) non-insulin-dependent diabetes is usually controlled with anti-diabetic oral medication (if not previously diagnosed, it may be misdiagnosed in pregnancy as gestational diabetes).

Gestational diabetes mellitus: carbohydrate intolerance of varying degrees of severity with the onset or first recognition during pregnancy and which resolves after pregnancy.

INTRODUCTION

Diabetes has been recognised for more than 2000 years. The word comes from Greek for siphon, referring to the speed of water passing through the body – polyuria. Although the value of diet modifications has long been recognised, there was no treatment until insulin was discovered in 1922, for which the researchers from Toronto (Banting, Best and others) received the Nobel prize (Hadden, 2003). As women with diabetes began to survive, they were able to become pregnant, and although up until the 1940s this was still considered dangerous, improvements in their care increased the success rate of these pregnancies. However, despite the St Vincent's Declaration written by the WHO and the International Diabetes Federation in 1989, which included the aim that pregnancy outcomes in diabetic women should approximate those in women without diabetes (Diabetes Care and Research in Europe, 1990), in 2007 the Confidential Enquiry into Maternal and Child Health (CEMACH, 2007) published findings showing the risks continued for both mother and baby.

There is clear evidence to underpin caring for those with Type 1 diabetes, although this is not always achieved. Type 2 diabetic women are a more unusual (although fast growing) group, and therefore there has been less experience and less evidence of how to care for them. However, Type 2 diabetes needs to be recognised to be as serious as Type 1 in pregnancy (Keely and Montoro, 2008).

In addition to the ongoing risk, there is evidence that the number of women with all types of diabetes is increasing, probably resulting from lifestyle changes such as in creasing obesity, the reduction in activity levels and changes of diet (Amos, *et al.*, 1997; National Institute for Health and Clinical Excellence (NICE) 2008). Births to women with Type 1 or 2 diabetes constitute about 0.38% of all births in England, Wales and Northern Ireland (approximately 1:264) (CEMACH, 2007). Type 2 incidence varies widely throughout the counties studied, probably reflecting the varying ethnic diversity of the population. Gestational diabetes may complicate up to 3.5% of pregnancies (NICE, 2008), although it must be remembered that follow-up studies of these women have suggested that as many as 20–50% of women diagnosed with gestational diabetes may have had pre-existing undiagnosed diabetes prior to pregnancy (Maresh, 2002).

There is therefore an ongoing need for increased awareness of the effects of diabetes on pregnancy and for knowledgeable midwives to care for these women. An understanding of carbohydrate metabolism in normal pregnancy is necessary to underpin this.

PHYSIOLOGY AND PATHOPHYSIOLOGY

The need to provide adequate nutrients to support fetal growth and development brings about major changes to the metabolism of a pregnant woman, in particular, changes to carbohydrate and fat metabolism. The fetus needs nutrients for the tremendous growth and development that takes place *in utero* as well as requiring adequate stores of energy and substrates for the transition to extra-uterine life. This fetal demand is balanced against the maternal need for energy and nutrients for the physiological demands of pregnancy, labour and lactation (*see* Figure 1.1). Any compromise of metabolic function, which is closely linked to hormonal changes, such as a lack of insulin, will affect the health of the mother and fetus/baby.

Diabetes is caused by an absence or limitation of insulin, a key hormone for carbohydrate metabolism. Metabolism is a general term for the chemical reactions in the body that enable it to function. All the metabolic pathways in the body start with the digestion and absorption of carbohydrates, fats and proteins. The body then uses these nutrients to provide the energy and raw materials it requires. The preferred fuel molecule for cellular activity is glucose, although fats and proteins can be utilised when

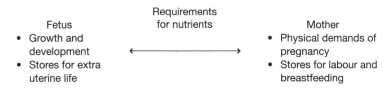

FIGURE 1.1: Metabolic tug of war

glucose is not available. Plasma glucose needs to be maintained within the normal range (4–8 mmol) and a store of glycogen maintained as emergency fuel (Blackburn, 2007).

Glucose is derived from the breakdown of carbohydrates. It is absorbed into the blood capillaries of the villi of the small intestine and transported via the portal circulation to the liver.

Glucose is used in a number of ways (*see* Figure 1.2):

▶ glucose is broken down to form adenosine triphosphate (ATP) (energy transfer molecule) and used for the metabolic activity of the liver and other body cells
▶ some glucose remains in the circulating blood to maintain blood glucose levels
▶ some excess glucose is converted to glycogen and stored in liver and skeletal muscle (glycogenesis)
▶ further excess glucose is converted to fat deposits.

Insulin is necessary for glucose to be utilised by cells.

When blood glucose levels fall, glucose can be generated from glycogen in the liver and muscle under the influence of the hormones adrenaline (in times of stress), thyroxine and predominantly glucagon (glycogenolysis). Glucose can also be generated from non-carbohydrate sources such as amino acids (protein) and fat (gluconeogenesis).

INSULIN AND GLUCAGON

Insulin is a small protein hormone secreted by the beta cells in the islets of Langerhans in the pancreas. When blood glucose levels rise more insulin is secreted. In simple terms insulin acts like a key to unlock the cell to allow glucose to enter the cell and be utilised. Insulin brings about changes in cell surface membrane permeability and enzyme activity to allow the uptake of glucose and amino acids into cells. The maintenance of stable blood sugar is regulated by insulin and glucagons, which act in opposition to each other (*see* Figure 1.3).

Glucagon is secreted by alpha cells in the islets of Langerhans, triggered by a fall in blood sugar levels. Glucagon activates enzymes in the liver, which catalyses the breakdown of glycogen to glucose.

Insulin is also involved in the regulation of amino acids and fats. With reduced insulin or loss of its action there is an increase in blood sugar and amino acids. Furthermore increased breakdown of fats will occur and ketones are produced.

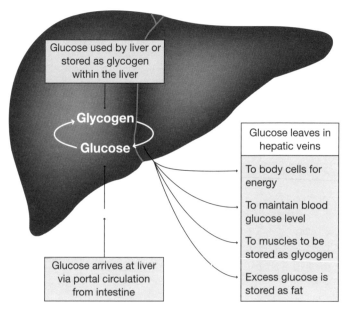

FIGURE 1.2: Utilisation of glucose in the liver

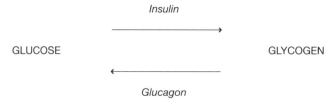

FIGURE 1.3: Insulin and glucagon

CARBOHYDRATE METABOLISM IN NORMAL PREGNANCY

Changes in carbohydrate and lipid metabolism occur in pregnancy to ensure a constant supply of nutrients (predominantly glucose) to the growing fetus. There is a difference in the focus of the changes between early and late pregnancy.

Early pregnancy

In early pregnancy there is a metabolic drive to laying down fat stores as a preparatory phase for the later demands of the pregnancy. Less insulin appears to be required in early pregnancy with accompanying enhanced insulin sensitivity (Catalano, 2003). There are a number of reasons for this. Firstly, the embryo and young fetus are utilising available glucose directly from the mother's bloodstream. Cells, particularly those that make up adipose tissue, develop an increased sensitivity to insulin, encouraging an enhanced uptake of nutrients and resulting in enhanced fat storage. Decreased amounts of food may be consumed in early pregnancy because of nausea in pregnancy (Catalano, 2003), although other writers suggest that food intake increases (Blackburn, 2007). It has been observed that pregnant women tend to eat frequent carbohydrate-based snacks in early pregnancy to combat feelings of nausea. Finally, significant tiredness resulting in activity decrease is noted by women in the early stages of pregnancy, thereby conserving energy use.

Overall, in early pregnancy an increased response to insulin lowers fasting blood glucose, which leads to an increased uptake of glucose and nutrients that in turn results in an increase in maternal fat stores.

Late pregnancy

From 20 weeks to term insulin secretion increases progressively, as does insulin resistance (Catalano, *et al.*, 1993). Insulin resistance means that a normal response by the cells to a given amount of insulin is reduced and as a result, higher levels of insulin are needed. Returning to the analogy that insulin is the key that unlocks the cell to allow glucose to enter, in insulin resistance the lock is stiff and needs more insulin to prise it open. Insulin resistance means that blood glucose levels do not drop as rapidly as usual after a meal. The mechanism for increased insulin resistance is poorly understood, but it appears to be mediated by increasing levels of placental hormones (Butte, 2000). Glucose is kept in the plasma longer and can be carried via the placenta to ensure a consistent supply to the fetus. High glucose levels in the renal circulation, along with an increased glomerular filtration rate, mean that glucose can spill into the urine of a pregnant woman (Coad and Dunstall, 2005).

Placental glucose transport to the fetus is not dependent on insulin. During the post-absorptive state when the supply of glucose has diminished, plasma glucose levels fall as the fetus drains the supply. Glucose supply to the mother's central nervous system is preferentially maintained (Blackburn, 2007).

Effects on fat metabolism

Changes in hormonal levels as pregnancy advances also have an effect on fat metabolism. To conserve glucose for the fetus, fat is used more readily as an alternative to glucose. Fats are the body's most concentrated source of energy and are broken down into free fatty acids and glycerol. Pregnant women may experience more rapid development of ketosis and thus should avoid long periods without food. Ketones can cross the placenta and have been implicated in neurological impairment in the fetus (Butte, 2000). Diets that restrict calorie intake are not recommended in pregnancy: instead, a mixed diet that includes complex carbohydrates, protein and fat should be taken.

TYPE 1 DIABETES MELLITUS

Type 1 diabetes is caused by a lack of insulin. The most common reason for Type 1 diabetes is the autoimmune destruction of the beta cells. Genetic and environmental factors are thought to influence susceptibility (Williams and Pickup, 2004). Type 1 diabetes usually develops in a younger age group and pregnant women with Type 1 diabetes may have managed their condition for a number of years. Symptoms of undiagnosed Type 1 diabetes can be severe and have a sudden onset. Without insulin the cells cannot utilise available glucose and blood sugar levels rise. High blood glucose levels pass into the kidneys and filter into the urine (glycosuria). Glucose pulls water after it, resulting in polyuria and dehydration. Thirst increases to maintain body fluids. Weight loss occurs as the body tries to mobilise energy from fats and protein. The breakdown of body fat causes an excess production of ketone bodies. These are acidic and when they accumulate in the blood, the pH drops, causing ketoacidosis (Waugh and Grant, 2006). Diabetes is treated by using insulin injections to control blood glucose levels to within the normal range and eating a diet containing a controlled amount of carbohydrates. The changes to carbohydrate metabolism in pregnancy present a challenge to women with Type 1 diabetes to maintain their normal blood sugars.

TYPE 2 AND GESTATIONAL DIABETES MELLITUS (GDM)

The CEMACH report (2005) has highlighted the increased trend of problems associated with Type 2 diabetes in pregnancy. Type 2 diabetes develops when there is a progressive deterioration of beta cell function with a consequent diminishing of insulin production alongside increasing insulin resistance. Type 2 diabetes has been traditionally observed in the elderly and treated with diet and oral hypoglycaemic agents. However, an increased rate of obesity and other lifestyle changes have amplified the incidence of Type 2 diabetes in the young and child-bearing population (Dunne, 2005). Type 2 diabetes has been perceived as a less severe form of diabetes but this is not true in pregnancy, as perinatal mortality and congenital malformation occur at a similar incidence as for Type 1 diabetes (CEMACH, 2005; Clausen, *et al.*, 2005; Dunne, 2005; Macintosh, *et al.*, 2006). There is also an increased incidence of hypertension, pre-eclampsia, operative delivery and post-partum haemorrhage associated with Type 2 diabetes (Dunne, 2005). Type 2 diabetes and GDM share similar risk factors, have a corresponding prevalence and have the same genetic susceptibility (Ben-Haroush, *et al.*, 2003).

Pregnancy represents a metabolic challenge with increased insulin resistance by the tissues, creating a demand for more insulin. For most women, insulin requirements are readily met. If the insulin requirements are not met, hyperglycaemia develops and diabetes becomes overt as GDM. GDM pregnancies feature exaggerated insulin resistance as well as impaired insulin production (Verhaeghe, 2004).

Early development of GDM and the need to treat it with insulin coincides with the greatest risk of undiagnosed Type 2 diabetes (Ben-Haroush, *et al.*, 2003). In the rare occurrence of a new diagnosis during pregnancy of Type 1 diabetes, the woman will usually be very ill with symptoms and ketoacidosis. Those with Type 2 are rarely symptomatic and the diagnosis of GDM may be made initially and later confirmed to be Type 2 diabetes following delivery. Women who have true gestational diabetes are at significantly increased risk of the development of Type 2 diabetes in the future (Hadden, *et al.*, 2004), and it has been suggested that 40–60% of women diagnosed with gestational diabetes will have Type 2 diabetes within 10–15 years (Nelson-Piercy, 2006; Walsh, 2004).

Figure 1.4 shows the interrelationship between genetics, lifestyle and insulin resistance. Insulin resistance is a feature of polycystic ovarian syndrome and contributes to a high incidence of obesity in these women. Insulin resistance prevents cells using sugar in the blood normally and the sugar is stored as fat instead. Women who have polycystic ovarian syndrome and, in particular, those who are obese are at increased risk of Type 2 diabetes and GDM if they are pregnant (*see* Chapter 11 for further information on polycystic ovarian syndrome).

Obesity and diabetes

The link between obesity and Type 2 diabetes is clear. What is less well understood is why obesity interferes with carbohydrate metabolism. One suggested mechanism is that fat cells produce substances (adipocytokines) that interfere with the signaling pathways in the cell and impair the cell's ability to respond to insulin (Powell, 2007).

The association between diabetes and obesity is compounded by inactivity. Physical exercise increases insulin sensitivity, improves glucose tolerance, corrects blood lipid abnormalities, lowers blood pressure and helps weight loss.

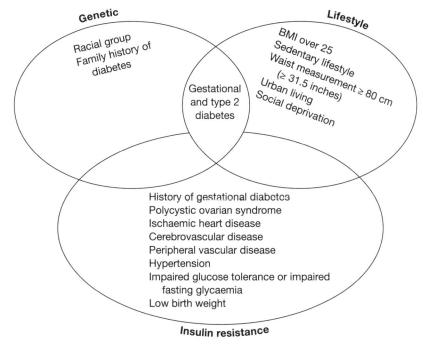

FIGURE 1.4: Interrelationship of genetics, lifestyle and insulin resistance

Sources: CEMACH (2005); Diabetes UK (2006); Fletcher, *et al.* (2002); Williams and Pickup (2004)

BLOOD TESTS
ORAL GLUCOSE TOLERANCE TEST (GTT)

There is much debate over the method, use and interpretation of this test, and local criteria may vary. It aims to diagnose gestational diabetes by measuring the blood glucose response to a carbohydrate load. After an overnight fast (8–14 hours), blood is taken to determine the woman's fasting blood sugar. The woman is then asked to drink a glucose-containing fluid (usually 75 g). After two hours a further blood test is taken for blood glucose estimation. Gestational diabetes is typically diagnosed when the fasting level is ≥ 6.1 mmol/L and the two-hour value is ≥ 7–8 mmol/L. The test is not physiological in that most food is taken in a mixed form of carbohydrates, fats and proteins. Results are difficult to interpret as there is a relatively wide normal distribution of carbohydrate indices in asymptomatic pregnant women.

MINI ORAL GLUCOSE TOLERANCE TEST

This test is used as a screening tool, either routinely or for those in a risk category from about 26–28 weeks' gestation. A glucose drink (usually 50 g) is given to the woman, and her blood is taken after one hour. An abnormal result (levels vary but usually > 7.7 mmol/L) will lead to a full oral glucose tolerance test as described above, and gestational diabetes will be diagnosed on those findings.

RANDOM BLOOD SUGAR

Some areas include a random blood sugar test as part of their routine booking bloods (or it may be offered to those with previous gestational diabetes) to screen for undiagnosed Type 2 diabetes. A level of 5.8–6.4 mmol/L (depending on when her last meal was) would lead to a full oral glucose tolerance test for diagnosis.

GLYCOSYLATED HAEMOGLOBIN

Glucose in the blood becomes bound irreversibly to the haemoglobin of red blood cells over an approximately 10-week period, forming glycosylated haemoglobin (HbA1c). The more glucose available in the blood, the more glycosylated haemoglobin will be present. Measurement of HbA1c therefore gives an indication of the levels to which the red cells have been exposed over the previous two months (Maresh, 2002). NICE (2008) does not recommend the use of this test for routine assessment during the second and third trimester of a woman with diabetes; however, at booking a raised HbA1c may highlight the need to offer increased screening for fetal anomalies (*see* the following section) or pre-eclampsia.

PREGNANCY COMPLICATIONS OF DIABETES
EFFECTS OF DIABETES ON THE WOMAN

Box 1.1 provides a summary of the maternal complications of diabetes in pregnancy.

BOX 1.1: SUMMARY OF MATERNAL COMPLICATIONS

- Hypoglycaemia
- Diabetic retinopathy
- Diabetic nephropathy
- Hypertension
- Diabetic ketoacidosis
- Infection and impaired wound healing
- Premature labour

Hypoglycaemia

The tight glycaemic controls that are advocated for pregnancy may lead to hypoglycaemia. Women may recognise hypoglycaemic symptoms which include autonomic nervous system reactions (including sweating, pounding heart, shaking and hunger) and those caused by the depletion of glucose in the brain (such as confusion, drowsiness, difficulty with speech and atypical behaviour). Most hypoglycaemic events occur in the first 20 weeks of pregnancy (Ang, *et al.*, 2006; Williams and Pickup, 2004).

Microvascular disease

Damage to the capillary blood vessels of diabetics includes retinopathy (eye), nephropathy (kidney) and neuropathy (nerve). These areas are particularly vulnerable because glucose is used by these cells in a way that is independent of insulin, unlike other body cells.

In *diabetic retinopathy* the arteries in the retina become weakened and leak, forming small, dot-like haemorrhages. These leaking vessels can lead to swelling or oedema in the retina and decreased vision. With further proliferative damage, circulation problems cause areas of the retina to become oxygen-deprived or ischaemic. Pregnancy can advance the progression of retinopathy (Perri, *et al.*, 2003), but if the retinopathy is treated there is usually a successful outcome. Both Type 1 and Type 2 diabetic women should ideally have been assessed for diabetic retinopathy pre-pregnancy and will be checked at least 2–3 times during the pregnancy (Maresh, 2002; Nelson-Piercy, 2006).

Microvascular injury to the kidney will damage the glomerular membrane and protein will leak into the urine. As kidney function deteriorates the loss of protein will cause fluid retention and the kidneys will be less efficient at removing waste products such as creatinine. This is known as *diabetic nephropathy* and will contribute to complications in pregnancy, including pre-eclampsia, hypertension, low birth weight and preterm delivery. A decline in renal function is common in pregnancy and is related to the pre-pregnancy renal function (Rosenn and Miodovnik, 2003). The renal function must be monitored closely throughout pregnancy and if it deteriorates then, whatever the gestation, delivery is recommended (Maresh, 2002). Women with this condition are usually admitted to hospital for close monitoring of their condition and that of the fetus. Intra-uterine growth restriction (IUGR) is a common complicating factor. Care must be taken not to confuse this condition with pre-eclampsia, since it has so many common features. Related hypertension can cause ongoing renal damage so antihypertensive medication is often used (Nelson-Piercy, 2006).

Hypertension

Hypertension is twice as common in those with diabetes than in the general population. In Type 2 diabetes hypertension is associated with central obesity, dyslipidaemia (high triglycerides) and atherosclerosis, which are all factors in increasing insulin resistance. In Type 1 diabetes, hypertension is associated with diabetic nephropathy. Control of blood pressure is important because hypertension worsens microvascular disease and predisposes the woman to coronary heart disease and stroke. Chronic hypertension is also a risk factor for the development of pre-eclampsia in pregnancy.

Diabetic ketoacidosis

(Note: ketoacidosis should not be confused with ketosis, which is one of the body's normal processes to metabolise body fat.) Ketoacidosis is a serious complication of diabetes and, although it is far more common in Type 1, it has been reported in Type 2 and even in women with gestational diabetes (Newton and Raskin, 2004). Development of ketoacidosis can be more rapid in pregnancy (Keely and Montoro, 2008). Uncontrolled hyperglycaemia occurs because of a lack of insulin exacerbated by the presence of catabolic counter-regulatory stress hormones, glucagons and catecholamines. An excess

breakdown of fats releases free fatty acids into the circulation. In the liver these fatty acids are partially oxidised and contribute to keto acids and acetone. The latter gives a distinctive smell on the breath. Keto acids produce a metabolic acidosis disturbing the pH of the blood, which is harmful to cell metabolism (Yogev, *et al.*, 2003). Acidosis stimulates the brain's respiratory centre, which causes the deep sighing and rapid breathing known as Kussmaul's respiration. Hyperglycaemia results in glycosuria and this triggers osmotic diuresis, dehydration and the loss of the important electrolytes potassium and sodium. *See* Box 1.2 for factors precipitating ketoacidosis in diabetic pregnancies.

BOX 1.2: FACTORS PRECIPITATING KETOACIDOSIS IN DIABETIC PREGNANCIES

- Hyperemesis and/or vomiting
- Infection
- Tocolytics
- Steroids given for lung maturity
- Insulin pump failure
- Failure to take insulin (non-compliance)
- Poor management

(Ang, *et al.*, 2006; Kamalakannan, *et al.*, 2003; Yogev, *et al.*, 2003)

Coma and death can occur if untreated (Williams and Pickup, 2004). Upon observation of the signs and symptoms (*see* Box 1.3) prompt treatment is necessary – diabetic ketoacidosis is an emergency which needs the mobilisation of the multidisciplinary team. Investigations are predominantly laboratory based, and blood samples will be sent for electrolyte assessment, septic screen, plasma ketone estimation, arterial blood gases and laboratory blood glucose levels, although these will also be done as a bedside test with a glucometer. It should be noted that blood glucose levels may not necessarily be high. Urine also needs to be tested for ketones (some laboratories do not offer plasma ketone testing) and all possible sites of infection need to be assessed.

Management is aimed at rehydration (with non-glucose fluid initially then, when the blood sugar is lowered, a glucose solution) and achieving normal blood glucose levels. To this end, fluid replacement may need to be guided by a central venous pressure (CVP) line and an indwelling urinary catheter. An arterial line may be necessary to monitor arterial blood gases and potassium levels. An infusion of insulin will be used, guided by frequent (approximately hourly) blood glucose estimations. Potassium replacement is also likely to be necessary.

Assessment of the fetal condition should be undertaken by cardiotocography (CTG), however, as always in an emergency situation, the emphasis is on stablising the woman's condition. A bradycardic trace may be observed, but as the woman's condition improves, so should that of the fetus (Hagay, *et al.*, 1994). Nevertheless diabetic ketoacidosis is associated with significant fetal loss.

The woman's understanding and avoidance of the precipitating factors (*see* Box 1.2) is important, and the midwife should ensure she has this knowledge.

BOX 1.3: SIGNS AND SYMPTOMS OF KETOACIDOSIS

- Dehydration
- Weakness
- Hyperventilation (Kussmaul's respiration)
- Abdominal pain
- Vomiting
- Confusion
- Ketone smell
- Coma (10%)

(Kamalakannan, *et al.*, 2003)

Infection

Infections are more common in women with diabetes. Humoral immunity is suppressed, neutrophil function is compromised and defects in antioxidants contribute to the impaired immunology of diabetes. Macrovascular and microvascular disease compromise circulation, leading to a delayed response to infection and impaired wound healing. Defects in immunity, increased hospitalisation and delayed wound healing mean that up to 80% of women with Type 1 diabetes will have at least one episode of infection during their pregnancy (Ang, *et al.*, 2006).

Urinary tract infection, which may precipitate premature labour, is of particular concern in pregnancy and may be due to incomplete bladder emptying caused by autonomic neuropathy and the high sugar concentration in the urine which favours the growth of some bacterial organisms (Shah and Hux, 2003; Williams and Pickup, 2004). Vaginal candida infection (pruritus vulvae) is a common complaint of diabetic women, and pregnancy exacerbates this.

Premature labour

One-third of babies of diabetic mothers are preterm – which is five times the rate of non-diabetic pregnancies (CEMACH, 2007). However, many of these result from elective early delivery of the baby. Nevertheless, the spontaneous premature labour rate is twice that of the general maternal population (CEMACH, 2007). This could be directly associated with complications such as macrosomia and/or polyhydramnios (Maresh, 2002). However, it has also been suggested that the risk of spontaneous preterm birth increases with increasing levels of pregnancy glycaemia (Hedderson, *et al.*, 2003).

Suppression of premature labour with beta-sympathomimetic drugs is generally contraindicated because of their gluconeogenic effect (NICE, 2008). The use of corticosteroids for fetal lung maturity also has the potential to cause extreme hyperglycaemia in the mother; therefore if it is considered necessary, it should be given only in well-controlled situations with IV regimes of insulin and attended by experienced and knowledgeable staff (Maresh, 2002; NICE, 2008).

EFFECT OF DIABETES ON THE FETUS

Many studies have confirmed an increased perinatal mortality and morbidity for babies of diabetic mothers (CEMACH, 2005; Crowther, *et al.*, 2005; Macintosh, *et al.*, 2006). Fetal risks include congenital abnormality, miscarriage, unexplained stillbirth, premature delivery and macrosomia. Neonatal problems for the baby of the diabetic mother include cardiomyopathy, jaundice, hypocalcaemia, hypoglycaemia and respiratory distress syndrome.[*]

It has been suggested that both Type 1 and Type 2 diabetic women have an increased miscarriage rate (Eriksson, 2004; CEMACH, 2007). It is possible that this is directly related to the increased rate of congenital abnormalities.

Congenital abnormality

The occurrence of major congenital abnormalities in babies of diabetic women is two-fold that of non-diabetic women (CEMACH, 2007). While the connection between maternal hyperglycaemia during the period of embryonic organogenesis (3–8 weeks) and congenital abnormality is well established, the aetiology is complex and poorly understood. Excessive production of free radicals, an imbalance of thromboxane and prostacyclin causing impaired tissue vascularisation, accumulation of sorbitol and trace metals and glucose damage to regulating genes have all been proposed (Moley, 2001). Abnormalities include neural tube defects, cardiovascular anomalies, skeletal malformations, and genitourinary and gastrointestinal defects. Good glycaemic control around conception and early pregnancy is advocated, as the risk of congenital abnormality is directly related to the maternal HbA1c level at this time.

Fetal anomaly screening

It is therefore important that a diabetic woman is offered a range of fetal screening and diagnostic tests throughout the pregnancy and is aware that her risk is increased if her HbA1c is raised. An increased HbA1c at about 14 weeks' gestation indicates an increased risk of congenital abnormality (Suhonen, *et al.*, 2000).

Ultrasound nuchal translucency screening may indicate cardiac anomalies and also be more reliable for Down's syndrome screening than serum screening, as alpha-fetoprotein (AFP) values are reduced in a diabetic pregnancy. When using serum screening, unconjugated oestriol is also lower in women with Type 1 diabetes, but other markers are the same (NICE, 2008).

Fetal assessment by ultrasound at 20 weeks is recommended, with particular attention to careful screening of the fetal spine, as neural tube defects (NTD) is the second most common anomaly. NICE (2008) recommends that this scan should include a four-chamber view of the fetal heart and outflow tracts. Fetal echocardiography at 20–22 weeks can be offered where abnormalities are detected or if there is a history of cardiac malformations.

---

[*] It is beyond the remit of this chapter to consider neonatal complications and their care, but it is worth noting that optimum glucose control by the mother during pregnancy will improve outcome for the neonate. As more effort is made to keep mother and baby together after delivery, the midwife is likely to be the primary carer, and referral to a good neonatal text and the NICE Guidelines (NICE, 2008), which contain a chapter on neonatal care, is recommended.

Macrosomia

Macrosomia is caused by the delivery of excessive glucose and other nutrients to the fetus. The hyperglycaemia stimulates the fetal islet cells to produce insulin (which, in the fetus, acts like growth hormone) and other growth factors that promote fat deposition (especially around the upper trunk), larger shoulders and the enlargement of organs (Blackburn, 2007). These infants are therefore at increased risk of delivery complicated by shoulder dystocia and may suffer trauma, including brachial plexus injury or a fractured clavicle. The enlarged organs require greater metabolic activity, and neonatal hypoglycaemia can arise as a rebound effect from the loss of glucose supply at birth.

During the second trimester, maternal diabetic control may determine whether the fetus accelerates growth in the third trimester (Raychaudhuri and Maresh, 2000). In the third trimester poor control can lead to macrosomia, polyhydramnios or premature labour (Maresh, 2002). However, although macrosomia occurs more often in association with poor diabetic control, it can also occur when control is excellent (Nelson-Piercy, 2006).

Fetal surveillance

Ultrasound plays an important part in assessing the well-being of the fetus of a diabetic woman. In the first trimester ultrasound is used for dating the pregnancy and is particularly relevant to these women as induction of labour is a very real option for them.

Growth scans from about 24–26 weeks gestation are recommended every 2–4 weeks (Maresh, 2002; NICE, 2008), and regular assessments of the volume of amniotic fluid may also be carried out. Routine Doppler assessment of fetal well-being is not usual unless the fetus is found to be growth restricted (NICE, 2008) or there are other maternal complications such as pre-eclampsia or vascular disease (Maulik, *et al.*, 2002). It is worth noting that 20% of pregnant diabetic women have evidence of vascular disease (Maresh, 2002).

Some authorities suggest a CTG may be done routinely 2–3 times a week from about 36 weeks' gestation (Maresh, 2002), although this may not be necessary with good maternal control and normal fetal growth. Intra-uterine death cannot be accurately predicted from the CTG (Nelson-Piercy, 2006) or indeed from other fetal assessment tests.

Fetal death

Late unexplained intra-uterine death has been a classic risk of pregnancy in a diabetic woman and is why routine induction of labour, often preterm, was introduced. Recent studies (CEMACH, 2007; NICE, 2008) from the UK suggest this risk is still present, even though most units offer an early delivery to these women. The perinatal mortality rate for diabetic pregnancy is 31.8/1000 births, which is three times that of the general population (Macintosh, *et al.*, 2006). Stillbirths occur most commonly after 36 weeks in diabetic women with poor glycaemic control, polyhydramnios and fetal macrosomia (Nelson-Piercy, 2006). Stillbirth is also more common in women with vascular complications of diabetes and pre-eclampsia in which the fetus is growth restricted.

Reduced uterine blood flow that results in chronic intra-uterine hypoxia, secondary to diabetic vascular damage, is thought to be responsible.

Assessing fetal well-being is important. The fetus can be at risk of asphyxia, increased fetal metabolic rate and increased oxygen requirements and ketoacidosis, and an increased incidence of all these is present if the mother's diabetes is complicated with vascular disease or pre-eclampsia (Luzietti and Rosen, 2003). Therefore, the timing and mode of delivery should be planned according to the individual condition of the mother and fetus, and waiting for spontaneous labour can be safe if diabetes is well controlled and there are no complications (Maresh, 2002), although it has been suggested that this should not exceed 40 weeks' gestation (Nelson-Piercy, 2006).

TYPE 1 DIABETES: CARE ISSUES

The greatly increased knowledge of the needs of a pregnant diabetic woman has enhanced her treatment and pregnancy outcome over the years. The CEMACH study (2007) which reported that many women are not accessing (or being able to access) this care is therefore a great disappointment. While much of this care is outside the midwife's normal remit – such as preconception counselling – it is nevertheless important for her to know all that optimal care could include, so the appropriate advice and referrals can be offered to all diabetic women.

PRECONCEPTION CARE

Although it has long been recognised as an important part of a successful pregnancy in a woman with Type 1 diabetes (*see* Box 1.4), preconception counselling is received by only about one-third of diabetic women (CEMACH, 2007).

BOX 1.4: PRE-PREGNANCY CARE AIMS TO:

- improve control – optimise HbA1c to < 6.1% (NICE, 2008)
- diagnose and treat pre-existing complications (for example, retinopathy, renal disease and hypertension)
- commence folic acid
- optimise health (for example, weight reduction, smoking cessation).

Preconception care may be offered in specific diabetic centres, specialised GP services or in a pre-pregnancy clinic, but increased easily accessible preconception counselling is vital (Maresh, 2002). However, many studies have reported that a substantial number of pregnancies are unplanned (CEMACH, 2007). Good glycaemic control around conception can increase the chance of pregnancy, reduce miscarriage rates and reduce occurrence of fetal congenital abnormalities, and it is recommended that contraception should be used until there is optimal control.

Folic acid supplement administration is recognised as an evidence-based practice during all pregnancies. Type 1 diabetic women are in a high-risk category for NTD and a higher dose of folic acid (5 mg daily) is recommended (NICE, 2008). However, folic acid may be being taken by less than half of diabetic women (CEMACH, 2007).

Counselling about the effects pregnancy might have on them should also be available to each individual diabetic woman. Information on contraindications to pregnancy, such as ischaemic heart disease, severe renal disease and untreated proliferative retinopathy (Nelson-Piercy, 2006) would allow her to make an informed choice before becoming pregnant, rather than being faced with difficult decisions in early pregnancy.

PREGNANCY CARE

Women with diabetes need to be cared for by a multidisciplinary team of obstetrician, diabetic physician, dietician and specialist midwife, and most units now offer a joint diabetic clinic where this expertise, together with any other needs (for example, ophthalmological examinations) can be accessed. The frequency of antenatal visits depends on the maternal diabetic control but every 1–2 weeks has been suggested (Maresh, 2002; NICE, 2008). Routine antenatal care is important, for example, screening for pre-eclampsia. A diabetic woman has an increased risk of developing pre-eclampsia independent of the risk associated with pre-existing renal disease or hypertension. It is suggested that the risk of pre-eclampsia may be associated with glycaemic levels at conception and in early pregnancy, and in fact may increase in direct relationship to the rise in HbA1c before 20 weeks' gestation (Nelson-Piercy, 2006).

Other aspects of routine antenatal care directly relevant to a woman with diabetes include regular abdominal palpation to screen for macrosomia and polyhydramnios, both common pregnancy complications for diabetic women (*see* the *role of the midwife* section for further information on estimation of fetal size). Identification of infection, which could lead to unstable diabetic control, is also important. Regular screening for common complications of a diabetic pregnancy, such as proliferative retinopathy, diabetic nephropathy and hypertension, are necessary (*see* section on *pregnancy complications of diabetes* at the beginning of this chapter).

Dietician involvement and nutritional advice may be necessary, even if the woman has managed her diabetes successfully for many years. Updating and educating her on the importance of diet in pregnancy can be considered, and if the pregnancy is complicated by hyperemesis, or even just morning sickness, this is particularly necessary. See the section on *role of the midwife* later in this chapter for further information.

Women with Type 1 diabetes require increasing amounts of insulin as pregnancy progresses, although in early pregnancy their requirements may fall (*see* section on *carbohydrate metabolism in pregnancy* at the beginning of this chapter). Insulin and the change of doses necessary in pregnancy are prescribed according to individual needs, although they usually include an intermediate-acting dose (once or twice a day) or a combination of rapid and intermediate-acting doses (biphasic). There is some evidence that four injections (i.e., a long-acting baseline and one for each meal) daily are better than two (Nachum, *et al.*, 1999) and this would allow maximum flexibility as well as perhaps achieving better glycaemic control (Nelson-Piercy, 2006). There is also evidence of rapid-acting insulin analogues being increasingly used (Nelson-Piercy, 2006) and these may be more convenient as they can be taken with, as opposed to before, a meal. The use of continuous subcutaneous insulin infusions may also be considered if there is difficulty in obtaining good glucose control. If there is a sudden decrease in insulin requirement in the third trimester, the placenta may be compromised and close surveillance of the fetus is necessary (Keely and Montoro, 2008).

It is recommended that women test their blood sugar levels before breakfast (fasting) and one hour after each meal, as well as before bed (NICE, 2008). Post-prandial glucose levels are suggested, as hyperglycaemia at this time is associated with accelerated fetal growth (Maresh, 2002) and also maternal HbA1c levels may be improved if these readings are targeted (Nelson-Piercy, 2006).

The aim of diabetic management during pregnancy is to achieve as near normo-glycaemia as possible. It has been suggested (NICE, 2008) that fasting blood sugars of 3.5–5.9 mmol/L and one hour post-meal blood sugars of < 7.8 mmol/L should be considered ideal. Glucagon kits need to be provided for women, with instructions for using them given to both the women and their partners, due to the increased risk of hypoglycaemia unawareness during pregnancy. Ketone testing strips should also be given to women, along with instructions for using them, as the risk of diabetic ketoacidosis is increased in pregnancy.

The reasons for an elective induction of labour at term in a diabetic pregnancy not only include avoiding intra-uterine death but also an attempt to deliver the baby before increased fetal growth results in shoulder dystocia or a Caesarean section for obstructed labour (Sacks and Sacks, 2002).

According to the most recent CEMACH figures (2007), the Caesarean section rate for Type 1 diabetic women is 67%, and the early induction of labour contributes at least in part to this rate (Nelson-Piercy, 2006). Early induction of labour may also result in a premature baby, and even at term the baby of a diabetic mother may exhibit signs of respiratory distress syndrome due to poor surfactant production.

The high number of planned preterm deliveries may reflect the increased surveil-lance of these women as well as their propensity to pre-eclampsia, previous Caesarean sections which could predispose to placenta praevia and other medical conditions.

Summary of pregnancy care issues for a diabetic woman

▶ Booking at a facility offering specialised diabetic care and a neonatal unit.
▶ Early booking and assessment of HbA1c.
▶ Fetal anomaly screening offered.
▶ Consultation with a dietician.
▶ Support for changing home blood glucose monitoring, and insulin dose and frequency changes.
▶ Provision of home glucagon kits and ketone testing equipment.
▶ Surveillance of maternal condition (e.g., blood pressure, renal function, retinal testing).
▶ Fetal surveillance.
▶ Assessing mode of delivery.

LABOUR CARE

Labour care should begin before labour starts, as evidence shows that a woman who achieves normoglycaemia for 12–24 hours pre-delivery will reduce the degree of hypoglycaemia in the neonate (Maresh, 2002). This may, in turn, avoid admission of the baby to a neonatal unit, with the consequential upsetting separation of mother and neonate. If a morning induced labour or elective Caesarean section is planned, consideration needs to be taken of the insulin level the night before.

Induction of labour

Induction of labour, especially with an unfavourable cervix, can be expected to take an unpredictable amount of time; therefore short-acting insulin and snacks should be given until labour begins (Maresh, 2002).

General labour care

During labour insulin requirements alter because of increased energy needs and the presence of oxytocin, which has an insulin-like effect (Blackburn, 2007). The aim is to stabilise maternal blood sugar at 4–8 mmol/L (Nelson-Piercy, 2006).

A suggested regime for labour is shown in Box 1.5, but although this may vary slightly – or indeed, substantially – the midwife needs to be aware of her local unit protocols as well as the evidence that underpins them.

BOX 1.5: SUGGESTED REGIME FOR TYPE 1 DIABETIC WOMEN IN LABOUR

- Intravenous infusion (IVI) 10% dextrose at 100/125 mL/hour via infusion pump.
- Insulin results in extracellular potassium entering cells, therefore potassium replacement is needed. This is usually given as part of the dextrose infusion.
- 20 units (0.2 mL of 100 units/mL) soluble insulin in 19.8 mL normal saline via infusion pump at a rate correlated to woman's blood sugar (sliding scale).
- Minimum of hourly blood sugar readings to determine insulin infusion rate.
- Additional fluids – Hartmann's solution used.

IVI glucose and insulin are part of most common regimes, but subcutaneous (SC) insulin may be possible for a woman with well-controlled Type l diabetes who wishes to mobilise (Maresh, 2002) and has a skilled and knowledgeable midwife looking after her exclusively.

Although insulin requirements in labour tend to be low (Maresh, 2002), blood sugars can fluctuate due to the physiological and psychological stresses of labour. As this can adversely affect the fetus, continuous electronic monitoring in labour is usual. There is evidence linking hyperinsulinaemia with fetal hypoxaemia (Luzietti and Rosen, 2003), but the most common cause of an abnormality in the CTG is maternal hyperglycaemia (Maresh, 2002). However, it must be remembered that CTG monitoring gives only limited information, although an optimal trace (a normal consistent baseline, good variability, accelerations and no decelerations) is reassuring. Fetal blood sampling can be a valuable adjunct but the blood sampled is peripheral and does not reflect the metabolic acidaemia in the tissues (Luzietti and Rosen, 2003).

It should also be noted that all urine passed should be tested for ketones. Diabetic ketoacidosis is unlikely to develop during a well-supervised labour, but even a small rise in ketones may cause fetal distress.

Shoulder dystocia is suggested to be more than twice as likely in the delivery of a diabetic woman (CEMACH, 2007), probably due to the propensity for the fetus to have increased upper torso or shoulder size (*see* section on *macrosomia* earlier in this chapter). There is therefore an increased risk of damage to these infants, in particular with shoulder dystocia and Erb's palsy (although some Erb's palsy have been reported with Caesarean section delivery) (CEMACH, 2007). Caesarean sections undertaken during labour are probably often a reflection of the concern over disproportion – any delay in labour is more likely to be treated with a Caesarean section rather than with oxytocin (Maresh, 2002).

Immediate post-delivery
Following the third stage, the withdrawal of the placental hormones that were driving the increased insulin resistance causes demand for insulin to drop dramatically and all intravenous infusions should be reduced or stopped. If the woman used insulin pre-pregnancy, her previous regime should be recommended, although if the woman has had a Caesarean section her diet may be limited and this needs to be taken into account when determining insulin requirements. Frequent blood sugar estimation will identify when she has returned to her pre-pregnancy condition. Those women who did not use insulin pre-pregnancy can stop insulin immediately after delivery and if their blood sugar is normal they need only a single final blood sugar check about 6–8 hours post-delivery to ensure hyperglycaemia is not present.

Baby
The needs of the baby of a diabetic woman can be complex and cannot be addressed in detail here (*see* footnote, p. 12). However, as a minimum the general condition of this infant needs to be frequently observed and regular blood sugar estimations and early and frequent feeds should be instigated.

POSTNATAL CARE
Breastfeeding
Breastfeeding should be encouraged, not only for its many known benefits, but also because there is evidence that this may help protect the baby from developing child-hood obesity and insulin resistance (Dabelea, *et al.*, 2000; Schaefer-Graf, *et al.*, 2006; Vohr, *et al.*, 1999). As about one-third of babies of diabetic mothers are admitted to a neonatal unit (CEMACH, 2007) and Caesarean section is common with diabetic women, enabling breastfeeding will be a challenge for midwives, but it is a very important part of their work. Breastfeeding is to be encouraged but, as it uses extra calories, it is suggested that an increase of carbohydrates may be necessary. A dietician will be an important resource for the mother and midwife on the postnatal ward.

Wound healing
Even following a spontaneous vaginal delivery with no perineal trauma, the ability to heal effectively following childbirth is necessary, and diabetes is well known to compromise healing (Boyle, 2006). Diabetic women often have Caesarean sections or deliver large babies, which predisposes them to perineal trauma, so they will have additional healing to do.

Post-partum thyroiditis

Post-partum thyroiditis is common in those with Type 1 diabetes (Keely and Montoro, 2008) and a diabetic woman should be screened for it, especially if she is symptomatic (*see* Chapter 10).

Contraception

Considering contraception for a diabetic woman can be seen as part of the preconception care for her next pregnancy. As a diabetic, she will have special needs, and a practitioner knowledgeable in this specific area should be accessed, but the midwife – as part of her role as a health promoter – needs to be aware, and ensure the mother is aware, of its importance.

TYPE 2 DIABETES: CARE ISSUES

At present, care of women with Type 2 diabetes is a very small part of any midwife's role, but as the number of younger women diagnosed with Type 2 diabetes grows, and the ability to distinguish between gestational diabetes and Type 2 increases, midwives will find they meet many more of these women.

MATERNAL SCREENING

It is possible to have hyperglycaemia for a long time without clinical symptoms and diagnosis (Nelson-Piercy, 2006). It is also estimated that 10–30% have established eye or renal disease by the time they are diagnosed with Type 2 diabetes (Nelson-Piercy, 2006). This has serious relevance to women who unknowingly conceive with a high blood sugar and begin pregnancy with undiagnosed medical conditions.

Random blood sugar estimation, if done at booking, may identify women with undiagnosed Type 2 diabetes (although this is some time after conception and the vital organogenesis period). Few units offer this routinely at present, but this may change as the number of Type 2 diabetic women increase.

PRECONCEPTION CARE

Traditionally women taking oral antihyperglycaemic and hypoglycaemic drugs were changed to insulin – ideally in the preconception period, or as early in pregnancy as possible – as these tablets were seen as possibly teratogenic. However, a new generation of diabetic tablets has been identified as potentially safe for the developing fetus, as they do not cross the placenta and provide a comparable perinatal outcome (NICE, 2008). Women with Type 2 or gestational diabetes may now receive oral medication (metformin) during the preconception period and during pregnancy. Nevertheless, a change to insulin is still often recommended, or becomes necessary during pregnancy, as better glycaemic control is usually possible with insulin (Maresh, 2002).

It has been found that women with Type 2 diabetes presented for care later than those with Type 1 (Cundy, *et al.*, 2000). An awareness that preconception care and special combined clinics are important for these women too is needed.

PREGNANCY CARE

In a study of known Type 2 diabetic women, 19% were taking insulin at booking but 96% needed it as pregnancy progressed (Cundy, *et al.*, 2000). This highlights the importance of these women receiving the increased care recommended for Type 1 diabetic women.

Maternal complications
As women with Type 2 diabetes are susceptible to the same range of complications, albeit often to a lesser degree than those with Type l diabetes, see the section on *pregnancy complications of diabetes* earlier in this chapter.

Fetal screening
Type 2 diabetes is associated with an increased perinatal mortality nearly four times that of a non-diabetic woman, mostly due to late (28–40 weeks) fetal death, although there is also an increase in earlier fetal deaths, late neonatal deaths and death from genetic malformations (CEMACH, 2007). Type 2 diabetes is associated with increased maternal age and increased maternal weight, which are also risk factors for fetal/neonatal complications. Women with Type 2 diabetes should be offered the same range of fetal screening and diagnostic tests as those with Type l diabetes (*see* previous sections on *fetal surveillance* and *fetal anomaly screening*).

LABOUR CARE
If a woman with Type 2 diabetes is using insulin, her labour care will be the same as one with Type 1 diabetes (*see* the relevant section). The labour regime for women with Type 2 diabetes (or gestational diabetic women) not using insulin is to undertake regular blood sugar readings during labour (for example, every two to four hours) and if readings are persistently raised, an insulin regime such as the one described in Box. 1.5 may be necessary. It has been suggested that if these women are taking less than 20 units of insulin daily they may not need to start the insulin regime at the beginning of labour, but careful, frequent blood sugar readings are still necessary (Maresh, 2002).

Some of the areas discussed in the labour care section for Type l diabetes (for example, CTG monitoring and urine testing) are relevant for the woman with Type 2 or gestational diabetes, so the section on this topic should be read.

POSTNATAL CARE
If a woman with Type 2 or gestational diabetes has been taking insulin during pregnancy or labour this can be stopped after the delivery of the placenta, but careful, frequent blood glucose monitoring needs to be undertaken until her condition is stable. Many oral hypoglycaemics are contraindicated while breastfeeding.

GESTATIONAL DIABETES: CARE ISSUES
Although it was recognised as far back as 1823 that some women became diabetic during pregnancy and then 'recovered' after delivery, the term gestational diabetes came into general use only in the 1960s (Kalter, 2000).

POSSIBLE PREVENTION
It has been found that physical activity before and during pregnancy may decrease the risk of gestational diabetes (Dempsey, *et al.*, 2004). Diets rich in antioxidants (including vitamin C) may decrease the risk of gestational diabetes (Zhang, *et al.*, 2004). However,

although these suggestions are in themselves healthy ones, more evidence is needed before midwives can make informed recommendations about the specific prevention of gestational diabetes.

MATERNAL SCREENING

Untreated gestational diabetes can increase the risk of perinatal morbidity in all disease levels (Langer, *et al.*, 2005). Perinatal mortality rises even in those with impaired glucose tolerance (Maresh, 2005). Screening should therefore be offered to all appropriate women in the antenatal period.

There is currently no consensus in the literature regarding testing women for gestational diabetes. Some authorities believe that universal screening for gestational diabetes improves perinatal outcomes (Griffin, *et al.*, 2000). However, many areas test only women with identified risk factors (*see* Box 1.6), and, indeed, this is recommended by NICE (2008). However, it must be remembered that screening by risk groups may mean that 44–55% of gestational diabetics remain undiagnosed (Carr, 1998).

Others identify women at low risk and test all others. Those considered at low risk are < 25 years old, have a normal weight, belong to an ethnic group with a low prevalence of gestational diabetes, have no known first-degree relative with diabetes and no history of abnormal glucose tolerance or poor obstetric outcome (Metzger and Coustan, 1998).

BOX 1.6: RISK FACTORS FOR GESTATIONAL DIABETES

Pre-pregnancy
- Certain high-risk ethnic groups
- Short stature < 150 cm
- Raised BMI
- Previous poor obstetric outcome: congenital abnormality, stillbirth, macrosomia, shoulder dystocia, Caesarean section
- Previous history of gestational diabetes or glucose intolerance
- Diabetes in a first-degree relation
- Polycystic ovarian syndrome

Pregnancy
- A large pregnancy weight gain, or pregnancy weight > 91 kg
- Increased blood pressure in pregnancy
- Multiple pregnancy
- Current glycosuria (on two separate occasions)

Many women have more than one risk factor and often these are related, for instance, obesity and increased blood pressure. Ethnic origin and obesity are considered the most important independent variables associated with the development of gestational diabetes.

(Dornhorst and Chan, 1998)

It has been suggested that early-onset gestational diabetes has more complications and results in poorer outcomes (Bartha, *et al.*, 2000). However, it is possible that a diagnosis of gestational diabetes may also be one of previously undiagnosed Type 2 diabetes.

PREGNANCY CARE

There remains controversy about screening for gestational diabetes but there is no doubt about the management once it is diagnosed (Nelson-Piercy, 2006). Box 1.7 lists the main management options for gestational diabetes.

BOX: 1.7: MANAGEMENT OPTIONS FOR GESTATIONAL DIABETES

- Diet
- Exercise
- Blood sugar monitoring
- Stress reduction
- May require medication

Most women with gestational diabetes are managed with diet alone (Dornhorst and Frost, 2003). The optimal diet for pregnant diabetic women has not been definitely established in controlled clinical trials. *See* Box 1.8 for the principles of a diabetic diet, which closely resemble those identified as a healthy diet for anyone.

BOX 1.8: PRINCIPLES OF A DIABETIC DIET

The general principle is to aim for three meals and three snacks daily, with 10–20% protein and < 10% saturated fat, 50% carbohydrates and total calories of about 1800–2000 (with perhaps a reduction in the obese, although during pregnancy this must be carefully managed by a dietician). Increasing the fibre content of meals may reduce post-meal hyperglycaemia.

Women diagnosed with gestational diabetes need to commence home blood glucose monitoring. This, together with attention paid to diet and exercise, is all many women need, but it is suggested that 10–20% of women will need oral hypoglycaemic drugs or insulin. It is recommended that women should begin medication if their blood sugars are abnormal or if the fetal abdominal circumference measurement is more than the 70th centile after 29–33 weeks of gestation.

Obese women with gestational diabetes may benefit from insulin. A study considering women with a BMI > 30 showed an achievement of optimum glycaemic control associated with improved outcome only in those treated with insulin (Langer, *et al.*, 2005). Exercise may help avoid insulin treatment for overweight (BMI > 25) women. In a study by Brankston *et al.* (2004), those including exercise along with diet modification needed less insulin and experienced a longer delay before needing insulin.

Fetal screening

The association of congenital abnormality and diabetes is suggested to lie in the organogenesis period (*see effect of diabetes on the fetus* section earlier in this chapter). Studies have shown higher numbers of fetal congenital abnormalities in pregnancies of Type 1 diabetic women who had high blood sugars around conception and in the very early days of pregnancy, compared to those who had blood sugars within normal limits at this time. In true gestational diabetes there will not be high blood sugar during early pregnancy, although there may be hyperglycaemia in a woman with undiagnosed Type 2 diabetes.

A continuum of risk probably exists, from mild gestational diabetes easily controlled with diet to gestational diabetes that is difficult to control and needs relatively large amounts of insulin. This more severe form of the disease is associated with increased adverse outcomes such as prematurity, Caesarean section and admission to a neonatal unit (Sendag, *et al.*, 2001). The more severe form of gestational diabetes is also more likely to be undiagnosed but previously existing Type 2 diabetes.

Since it is impossible to tell during pregnancy whether a woman is an undiagnosed Type 2 diabetic, those diagnosed with gestational diabetes should be offered whatever fetal screening is appropriate, although in practice, since most testing for gestational diabetes is carried out at around 26 weeks' gestation, she will probably have already had the opportunity for fetal screening.

Maternal complications

There is a clear association of gestational diabetes and pre-eclampsia, and some studies have found a twofold to fourfold increased rate (Eriksson, 2004). Obesity is a confounding factor but there is also an independent risk (Ostlund, *et al.*, 2004). Both increased pre-eclampsia and gestational diabetes rates have been demonstrated in women with polycystic ovarian syndrome (Bjercke, *et al.*, 2002).

LABOUR CARE

See this section under *Type 2 diabetes* earlier in this chapter for information on this period.

POSTNATAL CARE

If a woman with GDM has needed an insulin infusion during labour, this should be stopped after delivery of the placenta, and blood sugar recordings should be done regularly until her condition is stable. If she did not need insulin, at about 6–8 hours following delivery a blood sugar should be taken to ensure it is within normal limits. In addition, all women diagnosed with gestational diabetes should be given a follow-up appointment for a glucose tolerance test (GTT), most commonly at six weeks postnatal (*see* following section).

A woman with gestational diabetes should receive education into her condition, and it is recommended that she seeks preconception care for the next pregnancy (Farrell, 2003). These women also need health advice from their midwife. Some lifestyle modifications, such as maintaining a healthy diet, losing weight and increasing exercise, may delay, reduce the severity or perhaps even prevent the onset of Type 2 diabetes

(Hadden, *et al.*, 2004; McElduff, 2003). Breastfeeding is very important for this woman – *see* the section on *breastfeeding* earlier in this chapter.

LONG-TERM CARE AND PROGNOSIS

Women with gestational diabetes, and some would suggest also those with impaired glucose tolerance, should be offered a glucose screening six weeks after delivery and annually thereafter (NICE, 2008). This will ensure that those with Type 2 diabetes undiagnosed before pregnancy will be identified. Women with gestational diabetes have a greatly increased risk of developing Type 2 diabetes over the next 10 years, and those with an increased BMI are at the greatest risk (Lauenborg, *et al.*, 2004). An Australian study found that more than 50% of women diagnosed with gestational diabetes progressed to overt diabetes (Walsh, 2004).

Although all women diagnosed with gestational diabetes should receive a careful follow-up to determine their diabetic status in the puerperium, it is particularly important for those who needed insulin in their pregnancy, as there is a high likelihood of a Type 2 diagnosis (Cundy, *et al.*, 2000).

ROLE OF THE MIDWIFE

There is a clear role for the diabetic specialist midwife to be a key member of the multi-disciplinary team (Maresh, 2002). As part of her role she will usually need to teach blood sugar monitoring, teach insulin administration and regimes if necessary, re-inforce dietary changes and organise parent education in one-to one sessions or small groups (or enhance the information women receive in general classes). However, the specific skills of the midwife are also very important, as routine antenatal care for these women is so important (screening for pre-eclampsia, infections or polyhydramnios, for example). It is worth noting that in ultrasound assessments of estimated fetal weight, accuracy decreases with the increase of birth weight (Ben-Haroush, *et al.*, 2004). A mid-wife's skilled clinical assessment may therefore be vital in diagnosing macrosomia.

The midwife is also the prime resource for all general pregnancy information and can be a normalising presence for a diabetic woman, especially one newly diagnosed with gestational diabetes who may be feeling particularly vulnerable.

Continuity of midwifery care may provide an improvement in some parameters such as shorter labours and decreased admissions to the neonatal unit with hypoglycaemia (Morrison, *et al.*, 2002).

As the midwife's role stretches into the puerperium, this will give her the opportunity of building on the health promotion teaching undertaken during pregnancy.

The dietician has a role in all diabetic pregnancies, whether it is to give new dietary advice to a woman diagnosed with gestational diabetes, or in reinforcing or perhaps adapting a previous diet programme for established diabetic women. Dietary advice is the remit of the dietician, but a midwife will be supporting women throughout their pregnancy, so she needs to have a basic knowledge in this area.

PSYCHOSOCIAL ISSUES

When examining those who had been given care that did not meet established standards, those whose ethnic origin was other than white were over-represented (CEMACH, 2007). This shows that midwives may need to target these women – in particular those who do not speak English – in order to ensure they receive care to enable the best possible outcome of their pregnancy.

The CEMACH report into diabetes in pregnancy (2007) has identified deprivation as being strongly associated with Type 2 diabetes. Since women identified as socially deprived often find it difficult to access services, midwives may need to be proactive in finding these women and ensuring they receive the care they need to improve their pregnancy outcome and maintain their own health.

Pregnancy is a time of emotional lability and those who have a stressful lifestyle, for example demanding jobs, family commitments or financial challenges, may not find achieving ideal diabetic control easy as stress may cause fluctuations in blood glucose (Maresh, 2002). Pregnancy has the propensity to be an extremely stressful time. While it is probably impossible to remove this altogether, midwives need to ensure that women in their care understand that stress can have an effect on their diabetic control, and perhaps exploring some relaxation and anti-stress strategies may be useful.

Gestational diabetes can have a profound effect on the woman diagnosed. Lawson and Rajaram (1994) found a combination of fear of the disease diabetes (with its potentially disastrous outcomes), the inconvenience of diet restriction and blood glucose monitoring and the prospect of a less than normal pregnancy led to the increase of fear, depression and anxiety. This study, as well as now being dated, was done in the US and appeared to find that very fragmented – and according to many of the women's statements – much unsympathetic care had been offered to diabetic women. It is to be hoped that care in the UK today is much more women-friendly. However, it is still valuable to remember how frightening the diagnosis of diabetes (in whatever form) may be to a woman, and how what are routine procedures for midwives may be worryingly alien for the woman.

A recent US study reported that a significant number of women with both Type 1 and gestational diabetes did not accurately record their blood glucose levels: for example, 80% added phantom values and 70% did not enter values that were perhaps considered undesirable (Kendrick, *et al.*, 2005). This may demonstrate how traumatic women find testing and/or the presentation of results at the diabetic clinic. Midwives have a role in ensuring that diabetic clinics are seen as a resource that is wholly directed towards supporting the woman, and is in no way judgemental of her efforts.

How women may react to the diagnosis of gestational diabetes will be influenced by many factors, including their background. A study of women living in Sweden comparing women born in Sweden with women born in the Middle East found a very different response to the disease (Hjelm, *et al.*, 2005). This underlines how important it is for the midwife to have the ability to support different women in a variety of ways to meet their psychosocial needs.

Although some studies report no increased anxiety after the initial diagnosis for gestational diabetes (Daniells, *et al.*, 2003), it is also clear that some women may view themselves and their child differently for some time after the birth. After screening positive for gestational diabetes, women in one study had lower perceptions of their own health (Rumbold and Crowther, 2002).

Long-term research done by Feig *et al.* and published in 1998 compared women diagnosed with gestational diabetes with matched controls without, at three to five years following the pregnancy. The women diagnosed with gestational diabetes worried more about their own health and rated their children as less healthy, although they still considered their children's health to be very good. However, it was found this increased worry did not lead to significant changes in preventative health behaviour directed at themselves. This is an area which needs further investigation in order to identify what educational input and ongoing support women need to ensure they know what a healthy lifestyle means and how to achieve it. This long-term work is beyond the remit of the midwife, but she can ensure that women have the initial educational input and identify appropriate resources for the long term.

One-third of term babies of diabetic women are admitted to a neonatal unit (CEMACH, 2007), and due to pregnancy complications many babies of diabetic women are born preterm. However, the recommendations are that wherever possible mothers and babies are not separated. Separation at birth can lead to an interruption to the normal mother–infant attachment, difficulty in initiating breastfeeding and great emotional distress for the parents. This will be compounded if the mother has reduced mobility from a Caesarean section. There is no doubt that babies of diabetic mothers will need additional observation and care, and that midwives' resources on postnatal wards can be severely stretched, but every effort needs to be made to ensure those babies who can be cared for without specialist neonatal resources are kept with their mothers.

COMMONLY USED DRUGS
INSULIN
This substance is vital for metabolism and must be given if production by the beta cells in the pancreas fails. It is inactivated by gastrointestinal enzymes, so it must be given regularly by subcutaneous injections or (in urgent situations) intravenous infusions. Insulin may have a short-acting, intermediate or long-acting effect, depending on its formulation, and dosage is based on individual blood glucose measurement.

METFORMIN HYDROCHLORIDE
This is an oral anti-diabetic (biguanides) drug which decreases gluconeogenesis and increases peripheral utilisation of glucose. There must be some residual functioning of the pancreatic islet cells present in order for it to be effective. Although at present metformin does not have UK marketing authorisation for pregnant and breastfeeding women, based on a number of studies NICE (2008) has advised it may be used in the preconception period or during pregnancy, where appropriate.

REFERENCES
Amos A, McCarty D, Zimmer P. The rising global burden of diabetes and its complications: estimates and projections to the year 2010. *Diabet Med.* 1997; **14** (Suppl. 5): S1–85.

Ang C, Howe D, Lumsden M. Diabetes. In: James DK, Steer PJ, Weiner CP, *et al.* editors. *High Risk Pregnancy Management Options.* 3rd ed. Philadelphia: Saunders Elsevier; 2006. pp. 986–1004.

Bartha J, Martinez-Del-Fresno P, Comino-Delgado R. Gestational diabetes mellitus diagnosed during early pregnancy. *Am J Obstet Gynecol.* 2000; **182**: 346–50.

Ben-Haroush A, Yogev Y, Hod M. Epidemic of gestational diabetes. In: Hod M, Jovanovic L, Di

Renzo GC, *et al.* editors. *Textbook of Diabetes and Pregnancy.* London: Martin Dunitz; 2003. pp. 64–89.

Ben-Haroush A, Yogev Y, Hod M. Fetal weight estimation. In: Diabetic pregnancies and suspected fetal macrosomia. *J Perinat Med.* 2004; **32**(2): 113–21.

Bjercke S, Dale P, Tanbo T, *et al.* Impact of insulin resistance on pregnancy complications and outcome in women with polycystic ovary syndrome. *Gynecol Obstet Invest.* 2002; **54**(2): 94–8.

Blackburn ST. *Maternal, Fetal and Neonatal Physiology.* 3rd ed. St Louis: Saunders; 2007.

Boyle M. *Wound Healing in Midwifery.* Oxford: Radcliffe Publishing; 2006.

Brankston G, Mitchell B, Ryan E, *et al.* Resistance exercise decreases the need for insulin in overweight women with gestational diabetes mellitus. *Am J Obstet Gynecol.* 2004; **190**(1): 188–93.

Butte NF. Carbohydrate and lipid metabolism in pregnancy: normal compared with gestational diabetes mellitus. *Am J Clin Nutr.* 2000; **71**(Suppl. 5): S1256–61.

Carr S. Screening for gestational diabetes mellitus. *Diabetes Care.* 1998; **21**(Suppl. 2): S14–18.

Catalano PM. Maternal metabolic adaptation to pregnancy. In: Hod M, Jovanovic L, Di Renzo GC, *et al.* editors. *Textbook of Diabetes and Pregnancy.* London: Martin Dunitz; 2003. pp. 50–63.

Catalano PM, Tyzbir ED, Wolfe RR, *et al.* Carbohydrate metabolism during pregnancy in control subjects and women with gestational diabetes. *Am J Physiol.* 1993; **264**(1 Pt. 1): E60–7.

Clausen TD, Hellmuth E, Mathiesen E, *et al.* Poor pregnancy outcomes in women with Type 2 diabetes. *Diabetes Care.* 2005; **28**(2): 323–8.

Coad J, Dunstall M. *Anatomy and Physiology for Midwives.* 2nd ed. Edinburgh: Elsevier Churchill Livingstone; 2005.

Confidential Enquiry into Maternal and Child Health (CEMACH) *Pregnancy in Women with Type 1 and Type 2 Diabetes in 2002–03. England, Wales and Northern Ireland.* London: CEMACH; 2005.

Confidential Enquiry into Maternal and Child Health (CEMACH) *Diabetes in Pregnancy: Are We Providing the Best Care? Findings of a National Enquiry: England, Wales and Northern Ireland.* London: CEMACH; 2007.

Crowther CA, Hiller JE, Moss JR, *et al.* Effect of treatment of gestational diabetes mellitus on pregnancy outcomes. *N Eng J Med.* 2005; **352**(24): 2477–86.

Cundy T, Gamble G, Townend K, *et al.* Perinatal mortality in Type 2 diabetes mellitus. *Diab. Med.* 2000; **17**(1): 33–9.

Dabelea D, Knowler W, Pettitt D. Effect of diabetes in pregnancy of offspring: follow-up research in the Pima Indians. *J Matern Fetal Med.* 2000; **9**(1): 83–8.

Daniells S, Greyner B, Davis W, *et al.* Gestational diabetes mellitus: is a diagnosis associated with an increase in maternal anxiety and stress in the short and intermediate term? *Diabetes Care.* 2003; **26**(2): 385–9.

Dempsey J, Sorensen T, Williams M, *et al.* Prospective study of gestational diabetes mellitus risk in relation to maternal recreational physical activity before and during pregnancy. *Am J Epidemiol.* 2004; **159**(7): 663–70.

Diabetes Care and Research in Europe. The St Vincent Declaration. *Diabet Med.* 1990; **34**: 655–1.

Diabetes UK. Position statement: early identification of people with Type 2 diabetes. 2006. Available at: www.diabetes.org.uk/Research/Research_position_statements/ (accessed 4 December 2008).

Dornhorst A, Chan S. The elusive diagnosis of gestational diabetes. *Diabet Med.* 1998; **15**: 7–10.

Dornhorst A, Frost G. Nutritional management in diabetic pregnancy: a time for reason not dogma. In: Hod M, Jovanovic L, Di Renzo GC, *et al.* editors. *Textbook of Diabetes and Pregnancy.* London: Martin Dunitz; 2003. pp. 340–58.

Dunne F. Type 2 diabetes and pregnancy. *Semin Fetal Neonatal Med.* 2005; **10**(4): 333–9.

Eriksson U. Abortion and congenital malfunctions. In: van Assche FA, editor. *European Practice in Gynaecology and Obstetrics: diabetes and pregnancy.* Amsterdam: Elsevier; 2004. pp. 59–68.

Farrell M. Improving the care of women with gestational diabetes. *MCN Am J Matern Child Nurs.* 2003; **28**(5): 301–5.

Feig D, Chen E, Naylor C. Self-perceived health status of women three to five years after the diagnosis of gestational diabetes: a survey of cases and matched controls. *Am J Obstet Gynecol.* 1998; **178**: 386–93.

Fletcher B, Gulanik M, Lamendola C. Risk factors for Type 2 diabetes mellitus. *J Cardiovasc Nurs.* 2002; **16**(2): 17–23.

Griffin M, Coffey M, Johnson H, *et al.* Universal vs risk factor-based screening for gestational diabetes mellitus: detection rates, gestation at diagnosis and outcome. *Diabet Med.* 2000; **17**: 26–32.

Hadden D. History of diabetic pregnancies. In: Hod M, Jovanovic L, Di Renzo GC, *et al.* editors. *Textbook of Diabetes and Pregnancy.* London: Martin Dunitz; 2003. pp. 1–12.

Hadden D, Kennedy A, Nugent A. Long-term implications of gestational diabetes for the mother. In: van Assche FA, editor. *European Practice in Gynaecology and Obstetrics: diabetes and pregnancy.* Amsterdam: Elsevier. 2004. pp. 97–108.

Hagay Z, Weissman A, Lurie S, *et al.* Reversal of fetal distress following intensive treatment of maternal diabetic ketoacidosis. *Am J Perinatol.* 1994; **11**: 430.

Hedderson M, Ferrara A, Sacks D. Gestational diabetes mellitus and lesser degrees of pregnancy hyperglycemia: association with increased risk of spontaneous preterm birth. *Obstet Gynecol.* 2003; **102**(4): 850–6.

Hjelm K, Bard K, Nyberg P, *et al.* Swedish and Middle-Eastern-born women's beliefs about gestational diabetes. *Midwifery.* 2005; **21**(1): 44–60.

Kalter H. *Of Diabetic Mothers and Their Babies.* Amsterdam: Harwood; 2000.

Kamalakannan D, Baskas V, Barton DM, *et al.* Diabetic ketoacidosis in pregancy. *Postgrad Med J.* 2003; **79**: 454–7.

Keely E, Montoro M. Type 1 and Type 2 diabetes. In: Rosene-Montella K, Keely E, Barbour L, *et al.* editors. *Medical Care of the Pregnant Patient.* 2nd ed. Philadelphia, PA: ACP Press. 2008. pp. 233–52.

Kendrick J, Wilson C, Elder R, *et al.* Reliability of reporting of self-monitoring of blood glucose in pregnant women. *JOGN.* 2005; **34**(3): 329–4.

Langer O, Yogev Y, Most O, *et al.* Gestational diabetes: the consequences of not treating. *Am J Obstet Gynecol.* 2005; **192**(4): 989–7.

Lauenborg J, Hansen T, Jensen D, *et al.* Increasing incidence of diabetes after gestational diabetes: a long-term follow-up in a Danish population. *Diabetes Care.* 2004; **27**(5): 1194–9.

Lawson E, Rajaram S. A transformed pregnancy: the psychosocial consequences of gestational diabetes. *Sociol Health Illn.* 1994; **16**(4): 536–62.

Luzietti R, Rosen K. Monitoring in labor. In: Hod M, Jovanovic L, Di Renzo GC, *et al.* editors. *Textbook of Diabetes and Pregnancy.* London: Martin Dunitz; 2003. pp. 418–29.

McElduff A. Scared care: gestational diabetes. *Aust Fam Physician.* 2003; **32**(3): 113–18.

Macintosh MCM, Fleming KM, Bailey JA, *et al.* Perinatal mortality and congenital anomalies in babies of women with Type 1 or Type 2 diabetes in England, Wales, and Northern Ireland: population based study. *BMJ.* 2006; **333**(7560): 177. Epub 2006 Jun 16.

Maresh M. Diabetes. In: de Swiet M. *Medical Disorders in Obstetric Practice.* 4th ed. Oxford: Blackwell; 2002. pp. 386–413.

Maresh M. Screening for gestational diabetes mellitus. *Semin Fetal Neonatal Med.* 2005; **10**(4): 317–23.

Maulik D, Lysikiewicz A, Sicuranza G. Umbilical arterial Doppler sonography for fetal surveillance in pregnancies complicated by pregestational diabetes mellitus. *J Matern Fetal Med.* 2002; **12**(6): 417–22.

Metzger B, Coustan D. Summary and recommendations of the 4th International Workshop on Gestational Diabetes Mellitus. The Organising Committee. *Diabetes Care.* 1998; **21**(Suppl. 2): B14–18.

Moley KH. Hyperglycemia and apoptosis: mechanisms for congenital malformations and pregnancy loss in diabetic women. *Trends Endocrinol Metab.* 2001; **12**(2): 78–82.

Morrison J, Neale L, Taylor R, *et al.* Caring for pregnant women with diabetes. *Br J Midwifery.* 2002; **10**(7): 434–9.

Nachum Z, Ben-Shlomo I, Weiner E, *et al.* Twice daily versus 4 times daily insulin dose regimes for diabetics in pregnancy: randomised controlled trial. *BMJ.* 1999; **319**: 1223–7.

National Institute for Health and Clinical Excellence (NICE). *Diabetes in Pregnancy: management of diabetes and its complications from pre-conception to the postnatal period: NICE guideline 63.* London: NICE; 2008. www.nice.org.uk/Guidance/CG63

Nelson-Piercy C. *Handbook of Obstetric Medicine.* 3rd ed. Abingdon: Informa Healthcare; 2006.

Newton C, Raskin P. Diabetic ketoacidosis in Type 1 and Type 2 diabetes mellitus: clinical and biochemical differences. *Arch Intern Med.* 2004; **164**: 1925–31.

Ostlund I, Haglund B, Hanson U. Gestational diabetes and preeclampsia. *Eur J Obstet Gynecol Reprod Biol.* 2004; **113**(1): 12–16.

Perri T, Loya N, Hod M. Diabetic retinopathy. In: Hod M, Jovanovic L, Di Renzo GC, *et al.* editors. *Textbook of Diabetes and Pregnancy.* London: Martin Dunitz; 2003. pp. 475–85.

Powell K. Obesity: the two faces of fat. *Nature.* 2007; **447**(7144): 525–7.

Raychaudhuri K, Maresh M. Glycemic control throughout pregnancy and fetal growth in insulin-dependent diabetes. *Obstet Gynecol.* 2000; **95**: 190–4.

Rosenn BM, Miodovnik M. Diabetic vascular complications in pregnancy: nephropathy. In: Hod M, Jovanovic L, Di Renzo GC, *et al.* editors. *Textbook of Diabetes and Pregnancy.* London: Martin Dunitz; 2003. pp. 486–94.

Rumbold A, Crowther C. Women's experiences of being screened for gestational diabetes mellitus. *Aust N Z J Obstet Gynaecol.* 2002; **42**(2): 131–7.

Sacks D, Sacks A. Induction of labor versus conservative management of pregnant diabetic women. *J Matern Fetal Med.* 2002; **12**(6): 438–1.

Schaefer-Graf U, Harmann R, Pawliczak J, *et al.* Association of breast-feeding and early childhood overweight in children from mothers with gestational diabetes mellitus. *Diabetes Care.* 2006; **29**: 1105–7.

Sendag F, Terek M, Itil I, *et al.* Maternal and perinatal outcomes in women with gestational diabetes mellitus as compared to non-diabetic controls. *J Reprod Med.* 2001; **46**(12): 1057–62.

Shah BR, Hux JE. Quantifying the risk of infectious diseases for people with diabetes. *Diabetes Care.* 2003; **26**: 510–13.

Suhonen L, Hiilesmaa V, Teramo K. Glycaemic control during early pregnancy and fetal malformations in women with Type 1 diabetes mellitus. *Diabetologia.* 2000; **43**(1): 79–82.

Verhaeghe J. Gestational diabetes mellitus: pathophysiology, screening and diagnosis and management. In: van Assche FA, editor. *European Practice in Gynaecology and Obstetrics: diabetes and pregnancy.* Amsterdam: Elsevier; 2004. pp. 13–28.

Vohr B, McGarvey S, Tucker R. Effects of maternal gestational diabetes on offspring adiposity at 4–7 years of age. *Diabetes Care.* 1999; **22**: 1284–91.

Walsh E. Gestational diabetes: what happens post-partum? *Aust N Z J Obstetr Gynaecol.* 2004; **44**: 277–8.

Waugh A, Grant A. *Ross and Wilson Anatomy and Physiology in Health and Illness.* 10th ed. Edinburgh: Churchill Livingstone; 2006.

Williams G, Pickup JC. *Handbook of Diabetes.* 3rd ed. Oxford: Blackwell; 2004.

Yogev Y, Ben-Haroush A, Hod M. Diabetic ketoacidosis in pregnancy. In: Hod M, Jovanovic L, Di Renzo GC, *et al.* editors. *Textbook of Diabetes and Pregnancy.* London: Martin Dunitz; 2003. pp. 495–501.

Zhang C, Williams M, Sorensen T, *et al.* Maternal plasma ascorbic acid (vitamin C) and risk of gestational diabetes mellitus. *Epidemiology.* 2004; **15**(5): 597–604.

CHAPTER 2

The cardiac system:
Physiology and principles of care

CONTENTS
→ Introduction
→ Physiology and changes to the cardiac system in pregnancy
→ General care principles in cardiac conditions

INTRODUCTION

Heart disease has become one of the major causes of death for child-bearing women in the UK over the last decade. Although the contribution of heart disease to maternal mortality figures in the UK and US remains fairly constant, the aetiology is changing as most women with cardiac conditions undertaking pregnancy now have congenital heart disease. Whereas previously these women may not have lived past infancy, with new surgery and drugs they may now reach child-bearing age in a reasonable state of health. In comparison, fewer children in the UK are now left with the lifelong legacy of rheumatic heart disease (RHD). However, RHD remains a problem worldwide and is frequently seen in the immigrant population in the UK. Heart disease that is acquired through genetic predisposition and lifestyle, such as coronary artery disease (previously a disease of older men), is now becoming increasingly prevalent in women of reproductive age, probably as a result of lifestyle changes, and this number will increase.

The increased pregnancy rate for women with heart disease has resulted in midwives seeing many more women with this potentially life-threatening condition (Lewis, 2007). An improvement in diagnostic skills, monitoring techniques and drugs, as well as an increased knowledge of cardiac function – both normal and in pregnancy – has led to better management of pregnancy in women with heart disease. Midwives need not only specialist knowledge but also normal midwifery skills to care for these women effectively.

Pregnancy outcome depends on the type of heart disease and how it affects the woman physically when she is not pregnant. This functional status is often assessed by the New York Heart Association (NYHA) Criteria (*see* Box 2.1).

The NYHA suggest a range of maternal mortality from 0.4% in classification I to 6.8% in classifications III and IV, and fetal mortality from none in class I to 30% in class IV. It has been shown that NYHA classes III–IV carry a significant maternal and perinatal mortality and morbidity (Sawhney, *et al.*, 2003; Siu, *et al.*, 2001).

Heart disease can be newly diagnosed in pregnancy, and the midwife may be the first health professional to see the woman. At booking, midwives should be aware of the possibility of undiagnosed heart disease and be aware that those with a family history of cardiac conditions or sudden death, those with signs of cardiac disease (such as hypertension, cyanosis or clubbing) or those with possible cardiac symptoms (*see* Box 2.2) may need referral. Unfortunately, many of the early signs and symptoms are the same as those appearing in a normal pregnancy, but the symptoms and signs that may have their origins in the cardiac system are often progressive. Heart and lung auscultation is important, and referral to a practitioner skilled in the assessment of physiological and pathological heart murmurs should be made if necessary.

BOX 2.1: NEW YORK HEART ASSOCIATION CLASSIFICATION OF SYMPTOMS

I Patients who are not limited by cardiac disease in their physical activity. Ordinary physical activity does not precipitate the occurrence of symptoms such as fatigue, palpitations, dyspnoea and angina.

II Patients in whom the cardiac disease causes a slight limitation in physical activity. Those patients are comfortable at rest but ordinary physical activity will precipitate symptoms.

III Patients in whom the cardiac disease results in a marked limitation of physical activity. They are comfortable at rest, but less than ordinary physical activity will precipitate symptoms.

IV Patients in whom the cardiac disease results in the inability to carry on physical activity without physical discomfort. Symptoms may be present even at rest, and discomfort is increased by any physical activity.

PHYSIOLOGY AND CHANGES TO THE CARDIAC SYSTEM IN PREGNANCY

The adaptations of a woman's body to sustain pregnancy are rapid and profound. Changes to the cardiovascular system support the growing fetus and accommodate the increased metabolic requirement of the mother. The haemodynamic changes are mediated by increased levels of oestrogen, progesterone and prostaglandins, with endothelial-derived relaxing factor (EDRF, nitric oxide) responsible for the earliest vasodilatory effects (Duvekot and Peeters, 1998; de Swiet, 2002). For most women the demands are met without a problem. However, for women with cardiac disease, pregnancy poses a cardiovascular challenge.

CHANGES TO THE CARDIOVASCULAR SYSTEM IN PREGNANCY

▶ ↑ Oxygen consumption
▶ ↑ Plasma volume
▶ ↑ Red blood cells
▶ ↓ Resistance in systemic circulation

- ↓ Pulmonary vascular resistance
- ↑ Pulmonary vascular blood flow
- Development of placental circulation
- Blood pressure: systolic – stays the same
  diastolic ↓
- ↑ Heart rate
- ↑ Stroke volume
- ↑ Cardiac output
- Reduced colloid osmotic pressure
- ↑ Oedema of hands, feet and ankles
- Heart moves upward and laterally
- ↑ Heart size

CHANGES TO RELATED BODY SYSTEMS IN PREGNANCY

- ↑ Tidal volume
- ↑ Uterine blood flow
- ↑ Renal blood flow with ↑ glomerular filtration rate
- ↑ Skin perfusion
- Endocrine changes, in particular ↑ oestrogen, progesterone

BOX 2.2: SIGNS AND SYMPTOMS OF CARDIAC DISORDER

Symptoms:
- breathlessness at rest, severe breathlessness or feeling faint at exertion
- difficulty in breathing when laying down (orthopnoea) or during the night (paroxysmal nocturnal dyspnoea)
- palpitations, chest pain (especially when brought on by exertion)
- haemoptysis

Signs:
- heart murmurs – either new or pre-existing, changing intensity, (e.g., mitral and aortic regurgitation murmurs decrease while mitral and aortic stenosis murmurs are amplified)
- neck vein distention
- change in heart sounds
- sustained dysrhythmia
- clubbing

THE HEART

The heart is simply a muscular pump divided into a left and right side. The right side of the heart pumps deoxygenated blood to the lungs (pulmonary circulation) where gas exchange occurs (i.e., the blood picks up oxygen and unloads carbon dioxide). The left side of the heart pumps blood around the body (systemic circulation) where the blood supplies nutrients and oxygen to the cells and picks up tissue waste.

Cardiac tissue

In order to pump effectively, the heart is a very muscular organ. The heart muscle is called the myocardium and is composed of specialised cardiac muscle which is unique to the heart. Cardiac muscle is capable of contracting without nervous stimulation. Electrical impulses spread a synchronous wave of contraction across the muscle cells that compose each chamber, producing enough force to eject blood. In pregnancy oestrogen acts on the myocardium to increase contractility (Blackburn, 2007; Bonow, *et al.*, 2006). The inner layer of the heart is called the endocardium. This layer lines the chambers and valves of the heart. Those with cardiac diseases are vulnerable to an inflammation of the endocardium known as *endocarditis* (*see* Chapter 3) and require antibiotic prophylaxis at times of surgical intervention, including dental work and at the time of birth. The outer layer of the heart is called the pericardium, and this consists of two layers with a thin film of serous fluid between them.

Chambers of the heart

The heart (*see* Figure 2.1) is divided into the right and left sides, with each side functioning as separate but synchronous pumps. Each side has an upper chamber – the atrium (atria plural) – which receives blood returning to the heart and then transfers it to the lower chamber. The ventricles pump blood away from the heart. The right ventricle pumps blood to the lungs via the pulmonary artery and the left ventricle pumps blood to the tissues of the body via the aorta.

The two halves are separated by the septum, consisting of myocardium covered by endocardium. This septum or partition is very important as it prevents mixing of de-oxygenated and oxygenated blood from the two sides of the heart. In the fetus before birth a shunt known as the foramen ovale exists between the left and right atrium. At birth, when the infant takes its first breath this flap normally closes. Two congenital defects known as *atrial septal defect* and *ventricular septal defect* can persist. Pregnant women may have these defects (*see* Chapter 3), although most are usually repaired.

The pregnant woman has a physiologically dilated heart. The ventricles increase in size by about 10–15% with an increase in pumping ability (Gelson, *et al.*, 2006; de Swiet, 1998) and there is a small increase in left atrial diameter (Blackburn, 2007).

Valves

Blood flows through the heart in one direction from an area of high pressure to an area of low pressure. The valves are designed to work like one-way doors – they let blood through and then close to prevent flow from regurgitating backwards. The progress of blood through the heart is determined by four cardiac valves:

▶ tricuspid valve (consists of three cusps) – separates the right atrium and ventricle (right atrioventricular valve)
▶ mitral valve (consists of two cusps) – separates the left atrium and ventricle (left atrioventricular valve)
▶ pulmonary valve – from the right ventricle to the pulmonary artery
▶ aortic valve – from the left ventricle to the aorta.

(*see* Figures 2.2 and 2.3)

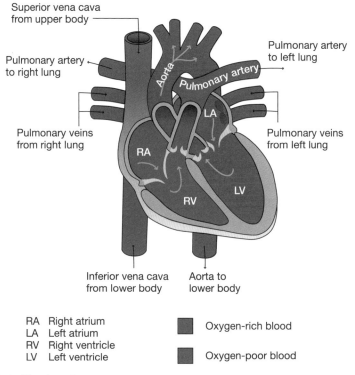

RA Right atrium
LA Left atrium
RV Right ventricle
LV Left ventricle

Oxygen-rich blood

Oxygen-poor blood

FIGURE 2.1: The heart

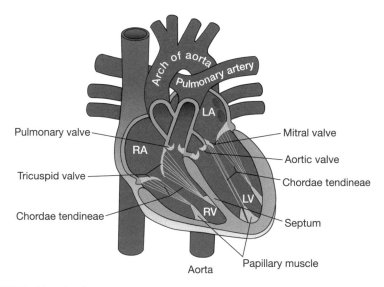

FIGURE 2.2: Heart valves

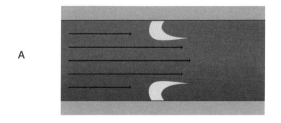

A

Valve opened

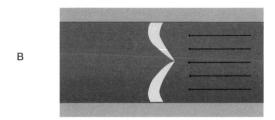

B

Valve closed; does not open in opposite direction

FIGURE 2.3: Mechanism of valve action

The edges of the atrioventricular valve cusps, which are pocket-like flaps of delicate tissue, are fastened by tough, thin fibrous cords (chordae tendineae) that prevent the valves being forced to open in the opposite direction by the increasing ventricular pressure. The aortic and pulmonary valves consist of three half-moon-shaped cusps. When the valves are closed the cusps are aligned and separate the vessels from the ventricles. During the period of systole (when the ventricles pump), the aortic and pulmonary valves open wide and blood flows into the vessels. When the ventricle relaxes (diastole) these valves close, backflow is prevented and the ventricles fill.

Valvular heart problems can involve narrowing (stenosis) or leakage (insufficiency or regurgitation). *Mitral valve prolapse* is relatively common in the child-bearing population. *Rheumatic fever* damages cardiac valves. *See* Chapter 3 for more detail on these conditions.

Blood supply to the heart

To sustain effective cardiac output the heart needs a good supply of oxygen to give the myocardium enough energy to contract effectively. In pregnancy an increased heart rate results in an elevated myocardial oxygen requirement, which may be significant in pregnant women with cardiac disease (Tomlinson, 2006).

The heart is supplied with arterial blood by the right and left coronary arteries that branch from the aorta immediately above the aortic valve. These coronary arteries receive about 5% of the blood pushed from the heart, with a large amount going to the left ventricle.

Coronary heart disease can cause myocardial ischaemia (reduced circulation of oxygenated blood to the heart muscle). Atherosclerosis is a progressive, degenerating arterial disease that leads to the gradual blockage of effected vessels. Blockages caused by atheromatous plaques, a feature of the disease, can be complicated by clot formation. The tissue beyond these narrow points becomes ischaemic (lacking oxygen). Ischaemic pain caused by these blockages is called angina and when a coronary artery becomes blocked it is known as *myocardial infarction* (*see* Chapter 3).

Electrical activity in the heart

Small groups of specialised neuromuscular cells in the myocardium initiate and conduct impulses allowing for co-ordinated and synchronous contraction of heart muscle. These are:

◗ sinoatrial node (SA node)
◗ atrioventricular node (AV node)
◗ bundle of His (atrioventricular bundle)
◗ Purkinje fibres.

The heart is influenced by autonomic nerves processed by the cardiovascular centre in the medulla oblongata (brain stem). The autonomic system consists of parasympathetic (which reduces rate and force of heartbeat) and sympathetic (which act to increase heart rate) nerves. *See* Box 2.3 for the factors that can affect heart rate.

The SA node acts as the pacemaker for the heart. The other zones – the AV node, the bundle of His and Purkinje fibres – are latent pacemakers that can take over, although at a lower rate, should the SA node fail. Complete *heart block* occurs when the conducting tissue between the atria and ventricles is damaged and the ventricles then beat at only 30 beats per minute. An artificial pacemaker is required to restore the normal heart rate. Occasionally an area of the heart, such as the Purkinje fibres, becomes overexcited and depolarises at a more rapid rate. This is known as *ectopic beats*. If the ectopic focus continues to charge rapidly the heart rate goes up. This can be associated with heart disease but more frequently occurs in response to anxiety, excess caffeine or smoking and alcohol. Ectopic beats are common in pregnancy (Adamson, *et al.*, 2007). Pregnant women may experience skipped beats, momentary pressure in the neck or chest or extra beats suggestive of arrhythmias. This is usually due to increased sympathetic nervous system activity. Occasionally cardiac problems may present during pregnancy so investigation is recommended (Blackburn, 2007).

Effective cardiac function depends on synchronous excitation with the atria contracting in sequence with the ventricles. Random unco-ordinated excitation and contraction of cardiac muscle cells is known as fibrillation. *Ventricular fibrillation* causes death but can be corrected using electrical defibrillation.

Cardiac cycle

The cardiac cycle is the sequence of events that takes place during one heartbeat, which normally takes about 0.8 seconds.

Stages include:

▶ atrial systole – contraction of the atria
▶ ventricular systole – contraction of the ventricles
▶ complete cardiac diastole – relaxation of atria and ventricles.

BOX 2.3: FACTORS AFFECTING HEART RATE

- Gender – oestrogen acts to increase heart rate in females
- Pregnancy – heart rate progressively rises during pregnancy (10–20 beats per minute)
- Age
- Circulating hormones, such as adrenaline and thyroxine
- Activity and exercise
- Temperature – increases in pregnancy as a result of fetal metabolism
- Baroreceptors
- Emotional stress

Heart sounds and murmurs

Heart sounds correspond to events in the cardiac cycle and are easily distinguishable as 'lub – dup, lub – dup, lub – dup'. The first 'lub' is low pitched, soft and relatively long and is due to the closure of the atrioventricular valves and heralds the start of ventricular systole. The second high-pitched, shorter and sharper sound, 'dup', is the closure of the aortic and pulmonary valves and thus corresponds with atrial systole.

Abnormal heart sounds and murmurs are usually (but not always) associated with cardiac disease. However, pregnant women may have an innocent *systolic murmur* that is indicative of increased cardiac output. A loud third heart sound is heard in up to 90% of pregnant women (Adamson, *et al.*, 2007; Robson, 1996).

When blood flows smoothly it does not produce any sound (laminar flow). When the flow becomes turbulent, a sound can be heard due to surrounding vibrations. The most common cause of turbulence is valve malfunction where the valve is stenosed (stiff or narrowed) (e.g., *aortic stenosis*) or incompetent (doesn't close completely). Incompetent valves result in a backflow of blood known as regurgitation (e.g., *aortic regurgitation*), which is sometimes described as a leaky valve.

Cardiac output

Cardiac output is the amount of blood ejected from the heart. It depends on the heart rate and stroke volume.

$$\text{CARDIAC OUTPUT} = \text{STROKE VOLUME} \times \text{HEART RATE}$$

The body's capacity to increase cardiac output is illustrated in exercise when both heart rate and stroke volume increase. Stroke volume is determined by the volume of blood in the ventricles before they contract. This is known as *ventricular end diastolic volume* (VEDV) or sometimes called preload. This preload depends on the extent of venous return. An increase in VEDV will result in stronger myocardial contraction.

Venous return is normally enhanced when lying flat, although in a pregnant woman compression of the inferior vena cava in the supine position decreases venous return. Muscle contraction around vessels, when walking for example, helps propel blood towards the heart.

During inspiration of air the expansion of the chest creates a negative pressure within the thorax, drawing blood towards the heart. Deep-breathing exercises when recovering from surgery such as Caesarean section is recommended to improve venous return and prevent clot formation. Box 2.4 summarises factors affecting stroke volume.

In pregnancy, stroke volume, heart rate and consequently cardiac output increases. Heart rate and increased blood volume are the main factors in determining the increasing cardiac output of pregnancy (Blackburn, 2007; de Swiet, 2002). Women with multiple pregnancies have a greater increase in cardiac output than do those with singleton pregnancies (Adamson, *et al.*, 2007). Pregnant women often experience reduced exercise tolerance, tiredness and dyspnoea, and women with heart disease may not tolerate this dramatic increase in cardiac output.

BOX 2.4: FACTORS AFFECTING STROKE VOLUME

- VEDV
- Venous return
  - position
  - skeletal muscle pump
  - respiratory effort
- Strength of myocardial contraction
- Blood volume – markedly increased in pregnancy
- Arterial blood pressure

FLUID DISTRIBUTION

In pregnancy there is pooling of fluid in feet and ankles, seen as oedema. The gravid uterus creates a mechanical impedance to blood flow through the inferior vena cava. Venous distensibility contributes to reduced venous return to the heart. This increase in venous pressure causes leakage of fluid from the vascular bed into the interstitium, giving rise to oedema (Tomlinson, 2006). Reduced plasma colloid pressure due to physiological haemodilution contributes to this tendency to oedema. Pregnant women are particularly susceptible to *pulmonary oedema* (fluid in the lungs) when given too much intravenous fluid, especially when they have pre-eclampsia, which increases pulmonary capillary permeability (leaky vessels) (Adamson, *et al.*, 2007).

SYSTEMIC VASCULAR RESISTANCE (SVR)

SVR is dictated by the diameter of the vessels. It is a reflection of the ratio between the mean arterial pressure and cardiac output (Duvekot and Peeters, 1998). The blood vessel diameter is altered by the contraction of the smooth muscle in the tunica media of the blood vessel wall. The less the contraction, the larger the diameter and the least resistance to flow and vice versa. In pregnancy there is a marked reduction in SVR, especially in the peripheral vessels. SVR falls to about 70% of its pre-pregnancy value by about eight weeks' gestation (Gelson, *et al.*, 2006; de Swiet, 1998).

Factors contributing to reduction in systemic vascular resistance in pregnancy:

▶ remodelling of spiral arteries. The walls of the spiral arteries of the uterus lose their muscular and elastic elements. They become almost completely dilated and are no longer responsive to circulating pressor agents or influences of the autonomic nervous system (de Swiet, 2002)

▶ vasodilatation due to progesterone, vasoactive prostaglandins, relaxin and EDRF (nitric oxide) (Duvekot and Peeters, 1998)

▶ heat production by the fetus results in vasodilatation of vessels in heat-losing areas such as the hands (Blackburn, 2007).

This relative vasodilatation of pregnancy increases not only uterine blood flow but blood flow to other organs such as the breasts, skin and kidneys (Duvekot and Peeters, 1998). Enhanced renal blood flow increases the glomerular filtration rate. Skin perfusion increases significantly in pregnancy, peaking around 20 to 30 weeks' gestation and accounting for the glow of pregnancy attributed to that time. There is an increase in skin temperature, clammy hands and skin capillary dilation. This facilitates the dissipation of excessive heat created by the fetal metabolism. Increased peripheral flow can also be seen in the mucous membranes of the nasal passages, leading to nasal congestion. Neck veins pulsate more vigorously and vein distension is evident from about 20 weeks' gestation (Blackburn, 2007; de Swiet, 2002)

Pregnancy gives rise to changes in structure of the vessel walls. This includes an increase in aortic size and compliance. Oestrogens can interfere with collagen deposition, weakening vessel walls and predisposing to dissection such as *aortic dissection* (Bonow, *et al.*, 2006) This can be a particular problem for women with *Marfan's syndrome* (*see* Chapter 3), which is a disorder of connective tissue.

BLOOD PRESSURE

Blood pressure is the force exerted on the wall of a blood vessel by the blood. The pressure varies rhythmically with the beating of the heart. It reaches maximum pressure as the left ventricle expels blood into the aorta (systolic) and falls when the aortic valve closes and the heart is filling (diastolic). It reaches minimum pressure just before the next heartbeat.

Blood pressure depends on:

▶ cardiac output (stroke volume × heart rate)
▶ systemic vascular resistance.

Blood pressure is controlled by:

▶ the cardiovascular centre in base of brain via the autonomic nervous system
▶ the diameter of vessels (vasomotor tone) – altered by relaxation or constriction of smooth muscle in walls of vessel
▶ baroreceptors that detect changes from sitting to standing and adjust the heart rate
▶ chemicals carried in the blood, such as adrenaline, noradrenaline and histamine

▶ chemoreceptors that are sensitive to changes in oxygen and carbon dioxide
▶ EDRF (nitric oxide), which plays a key role in vasodilatation of pregnancy
▶ the kidney – antidiuretic hormone, renin-angiotensin balance.

Despite increases in both blood volume and cardiac output during pregnancy, blood pressure does not increase; in fact, diastolic blood pressure falls. Mean arterial pressure decreases by the eighth week of gestation and women may complain of fatigue, headache and dizziness (Duvekot and Peeters, 1998). This is secondary to changes in peripheral vascular resistance caused by the vasodilatory effects of EDRF (nitric oxide) and other hormones, including progesterone (Blackburn, 2007). Diastolic pressure decreases 10–15 mmHg, particularly during the first half of pregnancy, and then rises progressively until it is slightly higher than pre-pregnancy values at term. Systolic pressure remains stable until 36 weeks when there is a slight rise (Gelson, *et al.*, 2006).

CHANGES TO HAEMODYNAMICS IN LABOUR AND POST-PARTUM

Cardiac output increases in labour (*see* Box 2.5). In labour without analgesia there is a 30% rise in cardiac output during contractions. Effective epidural analgesia may offset this increase (Gelson, *et al.*, 2006). Uterine contractions can lead to marked increases in both systolic and diastolic blood pressure (Bonow, *et al.*, 2006). Each contraction pushes about 400 mL of additional blood into the circulation (Blackburn, 2007).

With the delivery of the baby and placenta and a degree of blood loss, the immediate postnatal period is a time of changing haemodynamics. Despite blood loss at delivery, cardiac output remains significantly elevated above pregnancy levels for 1–2 hours post-partum with peak cardiac output occurring immediately after delivery (Blackburn, 2007). This rise is due to:

▶ a decrease in gravid uterus pressure and improved venous return via the inferior vena cava
▶ transfusion of blood from the placental bed going back into the maternal circulation, which can cause volume overload
▶ reduced amount of vascular bed due to the delivery of the placenta.

(Blackburn, 2007; Bonow, *et al.*, 2006; Uebing, *et al.*, 2006)

Post-partum haemorrhage, with potential for substantial loss of blood volume, can compromise cardiac function (Uebing, *et al.*, 2006). Oxytocic drugs, including Syntocinon and ergometrine, that promote uterine contraction also have major haemodynamic effects. Oxytocin can induce vasodilatation and arterial hypotension and ergometrine can cause arterial hypertension (Uebing, *et al.*, 2006).

Diuresis to get rid of extracellular fluid occurs following the birth. Without this diuresis, pulmonary oedema can develop in women with pre-eclampsia or heart disease. Cardiac output gradually decreases to non-pregnant values by 6–12 weeks postnatal (Blackburn, 2007).

BOX 2.5: INCREASES IN CARDIAC OUTPUT IN LABOUR

- First stage 12–30%
- Second stage 50%
- Third stage 60–80%

(Blackburn, 2007)

GENERAL CARE PRINCIPLES IN CARDIAC CONDITIONS

Although the care of a woman with heart disease will be individualised, both according to the specific condition and also to her particular situation, there are a few principles of care that apply generally. *See* Chapter 3 for additional issues specific to individual conditions.

PRECONCEPTION CARE

All women with heart disease should receive good preconception care and for some women the assessment may result in advice against pregnancy. Cardiac conditions that may lead to this advice include primary and secondary pulmonary hypertension, shunt lesions complicated by Eisenmenger's syndrome, complex cyanotic congestive heart disease, aortic coarctation complicated by aortic dissection or dilation, or poor residual left ventricular function. However, knowledge and supportive therapy is growing rapidly and all women should receive a skilled cardiology assessment from a team with up-to-date experience of pregnancy and heart disease. Nevertheless, the Confidential Enquiry into Maternal Deaths (Lewis, 2007) shows the very real risk many women may take in undergoing pregnancy.

Women with a history of heart disease should receive preconception advice before each pregnancy. Most congenital heart conditions, even following successful repairs in childhood, need full evaluation between pregnancies, even if the previous pregnancy was uneventful. A successful repair of a condition in childhood does not mean it will continue to perform well into and through adult life, and the physiological changes in pregnancy may compromise a woman's cardiovascular system whether she has had a previous repair of a congenital defect or has a benign condition. It is undoubtedly true that each year women die following heart disease complicating pregnancy, but the amount of stress a pregnancy puts on an abnormal heart condition is largely unknown, although there is evidence in certain specific conditions (Warnes, 2006a). In addition, many conditions are progressive, and prostheses can wear out. A full assessment of her condition, possible surgery pre-pregnancy (and use of biological valves rather than mechanical valves in order to avoid coagulation issues) (Warnes, 2006b) may improve pregnancy success rate. Surgical correction of the anomaly, if done before pregnancy, can give a better outcome. Predictors of adverse outcomes include poor maternal functional status, myocardial dysfunctions, significant aortic or mitral valve stenosis and a history of arrhythmias or cardiac events.

Issues commonly addressed during the preconception period include:

▶ assessment of the present status of the heart disease. Allied to this may be suggested improvements, e.g., surgery or changes to medication

- exploration, if possible, of potential future deterioration of the condition that may be caused by pregnancy
- depending on the condition, a discussion of the possibility of inherited heart disease and the options for fetal assessment
- discussion of the effect heart disease could have on the pregnancy, such as fetal intra-uterine growth restriction (IUGR) and/or necessary premature birth
- discussion of how to optimise health in general, for example by a decrease in weight, smoking cessation, etc., as necessary, and commencement of folic acid.

GENERAL CARE IN PREGNANCY

Ideally, all women with cardiac disease should be cared for by a multidisciplinary team, which should include a cardiologist, an obstetrician, an anaesthetist, a fetal-medicine specialist, a haematologist, a neonatologist, a specialist midwife and a cardiac nurse. If preconception counselling and assessment has not been done, an early referral should be made by the midwife as soon as she is aware of the woman's pregnancy.

All members of the team should contribute to ensuring a plan of care is identified and modified as necessary for pregnancy, labour and the puerperium.

The provision of a 'high risk' midwifery team will greatly enhance this woman's care. Normal midwifery assessment is important. Most cardiac conditions carry an increased risk of pre-eclampsia, so evaluations of blood pressure and urine as usual will be necessary.

Ongoing assessment of a woman's cardiac health should be undertaken as frequently as her condition needs and this may include a regular assessment of her heart rhythm, auscultation of the heart sounds and listening to lung bases, as well as the use of technology such as echocardiograms, magnetic resonance imaging (MRI) or electrocardiograms (ECGs).

Evaluation of drugs taken and their dose will continue throughout the antenatal period and be dealt with on an individual basis. Women need expert help in managing their drug regime and to avoid being tempted to stop certain medications if they carry a fetal risk. The risk to the mother or fetus from the disease being treated by the drugs may be greater than the potential risk to the fetus from the drug. Many cardiac conditions include a need for anticoagulation medication. Heparin (subcutaneously or IV) preconception and around delivery is used, as warfarin (which can be given orally) crosses the placenta. The risk of oesteopenia from long-term heparin use and the difficulty of titrating doses in pregnancy means a low molecular weight heparin (LMWH) may be prescribed, although this has not been studied fully yet (Trimm, et al., 2007).

There may be a danger to the fetus of inherited cardiac conditions, and this risk is inherited from both parents (Burn, et al., 1998). The level of risk varies depending on the specific anomaly but is roughly 23%. Some drugs taken by women with cardiac disease also carry a risk of teratogenicity, and for this reason an increased number of tests should be offered to screen for fetal cardiac anomalies if this is the woman's decision.

Ultrasound to identify nuchal translucency should be offered to all women (NICE, 2008), and raised levels are not only associated with Down's syndrome, but also with fetal cardiac anomalies (Ghi, et al., 2001). There is an association between increased nuchal translucency and cardiac defects both for fetuses with chromosomal abnormalities and for those without (Hyett, *et al.*, 1999), but there is no increased risk of any particular type of heart condition (Atzei, *et al.*, 2005). It has been suggested that effective referral of all those considered at risk (*see* Box 2.6) could optimise the detection rate (Gardiner and Daubeney, 2006).

Fetal echocardiography (transvaginal or transabdominal imaging studies from late in the first trimester to beyond the second trimester) is the normal diagnostic tool used. This may provide information for the mother (who may consider termination) or enable management plans to be made for the delivery to be at the best time and place and with relevant professionals available for a compromised baby. An early fetal echocardiography (14–16 weeks) is recommended, but many conditions may be missed at this early stage, and it is more commonly done – or repeated – at 18–22 weeks (Yu and Teoh, 2006). The usual 20-week ultrasound should also be carried out. Fetal MRI may detect structural brain lesions caused by cardiac abnormalities (Miller, *et al.*, 2004) but this test will be appropriate for only a minority of women.

BOX 2.6: RISK FACTORS NEEDING REFERRAL FOR FETAL CARDIAC ASSESSMENT

Booking:	family history/maternal congenital heart disease
	pre-existing diabetes
	connective tissue disease
	teratogenic drugs (e.g., lithium)
Antenatal:	extra-cardiac anomalies
	fetal cardiac arrhythmia
	aneuploidy
	monochorionic fetal pregnancy
	raised nuchal translucency
	suspicious cardiac scan
	two 'soft' markers suspicious of aneuploidy

(Based on Gardiner and Daubeney, 2006)

Regular assessment of fetal growth will usually be more frequent than normal, as IUGR (secondary to compromised maternal output) is common in women with cardiac conditions. Serial ultrasound for growth is undertaken if there is concern or if the woman has recognised risk factors for IUGR (increased blood pressure, cyanotic heart disease or is taking beta blockers).

As well as ultrasound growth studies, fetal assessment may include a specific Doppler examination of fetal pulmonary veins (Harman and Baschat, 2003) as well as the more usual umbilical arteries. A 20-week uterine artery Doppler (via transvaginal ultrasound) to screen for uteroplacental insufficiency (Papageorghiou, *et al.*, 2001) may be used. Umbilical artery Doppler velocimetry is known to be associated with placental function (Madazli, *et al.*, 2003) and this should be undertaken regularly throughout pregnancy to assess fetal well-being and underpin the timing of delivery (Yu and Teoh, 2006).

GENERAL CARE IN LABOUR AND IMMEDIATE POSTNATAL PERIOD

Premature labour

Should premature labour happen unexpectedly when unfractionated heparin is being used, protamine sulphate can reverse the anticoagulant effect. The usual drugs used to stop premature labour (ritodrine or salbutamol) are contraindicated with cardiac disease.

The use of steroids for fetal lung maturation is usual practice when possible before a premature delivery, but care is needed as this is associated with fluid retention which may lead to cardiac failure (Durbridge, *et al.*, 2006).

Timing and mode of delivery

In general, Caesarean section is rarely needed unless for obstetric reasons (*see* individual conditions for exceptions, Chapter 3) and a vaginal delivery is suggested for most cardiac conditions (Durbridge, *et al.*, 2006). A Caesarean section is associated with increased blood loss, infection, increased puerperal fluid shifts and increased metabolic demands (Van Mook and Peeters, 2005). However, a Caesarean section may be necessary for some women.

The ideal time of delivery would be following the spontaneous onset of labour, but most women with heart disease will have had close monitoring during pregnancy and the findings may indicate the need for induction of labour or a planned Caesarean section. These can frequently be preterm if the woman's condition or that of the fetus deteriorates.

Analgesia and anaesthesia

Cardiac stress can be caused by pain or exertion (such as pushing), as pain and anxiety increases the cardiac output (*see* section on *Changes to haemodynamics in labour and post-partum* earlier in this chapter). Regional analgesia is therefore usually recommended for women with cardiac disease during labour. It may also allow for a controlled second stage with a minimum of exertion by the woman. The common side effects, however, need to be considered, and peripheral vasodilation can cause decreased preload and therefore a reduced cardiac output. Excessive fluid infusion can lead to cardiac failure. Regional analgesia (or anaesthetic, if a Caesarean section is planned) needs to be undertaken by a skilled and experienced anaesthetist.

Anticoagulation may contraindicate a spinal or epidural insertion, and if the intention is for a vaginal delivery, then plans need to be made during pregnancy to cover all eventualities. If the woman has a condition that means that effective anticoagulation is a priority (for example, mechanical heart valves or a history of thromboembolism) then a planned Caesarean section under general anaesthetic may be considered. General anaesthetic has increased risks (for example, an increased blood loss) but it also may have benefits for a woman with cardiac disease, for instance, if she was to need cardiac interventions such as cardioversion during the operation or immediately after it.

Position

Aortocaval compression (when lying flat, or sometimes even semi-recumbent, on the back) must be avoided. The recommended positions are lateral (preferably left lateral) or upright. If it is necessary to be supine, for example for an instrumental delivery or suturing, then a wedge is necessary and elevated legs should be avoided.

Oxytocin

Oxytocin can usually be used to induce or augment labour (*see* section on drugs in Chapter 3) but care is needed. When fluid overload is a concern, the infusion is often made up in a smaller volume of fluid and the dosage altered appropriately.

Fluid balance

Fluid balance is of vital importance to women with cardiac disease, and hypovolaemia and hypervolaemia must be avoided. To this end, careful records need to be kept of input and output as far as possible.

Maternal and fetal monitoring

A woman with cardiac disease needs continuous observation, including regular blood pressure, pulse and saturation recordings, at a minimum. She may also need continuous ECG and haemodynamic monitoring according to her individual needs. A central venous pressure (CVP) line, providing information regarding intravascular filling, may be necessary to assess, monitor and shape fluid management. Arterial lines are not common on delivery suites at present in the UK, but they are being introduced to maternity high-dependency areas more frequently, and this will probably increase with growing demand. Arterial lines can be valuable in providing continuous blood pressure monitoring and when frequent arterial blood gas samples are necessary.

To be safe and effective all invasive monitoring needs to be undertaken by a midwife trained in using it. Infection control is always important in these vulnerable women, but particular emphasis on this is necessary when using invasive monitoring as this is a very high-risk situation for infection. Poor uteroplacental perfusion in very many women with cardiac disease means continuous cardiotocograph (CTG) fetal monitoring is recommended.

Second stage

The Valsalva manoeuvre decreases cardiac output and has an influence on blood pressure; therefore it should be avoided in women with cardiac disease. A short second stage is usually recommended and this may result in elective instrumental delivery. Because of the potential danger of hypovolaemia in many conditions, volume preloading to allow for loss at delivery or surgery is sometimes recommended.

Third-stage management

The use of uterotonics for management of the third stage may be problematic. Oxytocin affects the blood pressure and increases cardiac output (Durbridge, *et al.*, 2006) and also can cause decreased cardiac contractibility and heart rate (Mukaddam-Daher, *et al.*, 2001). If it is used it should be by a slow IV infusion. Ergometrine is contraindicated in most women with heart disease, as it causes peripheral vascular constriction and coronary vasospasm. Hemabate (carboprost/PGF2) and misoprostol are both also contraindicated when myocardial ischaemia is present.

Immediate postnatal period

Following the birth of the baby, when the uterus contracts and the placenta separates there is an increased intravascular volume of about 500 mL and approximately this amount is also thought to be lost as delivery blood loss. Cardiac output can also show peaks at 15 and 30 minutes post-delivery (Durbridge, *et al.*, 2006). Careful observation therefore needs to be made of women who may be compromised by fluid swings that could lead to congestive heart failure. O_2 saturation levels should be continuously monitored as a reduction may indicate pulmonary oedema. Hypoxia increases pulmonary vascular resistance (Rosenthal and Nelson-Piercy, 2000), so oxygen administration may be required. It has been observed that one to two hours post delivery, the cardiac output and stroke volume is still elevated, and there is evidence that changes in the haemodynamic status persists for some time into the puerperium (Ramsay, 2006). CVP or arterial lines may be continued from labour or inserted to guide fluid administration or monitor the woman's condition at this time.

Normal observations, such as pulse, respirations, blood pressure, oxygen saturation and fluid balance, need to be done frequently. Adequate analgesia continues to be important, as pain may result in tachycardia, and regional analgesia may continue from labour, but using opiates, which produce less systemic vasodilation. Position should be considered during the first few hours postnatal – left lateral, if the woman is vulnerable to changes in preload; sitting up, if the woman is at risk of pulmonary oedema (Ramsay, 2006).

The thromboembolic risk is highest at delivery and it is still high at three hours postnatal. Therefore careful attention needs to be paid to thromboprophylaxis (LMWH) or IV heparin if the woman is at high risk), wearing thromboembolic deterrent (TED) stockings and encouraging exercises/mobility, where appropriate.

Risks in the immediate postnatal period include pulmonary oedema, hypertension, alteration in the cardiac shunting of blood, arrhythmias, cyanosis, ventricular ischaemia, thromboembolism and infection (Ramsay, 2006). Some drugs are contraindicated for breastfeeding and this should be investigated on an individual basis.

CARE IN THE LATER PUERPERIUM

For many women a close level of care is necessary well into the puerperium, as changes in the cardiac output and plasma volume continue for at least two weeks (Ramsay, 2006).

REFERENCES

Adamson DL, Dhanjal MK, Nelson-Piercy C, *et al.* Cardiac disease in pregnancy. In: Greer IA, Nelson-Piercy C, Walters B, editors. *Maternal Medicine.* Edinburgh: Churchill Livingstone Elsevier; 2007. pp. 14–39

Atzei A, Gajewska K, Huggon I, *et al.* Relationship between nuchal translucency thickness and prevalence of major cardiac defects in fetuses with normal karyotype. *Ultrasound Obstet Gynecol.* 2005; **26**: 154–7.

Blackburn ST. *Maternal, Fetal and Neonatal Physiology.* 3rd ed. St Louis, MO: Saunders; 2007.

Bonow RO, Carabello BA, Chatterjee K, *et al.* Guidelines for the management of patients with valvular heart disease: executive summary: a report of the American College of Cardiology/ American Heart Association Task Force on Practice. *Circulation.* 2006; **114**: 1–78.

Burn J, Brennan P, Little J, *et al.* Recurrence risks in offspring of adults with major heart defects: results from first cohort of British collaborative study. *Lancet.* 1998; **351**: 311–16.

Criteria Committee of the New York Heart Association. *Nomenclature and Criteria for Diagnosis of Diseases of the Heart and Great Vessels.* 9th ed. Boston, Mass: Little, Brown and Co; 1994. pp. 253–56.

de Swiet M. The cardiovascular system. In: Chamberlain G, Broughton Pipkin F, editors. *Clinical Physiology in Obstetrics.* 3rd ed. Malden, MA: Blackwell; 1998. pp. 33–69.

de Swiet M. Heart disease in pregnancy. In: de Swiet M, editor. *Medical Disorders in Obstetric Practice.* 4th ed. Oxford: Blackwell; 2002. pp. 125–58

Durbridge J, Dresner M, Harding K, *et al.* Pregnancy and cardiac disease – peripartum aspects. In: Steer P, Gatzoulis M, Baker P, editors. *Heart Disease and Pregnancy.* London: RCOG Press; 2006. pp. 285–98.

Duvekot JJ, Peeters LLH. Very early changes in cardiovascular physiology. In: Chamberlain G, Broughton Pipkin F, editors. *Clinical Physiology in Obstetrics.* 3rd ed. Oxford; Malden, MA: Blackwell; 1998. pp. 3–32.

Gardiner H, Daubeney P. Antenatal diagnosis of fetal cardiac defects. In: Steer P, Gatzoulis M, Baker P, editors. *Heart Disease and Pregnancy.* London: RCOG Press; 2006. pp. 129–42.

Gelson E, Ogueh O, Johnson M. Cardiovascular changes in normal pregnancy. In: Steer P, Gatzoulis M, Baker P, editors. *Heart Disease and Pregnancy.* London: RCOG Press; 2006. pp. 29–44.

Ghi T, Huggon I, Zosmer N, *et al.* Incidence of major structural cardiac defects associated with increased nuchal translucency but normal karyotype. *Ultrasound Obstet Gynecol.* 2001; **18**: 610–14.

Harman C, Baschat A. Comprehensive assessment of fetal wellbeing: which Doppler tests should be performed? *Curr Opin Obstet Gynecol.* 2003; **15**: 147–57.

Hyett J, Perdu M, Sharland G, *et al.* Using fetal nuchal translucency to screen for major congenital cardiac defects at 10–14 weeks of gestation: population based cohort study. *BMJ.* 1999; **318**: 70–1.

Lewis G, editor. The Confidential Enquiry into Maternal and Child Health (CEMACH). *Saving Mothers' Lives: reviewing maternal deaths to make motherhood safer 2003–2005. The Seventh Report on Confidential Enquiries into Maternal Deaths in the UK.* London: CEMACH; 2007.

Madazli R, Somunkiran A, Calay Z, *et al.* Histomorphology of the placenta and the placental bed of growth restricted fetuses and correlation with the Doppler velocimetries of the uterine and umbilical arteries. *Placenta.* 2003; **24**: 510–16.

Miller S, McQuillen P, Vigneron D, *et al.* Preoperative brain injury in newborns with transposition of the great arteries. *Ann Thorac Surg.* 2004; **77**: 1698–1706.

Mukaddam-Daher S, Yin Y, Roy J, *et al.* Negative inotropic and chronotropic effects of oxytocin. *Hypertension.* 2001; **38**: 292–6.

National Institute for Health and Clinical Excellence (NICE). *Antenatal Care: routine care for the healthy pregnant woman: NICE guideline 62.* London: NICE; 2008. www.nice.org.uk/ Guidance/CG62/NiceGuidance/pdf/English

Papageorghiou A, Yu C, Bindra R, *et al.* Multicentre screening for pre-eclampsia and fetal growth restriction by transvaginal uterine artery Doppler at 23 weeks of gestation. *Ultrasound Obstet Gynecol.* 2001; **18**: 441–9.

Ramsay M. Management of the puerperium in women with heart disease. In: Steer P, Gatzoulis M, Baker P, editors. *Heart Disease and Pregnancy*. London: RCOG Press; 2006. pp. 299–312.

Robson SC. Maternal respiratory and cardiovascular changes during pregnancy. In: Hillier SG, Kitchener HC, Neilson JP. editors. *Scientific Essentials of Reproductive Medicine*. London: WB Saunders; 1996. pp. 443–54

Rosenthal E, Nelson-Piercy C. Value of nitric oxide in Eisenmenger syndrome during pregnancy. *Am J Obstet Gynecol*. 2000; **183**: 781–2.

Sawhney H, Aggarwal N, Suri V, *et al.* Maternal and perinatal outcome in rheumatic heart disease. *Int J Gynaecol Obstet*. 2003; **80**(1): 9–14.

Siu S, Sermer M, Colman J, *et al.* Prospective multicenter study of pregnancy outcomes in women with heart disease. *Circulation*. 2001; **104**: 515–21.

Tomlinson M. Cardiac disease. In: James D, Steer P, Weiner C, *et al.*, editors. *High Risk Pregnancy: management options*. 3rd ed. Philadelphia, PA: Elsevier Saunders; 2006. pp. 798–827.

Trimm J, Hung L, Rahimtoola S. Artificial heart valves. In: Oakley C, Warnes C, editors. *Heart Disease in Pregnancy*. 2nd ed. Oxford: Blackwell; 2007. pp. 104–21.

Uebing A, Steer PJ, Yentis SM, *et al.* Pregnancy and congenital heart disease. *BMJ*. 2006; **332**(7538): 401–6.

Van Mook W, Peeters L. Severe cardiac disease in pregnancy. Part II: impact of congenital and acquired cardiac diseases during pregnancy. *Curr Opin Crit Care*. 2005; **11**: 435–8.

Warnes C. Long-term outcome of pregnancy with heart disease. In: Steer P, Gatzoulis M, Baker P, editors. *Heart Disease and Pregnancy*. London: RCOG Press; 2006a. pp. 319–26.

Warnes C. Prosthetic heart valves. In: Steer P, Gatzoulis M, Baker P, editors. *Heart Disease and Pregnancy*. London: RCOG Press; 2006b. pp. 157–68.

Yu C, Teoh T. Fetal care and surveillance in women with congenital heart disease. In: Steer P, Gatzoulis M, Baker P, editors. *Heart Disease and Pregnancy*. London: RCOG Press; 2006. pp. 143–56.

CHAPTER 3

Common cardiac conditions,drugs and methods of assessment

CONTENTS

→ Cardiac transplant
→ Ischaemic heart disease: coronary arterial disease (CAD) and myocardial infarctions (MI)
→ Pericarditis
→ Drugs commonly used in cardiac disease
→ Methods of assessing, monitoring and diagnosing cardiac conditions

RHEUMATIC HEART DISEASE
RHEUMATIC FEVER

Rheumatic fever was once endemic but is now unusual in developed countries. The main complication – rheumatic heart disease (RHD) – is, however, still a significant problem in many parts of the world, and areas in the UK with a high immigrant population will continue to see many pregnant women with RHD that complicates their pregnancy. It is possible they will not have been diagnosed, and as women with poor English and from socially deprived areas are often the least able to access medical care, midwives need to be particularly vigilant in ensuring these women receive appropriate assessment and care.

Rheumatic fever mainly damages cardiac valves. It is an autoimmune disease occurring 2–4 weeks after a throat infection caused by *Streptococcus pyogenes*. The antibodies that fight the infection cause the tissue of the heart, in particular the valves, to become inflamed and oedematous. When the damaged areas heal they leave thick fibrous tissue which disturbs the shape of the heart valves, leading to stenosis and/or incompetence.

In pregnancy RHD can lead to congestive heart failure (CHF) and pulmonary oedema, with or without arrhythmias. Management during pregnancy is aimed at preventing CHF. Volume status should be carefully monitored and activity may need to be reduced. Bacterial endocarditis is a possible complication, so prophylactic antibiotics may be necessary. As it may reoccur in pregnancy, rheumatic fever prophylaxis may also be considered for women with RHD.

MITRAL STENOSIS

Mitral stenosis is the most common valvular heart lesion in child-bearing women. As the name implies, it involves a narrowing of the opening of the mitral valve (*see* section on *valves* in Chapter 2). This narrowing impedes blood flow from the left atrium to the left ventricle. Pressures back up in the left atrium leading to pulmonary congestion (*see* Figure 3.1). The left atrium increases in size and is prone to develop atrial fibrillation. Symptoms depend on the size of the orifice (normal is 2.5–4 cm^2) and exercise is usually possible if >2.5 cm^2, but with measurements of 1.5–2.4 cm^2 exercise may result in dyspnoea. Preconception care is based on individual needs, but there is always a risk of thromboembolic disease and CHF. If her condition is severe the woman should consider surgery before becoming pregnant.

Pulmonary oedema may be treated with digoxin and diuretics but emergency surgery may be required. Atrial fibrillation may be treated with digoxin, verapamil or beta blockers. Serial echocardiograms (ECHOs) can monitor left atrium dilation, thrombus formation and early signs of ventricular compromise. Fetal risks depend on the severity of the disease – IUGR or even fetal death is possible from maternal atrial fibrillation or decreased cardiac output.

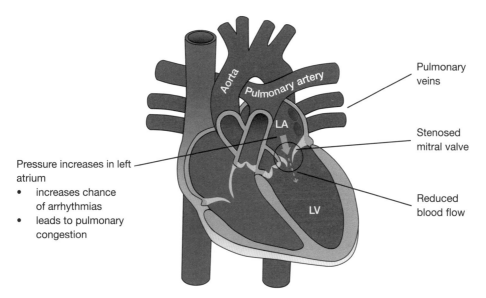

FIGURE 3.1: Mitral stenosis

In labour central haemodynamic monitoring with careful fluid management, including fluid restriction and diuretics, may be necessary. Cardiac monitoring is used as tachycardia leads to shortened ventricular filling, which could in turn lead to pulmonary congestion. Administering antibiotics is usual. The highest risk in labour is the late second stage and the first 15 minutes postnatal – cardiac output can increase up to 45% in the second stage and another 15% during contractions.

There is a risk of pulmonary oedema and pulmonary artery hypertension in the first 48 hours postnatal, even with good care. There is also a continuous risk of endocarditis or stroke due to clots forming in the dilated fibrillating left atrium.

AORTIC REGURGITATION

Aortic regurgitation occurs when the aortic valve does not close properly and blood leaks back into the left ventricle (*see* Figure 3.2). This backflow can lead to a left ventricular volume overload, with the heart having to work harder with each heartbeat, and may result in heart failure. It can be due to congenital abnormality of valves, rheumatic fever, endocarditis or systemic vasculitis – for example, rheumatoid arthritis or systemic lupus erythematosus (SLE) (Elkayam and Bitar, 2005). It is usually well tolerated in pregnancy. If symptomatic with left ventricular dysfunction, drug therapy may be needed. Antibiotics are usually prescribed for labour. In the postnatal period a residual valve dilation may result from the pregnancy, and this will need observation, monitoring and, perhaps, surgery.

AORTIC STENOSIS

Aortic stenosis, as the name implies, is a narrowing of the aortic valve opening (*see* Figure 3.3). It can be caused by a congenital defect whereby the aortic valve has two

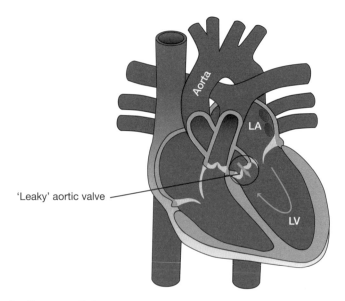

FIGURE 3.2: Aortic regurgitation

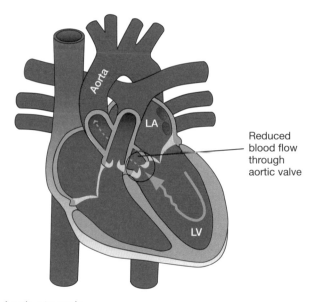

FIGURE 3.3: Aortic stenosis

cusps instead of three, or it may occur following damage to the valve from an episode of rheumatic fever. However, complications from aortic stenosis are rare in pregnancy.

In the preconception period the severity of the lesion and left ventricular function should be evaluated. If it is severe, the woman may be counselled against becoming pregnant as the mortality rate is high. Case reports of successful surgery (e.g., balloon dilatation of valve) during pregnancy have been reported for those with significant symptoms as a palliative measure. This allows deferment of valve replacement until after birth (Myerson, *et al.*, 2005).

Clinical symptoms, in particular pulmonary oedema, usually occur after 20–24 weeks and diuretic medication may be necessary. Uteroplacental perfusion may be decreased and it may be necessary to treat hypotension (late in pregnancy or associated with haemorrhage), which could necessitate volume replacement.

Antibiotics are often prescribed in labour. Invasive monitoring may be used as fluid management is vital: a small reduction in circulating volume may decrease cardiac output and cause hypotension, while a small increase may lead to pulmonary oedema. For this reason an epidural may not be suitable, but avoidance of tachycardia is also important. This woman is also very susceptible to supine hypotension and may not tolerate pushing. In the third stage the blood loss needs to be carefully controlled, monitored and replaced. In the immediate postnatal period, as cardiac filling pressures increase, diuretics may be necessary to avoid pulmonary oedema.

PROSTHETIC VALVES

Prosthetic heart valves carry the risk of clot formation. In pregnancy this is an even greater problem due to the hypercoagulable changes of pregnancy and thus achieving adequate anticoagulation is problematic but essential. Anticoagulation in pregnancy increases the risk of haemorrhage, especially peripartum (and there is a potential loss of the fetus through abruption or fetal intracranial haemorrhage) and oral anticoagulation has the potential to cause fetal abnormalities. However, if no anticoagulation has been taken, then embolic complications are likely and the woman may need a clot removed from the heart under cardiopulmonary bypass, which has a high mortality. A cardiologist needs to carefully asses anticoagulation requirements (Ginsberg, *et al.*, 2003). (*See* section on *anticoagulants* on p. 70).

Mechanical valves are most commonly used and are long-lasting. Tissue valves (bioprostheses) are less likely to cause thromoembolic risks, but they will degenerate and replacement surgery will become necessary. Some studies have shown a connection between pregnancy and more rapid degeneration of tissue valves; however, others have not (Warnes, 2007). All women with prosthetic valves need endocarditis prophylaxis.

INFECTIVE ENDOCARDITIS

Endocarditis is a serious complication of heart disease and is usually a bacterial or fungal infection. The usual infecting agent is *Streptococcus viridans* (Campuzano, *et al.*, 2003), but *Staphylococcus aureus* has also been identified (Cabell, *et al.*, 2002). Confidential Enquiries report that endocarditis causes between 1 and 3 deaths every three years, and about 50% of these women had a known cardiac anomaly (Lewis, 2007).

The risk is present for those with prosthetic cardiac valves, prior bacterial endocarditis (Horstkotte, *et al.*, 2004), complex cyanotic congenital heart disease or surgically constructed systemic pulmonary shunts. Besides those with congenital heart disease (Stuart, 2006), other groups of women at risk are those with drug addiction, periodontal disease (Joshipura, *et al.*, 2000), preterm rupture of membranes (Mercer and Arheart, 1995), prolonged labour, manual removal of the placenta and local infection (Stuart, 2006).

The diagnosis should be suspected in pregnant women with a pyrexia of unknown origin and heart murmur (Montoya, *et al.*, 2003). This can be confirmed with blood cultures demonstrating bacteraemia, especially *S. viridans* or *S. aureus* (although these have been shown to be negative in about 10% of cases) (Moreillon and Que, 2004), and an echocardiogram demonstrating anatomical lesions on the valves or another related abnormality.

It is not known whether antibiotic prophylaxis can prevent endocarditis (Stuart, 2006), and different authorities have different guidelines for prescribing antibiotics. Treatment is by the appropriate antibiotic given for a minimum of six weeks. In pregnancy, infection may lead to congestive cardiac failure and the need for valve replacement (Stuart, 2006).

MARFAN'S SYNDROME AND COMPLICATIONS

Marfan's syndrome is a rare genetic (autosomal dominant) disorder of the connective tissue (Pyeritz, 2000) involving skeletal, ocular, pulmonary and cardiovascular disorders, including mitral regurgitation. There is a risk of aortic rupture and dissection during pregnancy, most commonly in the third trimester or immediately postnatal (*see* Chapter 2, *Systemic vascular resistance*). The risk is greatest if there is pre-existing aortic dilation. All women with Marfan's syndrome should wear a medical alert information band or badge, and this is particularly important in pregnancy.

Many women are asymptomatic, so pre-pregnancy counselling is particularly important, as they may not obtain the investigations and information regarding possible outcomes before making the decision to become pregnant. The most important element of Marfan's syndrome is aortic aneurysm and aortic dissection, but other cardiac conditions such as prolapsing mitral valve or aortic regurgitation can also be involved. Pregnancy in all women with Marfan's syndrome must be considered high risk, but the risk of adverse outcome rises when the aortic root measurement is increased (Meijboom and Mulder, 2007). A family history of dissection (Silverman, *et al.*, 1995) increases any risk. Risk estimation is also dependent on the dissection site, with proximal dissection more predictable than distal dissections (Immer, *et al.*, 2003).

Those with Marfan's syndrome are probably already being treated with beta blockers (Meijboom and Mulder, 2007) and these should be continued during pregnancy. Beta blockers are taken to reduce the force against the aortic wall, and it is vital that the blood pressure is maintained at a low rate.

In pregnancy regular echocardiograms are recommended to measure the aortic diameter. MRI or computed tomography (CT) scans may also be used. If the diameters increase during pregnancy, surgery will be needed. If the pregnancy is not yet viable, it can be done with protective cardiopulmonary bypass techniques, but there is still a high risk of fetal loss (Parry and Westaby, 1996). If the pregnancy is viable, early delivery and then surgery is recommended (Swan, 2006).

The first sign of dissection may be cardiovascular collapse, but this could be preceded by syncope (transient loss of consciousness), chest and/or back pain. *See* section on *aortic dissection* following.

In labour blood pressure monitoring and control is vital and an arterial line is usually used to aid this. Caesarean section is common and this is often preterm. If a vaginal delivery is undertaken, epidural and instrumental delivery is recommended (Swan, 2006). Careful fluid balance with minimal variations in fluid shifts is necessary.

Ergometrine should be avoided because of the risk of increased blood pressure. If the woman has cardiac valve involvement, antibiotics are prescribed.

In the immediate postnatal period the risk of dissection remains, so close monitoring of blood pressure and fluid balance continues, together with cardiac assessment.

MITRAL VALVE PROLAPSE

Mitral valve prolapse is characterised by the displacement of an abnormally thickened mitral valve cusp (or flap) into the left atrium when the left ventricles contract. It is common in child-bearing women (Freed, *et al.*, 1999). It may be a benign, asymptomatic and even undiagnosed condition or be associated with many other cardiac anomalies. Symptoms include panic attacks, anxiety, faintness, palpitations, dyspnoea on exertion and chest pain. It may be part of Marfan's syndrome.

Common complications include mitral valve regurgitation (backflow of blood: *see* following section), infective endocarditis, cerebral ischaemia or sudden death, although the more dangerous complications are rarely seen in pregnant women as they are more usual in those > 45 years of age.

Mitral valve prolapse is difficult to diagnose during pregnancy, due to the normal changes of pregnancy. If the condition is uncomplicated, there are minimal risks to the pregnant woman or the fetus. If arrhythmias develop, these may be treated with digoxin or beta blockers. Antibiotics may also be necessary if there are complications.

MITRAL REGURGITATION

Although mitral regurgitation (*see* Figure 3.4) is commonly seen as a complication of mitral valve prolapse, there are multiple other causes, such as deformity of the valve, previous endocarditis or damage (for example, following surgery), or rheumatic fever. If it is serious, surgery may be necessary, ideally before pregnancy, but when

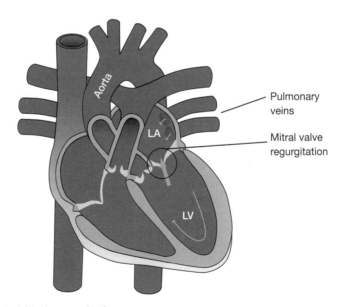

FIGURE 3.4: Mitral regurgitation

they are pregnant most women do well because of the reduced systemic resistance of pregnancy.

Assessment is made by serial echocardiograms. If left ventricular failure does occur, digoxin and diuretics are prescribed. Antibiotic prophylaxis for endocarditis is usual. In labour a rise in blood pressure needs to be avoided, and cardiac monitoring to detect atrial fibrillation is recommended.

AORTIC DISSECTION

Dissection occurs when the lining of the aorta tears and the blood flow escapes between the layers of the aortic vessel wall, creating a false lumen (*see* Figure 3.5). Rupture of the aorta can follow, resulting in death from excessive blood loss. It is not clear why tears develop but this may involve the degeneration of the collagen and elastin that make up the structure of the tunica media (middle layer of the vessel) in conditions such as Marfan's and Ehlers-Danlos syndromes. Hypertension is also a risk factor for aortic dissection in pregnancy.

Pregnancy is a risk factor for this life-threatening condition, especially in those with underlying pathology. It is not common, but in those aged under 40 years of age, 50% are seen in pregnancy (Ray, *et al.*, 2004). It usually occurs in the third trimester and presents with a stabbing, tearing chest pain, radiating to the back. There may be a loss of peripheral pulses, and the fetus may be compromised if the blood flow to the uterus is affected.

Aortic dissection is usually diagnosed by CT. A transoesophageal echocardiogram or MRI may also be used.

Medical treatment to lower the blood pressure may not be effective and can be dangerous to the fetus: surgery may be performed if the woman is less than 30 weeks

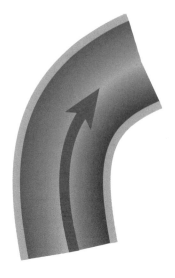
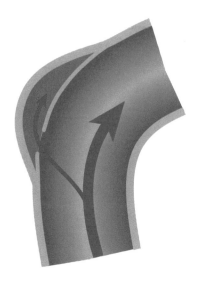

Normal   Dissection

FIGURE 3.5: Aortic dissection

pregnant (Immer, *et al.*, 2003). Later in pregnancy, a Caesarean section is carried out either at the same time or 24 hours before the repair. The aortic root is also vulnerable to sheer stress and dissection in the immediate postnatal period (Head and Thorne, 2005).

CONGENITAL HEART DISEASE
EISENMENGER'S SYNDROME AND PULMONARY HYPERTENSION

Eisenmenger's syndrome is defined as increased pulmonary vascular resistance as a result of uncorrected left-to-right shunt due to a ventricular septal defect, atrial septal defect or patent ductus arteriosus. The defect results in the mixing of deoxygenated blood with oxygenated blood and causes cyanosis.

Pulmonary hypertension is a progressive haemodynamic condition characterised by a rise in the blood pressure of the pulmonary arteries. It is not strictly congenital heart disease but is discussed together with Eisenmenger's because it has a similarly serious nature in pregnancy. The cause of pulmonary hypertension may be unknown (idiopathic) or secondary to a number of conditions, including congenital heart disease, HIV drugs and other diseases such as haemoglobinopathies or thyroid disorders. It may also be associated with some lung diseases or thrombotic or embolic disease (Parambil and McGoon, 2007).

Pulmonary hypertension may be diagnosed during the exploration of other conditions before symptoms appear, but the most common symptom is exertional dyspnoea. In pregnancy dyspnoea may be present even when resting.

In most cases these women will be advised not to become pregnant or to terminate the pregnancy. However, if a woman wishes to carry on with the pregnancy, she will need careful and intensive multidisciplinary care. In the antenatal period she will require close monitoring, probably hospital admission, with activity restriction or bed rest (Warnes, 2007), possible oxygen administration guided by saturation monitoring and effective anticoagulation therapy. Any congestive heart failure will need treatment, but diuretics can be difficult to administer as most of these women will not tolerate rapid fluid fluctuations.

Throughout pregnancy the fetus will receive intensive monitoring, as IUGR is common, but in those that proceed to delivery, maternal mortality is higher than fetal mortality (Parambil and McGoon, 2007).

Because of the woman's fixed low cardiac output, most authorities recommend delivery by Caesarean section under general anaesthetic (Bonnin, *et al.*, 2005) to avoid stresses of labour and the potential vasodilation of an epidural (these women are also usually anticoagulated). However, there is still debate about the best mode of delivery. In labour or at delivery haemodynamic monitoring is necessary, usually via a CVP line. Postnatal care requires close monitoring. There is a poor tolerance of hypovolaemia and hypervolaemia and a susceptibility to thromboembolism. Anxiety, effort and excitement can cause fainting and collapse (Daliento, *et al.*, 1998).

Most deaths will occur within 30 days postnatal, not during pregnancy or labour and delivery (Weiss, *et al.*, 1998), so this woman may need prolonged hospital admission and care.

ATRIAL SEPTAL DEFECTS

An atrial septal defect is a relatively common congenital heart condition and is more common in women than in men (Uebing and Gatzoulis, 2006). The flow is from left to right atrium and leads to an enlarged right atrium and ventricle and increased pulmonary blood flow (*see* Figure 3.6). It is frequently overlooked in childhood as it may produce few symptoms. However, it can progress in rare instances to pulmonary vascular disease, Eisenmenger's syndrome, right-sided heart failure and supraventricular arrhythmias.

Small defects may not need to be closed; however, if they are large or causing problems (for example, ischaemia or right heart enlargement) then closure may improve the symptoms and decrease the risk of right heart failure (Brochu, *et al.*, 2002). Treatment may be needed for atrial arrhythmias or thromboprophylaxis, but if there is no pulmonary hypertension or right ventricular dysfunction the pregnancy should be well tolerated (Uebing and Gatzoulis, 2006).

A short second stage is recommended, as the Valsalva manoeuvre may lead to emboli. Repaired ostium secundum and repaired sinus venous arterial septal defects do not need prophylactic antibiotics, but ostium primum defects do.

VENTRICULAR SEPTAL DEFECTS

Ventricular septal defects are very unlikely not to be repaired, but if they are not they will cause cyanotic heart disease and be classified as Eisenmenger's syndrome by the time the individual reaches adulthood. If they are repaired they may cause no problem, but any sequelae from the surgery has the potential to complicate pregnancy, and unrecognised pulmonary hypertension may become clinically obvious only when the woman is pregnant.

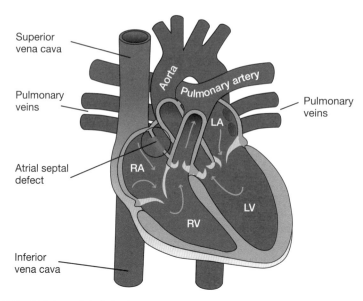

FIGURE 3.6: Atrial septal defect

PATENT DUCTUS ARTERIOSUS

Patent ductus arteriosus has usually been treated during childhood. If they are large and are not repaired, by adulthood there is a likelihood of Eisenmenger's syndrome and fetal loss. Surgery is possible during pregnancy. If unrepaired, close monitoring of the pregnancy will be offered and antibiotics are necessary as a prophylactic.

ATRIOVENTRICULAR SEPTAL DEFECT

An unrepaired atrioventricular septal defect will probably be Eisenmenger's syndrome by adulthood. It is often associated with chromosomal abnormalities such as Down's syndrome.

TETRALOGY OF FALLOT (R TO L SHUNT)

Tetralogy of Fallot (TOF) is the most common cyanotic congenital heart defect and consists of a ventricular septal defect, overriding aorta, pulmonary stenosis and right ventricular hypertrophy with consequent cyanosis (*see* Figure 3.7). Women with an uncorrected condition are rarely seen in pregnancy and those with a previous repair without residual defects and normal functional status should do well, although arrhythmias may be present. However, surgery may lead to pulmonary regurgitation, which could lead to right ventricular dysfunction, which may in turn result in ventricular tachycardia and sudden death (Gatzoulis, *et al.*, 2000).

Before pregnancy an evaluation of the past repair for residual defects such as ventricular septal defect should be made. The risks in pregnancy after repair depend on

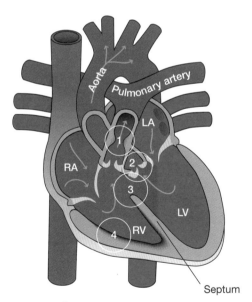

1. Pulmonary stenosis
2. Overriding aorta
3. Ventricular septal defect (VSD)
4. Right ventricular hypertrophy

FIGURE 3.7: Tetralogy of Fallot

the status of the repair. The presence of severe pulmonary regurgitation, right or left ventricular dysfunction or pulmonary hypertension will all increase the risk for mother and fetus (Veldtman, *et al.*, 2004).

Genetic testing should be offered to establish the condition of the fetus, especially if TOF in the mother is part of DiGeorge syndrome. In pregnancy care must be taken to prevent fatigue, and additional oxygen may be required. The fetus may be IUGR. Pregnancy assessment should concentrate on detecting signs of right or left heart dysfunction and arrhythmias.

During labour and delivery, central haemodynamic monitoring (although this has the potential to increase arrhythmias) is usual, and care must be paid to hydration, fluid management and blood pressure monitoring. Epidural and instrumental delivery may be used. Antibiotics are usually prescribed.

PULMONARY STENOSIS

Pulmonary stenosis is involved in about 10% of congenital heart disease. It may be an isolated obstruction of the right ventricle outflow or part of TOF (or its repair). The right ventricle has to pump harder to get blood past the blockage to the pulmonary artery (*see* Figure 3.8). The condition is usually asymptomatic, but if it is severe, right heart failure or atrial arrhythmias may develop (Uebing and Gatzoulis, 2006). Pregnancy is usually successful unless the right heart function is severely compromised (Elkayam and Bitar, 2005). If early right heart failure does occur, balloon valvuloplasty to dilate the stenosis may be undertaken, but this would ideally have been done before pregnancy. Antibiotic prophylaxis is usual in labour.

TRANSPOSITION OF THE GREAT ARTERIES

Transposition of the great arteries comprises 5–7% of all congenital heart defects. Most have had a surgical repair in childhood, and those with good or only slightly impaired

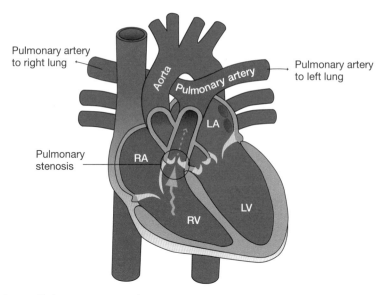

FIGURE 3.8: Pulmonary stenosis

right ventricular function and no arrhythmias are at relatively low risk in pregnancy (Drenthen, *et al.*, 2005). However, congenitally corrected transposition of the great arteries may be associated with other heart defects that can cause adverse effects and the success of the pregnancy will be dependent on the effect this has on the woman (Connolly, *et al.*, 1999).

Pre-pregnancy an assessment of ventricular function and effectiveness of arterial baffles (barriers put into the heart to redirect the blood flow) is undertaken, ideally by MRI, to ensure that the increased cardiac output of pregnancy can be tolerated. The woman may be at risk of the pregnancy causing a long-term deterioration of the ventricular function (Guedes, *et al.*, 2004), and she must be alerted to this possibility.

In pregnancy there is a risk of heart failure, arrhythmias and thromboembolism (some authorities suggest low-dose aspirin to reduce this risk). Reduced activity during pregnancy is recommended. Serial echocardiograms are usual, along with careful observation and treatment for congestive cardiac failure (Guedes, *et al.* 2004; Drenthen, *et al.* 2005).

During labour, cardiac monitoring is used, together with oxygen as necessary (monitoring saturation levels) and avoidance of volume overload. Epidural analgesia and a short second stage are recommended.

AORTIC COARCTATION (OR COARCTATION OF THE AORTA)

Aortic coarctation accounts for about 5 8% of congenital heart disease. It involves a narrowing of the aorta in the region where the ductus arteriosus existed in the fetal circulation (*see* Figure 3.9). The blockage results in an increase in blood pressure to the head and arms and a lowering of blood pressure in the lower body. Most women have been diagnosed and received surgery for this in childhood, but it can present for the first time in pregnancy. If repaired, maternal and fetal outcomes are generally good. However, the older the woman was when she had her repair, the higher the chance she has of developing hypertension in later life and in pregnancy. This condition is also often associated with other defects (Swan, 2006): for example, a predisposition to aortic dissection. Even after successful surgery she may be left with hypertension, aneurysms or recoarctation, all of which may impact on her pregnancy (Swan, 2006).

Before pregnancy, imaging with an echocardiogram and/or MRI is recommended to ensure that no aortic valve disease or related aneurysms are present. Imaging may also be carried out serially during the pregnancy.

An increased systolic blood pressure at booking should lead to investigation for undiagnosed cardiac disease, and the Confidential Enquiry into Maternal and Child Health (Lewis, 2004) relates a case of an increased systolic blood pressure being ignored and the woman later dying of undiagnosed aortic coarctation. If the echocardiogram, CT or MRI show severe coarctation, this may have dangerous consequences for the mother and fetus, often necessitating surgery and/or termination of the pregnancy (Swan, 2006).

During pregnancy, hypertension is common and may have been pre-existing, especially if the woman has not had regular cardiac follow-ups and/or preconception care. Blood pressure should be measured in both arms as the left may not reflect systemic blood pressure. An MRI may be necessary to assess for aneurysm (older methods of grafts predispose to this).

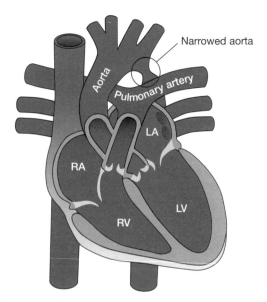

FIGURE 3.9: Aortic coarctation

In labour, swings in the blood pressure may lead to cerebral haemorrhage, and for this reason a carefully managed epidural and instrumental delivery is often recommended.

CARDIOMYOPATHY (VENTRICULAR DYSFUNCTION)

The most important of the cardiomyopathies in maternity care are hypertrophic obstructive cardiomyopathy (HOCM), dilated cardiomyopathies (DCM) and peri-partum cardiomyopathy (PPCM).

HYPERTROPHIC OBSTRUCTIVE CARDIOMYOPATHY

HOCM involves excessive thickening of the left ventricle muscle without any obvious cause. The thickened walls can obstruct or distort blood flow and arrhythmias can develop. HOCM (involving left ventricular diastolic dysfunction) has a 70% familial risk with autosomal dominant inheritance. Diagnosis is usually made by echocardio-gram to investigate symptoms or as part of familial screening following the diagnosis of a close relative. Usually women with HOCM will tolerate pregnancy well, but if they are symptomatic pre-pregnancy there is an increased risk of complications. Signs and symptoms in pregnancy may include chest pain, breathlessness, syncope, heart arrhythmias, heart failure or sudden death. Treatment may include medication (beta blockers or anti-dysrhythmics) or surgery (pacing or implantable defibrillators). The outcome relates to the presence and degree of the symptoms pre-pregnancy but is usually good. During labour it is particularly important to maintain stable fluid levels and avoid any conditions that restrict preload, such as supine position, haemorrhage or Valsalva manoeuvre. Anaemia, pain and dysrhythmia may lead to tachycardia and a high-risk situation that has the potential to end in the sudden death of the woman.

DILATED CARDIOMYOPATHIES

DCM involves dilation of the muscle walls of the heart, in particular, the left ventricle, which weakens the muscles and impairs contractibility. Arrhythmias may occur. Symptoms of DCM often fit New York Heart Association classifications III–IV, and pregnancy is usually not advised. It may be extremely dangerous for the woman if she continues with the pregnancy and expert counselling, assessment and management is vital. However, with this expert care, and if the woman's condition is stable, a successful pregnancy may be possible (Bernstein and Magriples, 2001). Assessment is made with echocardiology and/or stress tests preconception, and drug regimes may be changed. There is a risk of pulmonary oedema and congestive heart failure after 20 weeks, so diuretics and/or digoxin treatment may be necessary. There is also an increased risk of clot formation. In labour, haemodynamic monitoring, continuing at least until 24–48 hours postnatal, will be used.

PERIPARTUM CARDIOMYOPATHY

A rare complication of pregnancy, PPCM was defined in 1971 as the development of heart failure in the last month of pregnancy or within 3–5 months postnatal in the absence of other possible diagnoses, and echocardiography demonstration of impaired left ventricular systolic function. PPCM may occur earlier in pregnancy than the definition would allow, and any symptoms will need prompt attention to avert a possible disastrous outcome (Elkayam, *et al.*, 2005).

PPCM is responsible for a number of maternal cardiac deaths in the UK (Lewis, 2007). Although the mortality rate is high, it is declining, probably due to increased recognition and improved care, but long-term morbidity is common in those who do not die (Murali and Baldisseri, 2005). Overall 50–60% of women recover within six months but full cardiac function may never be restored, and in fact some women may need a heart transplant (Poppas and Miller, 2008). If recovery is made there may be a 25–50% reoccurrence in a future pregnancy (Elkayam, 2002). Future pregnancy prognosis will depend on the degree of recovery from PPCM and detailed assessment and counselling before another pregnancy is highly recommended. If the woman does become pregnant, she will need serial echocardiograms during pregnancy to assess her condition.

Risk factors are general and include advanced maternal age (>30 years old), greater parity, women of African origin, multiple pregnancy, hypertension and viral myocarditis. There are possible links to tocolytic treatment and cocaine abuse (Hibbard, *et al.*, 1999).

Signs and symptoms include chest pain, dyspnoea on exertion, orthopnoea, dependent oedema and fatigue, and these should prompt a rapid referral by the midwife. PPCM may also present as collapse within the defined time frame. It can be precipitated by fluid overload (for example, in Syntocinon use or epidural preloads) and is diagnosed by chest X-ray and echocardiography.

Management includes oxygen, diuretics, vasodilators and angiotensin-converting enzyme (ACE) inhibitors, thromboprophylaxis and other drugs as necessary. If the condition is very serious, the woman may need intubation and ventilation and treatment with invasive monitoring according to need.

DISORDERS OF ELECTRICAL CONDUCTION
WOLFF-PARKINSON-WHITE SYNDROME

Wolff-Parkinson-White syndrome is a congenital abnormality in about 0.2% of the population. It involves an additional conducting system between the atria and ventricles, giving rise to supraventricular arrhythmias. Normal anti-arrhythmic drugs may not work, but it may be possible to control paroxysmal supraventricular tachycardia by vagal control (e.g., respiratory effort) or it may resolve spontaneously. However, drugs (e.g., beta blockers) or direct current shock (defibrillation) may also be necessary (Downie, *et al.*, 2003). The best treatment is to ablate (destroy) the accessory pathway before pregnancy.

DYSRHYTHMIAS

A rise in dysrhythmias in pregnancy with reported palpitations is common and often non-threatening (see *Electrical activity in the heart* in Chapter 2). Palpitations may be due to sensitivity to oestrogen, anaemia, stress and anxiety, increased awareness of heartbeat due to the changing location of the heart within the chest, cold medicines, caffeine and cocaine. However, they may also be due to subclinical myocardial disease, especially in the last month of pregnancy. Assessment can be made via ambulatory Holter monitoring and an ECG. Treatment is according to the specific diagnosis.

CONDUCTION SYSTEM DISEASE

Those with pacemakers usually tolerate pregnancy well. In the absence of heart lesions, antibiotics may not be necessary.

CARDIAC TRANSPLANT

(See also the section on organ transplants and general pregnancy care issues in Chapter 5.)

As cardiac transplants are becoming more successful, an increase in the number of pregnancies in these women has likewise been reported. Heart/lung transplants with successful pregnancies have also been reported in the literature (Armenti, *et al.*, 2006).

The first sign of ischaemia in a transplanted heart may be dyspnoea (there is no perception of ischaemic pain in a transplanted heart). Transplants have increased sensitivity to vasoactive drugs and hypovolaemia (Kim, *et al.*, 1996). Hypertension (and pre-eclampsia) is greater in immunosuppressed women with cardiac transplants, and this could lead to pulmonary oedema. There is always a risk of rejection of the transplanted heart during pregnancy. There is also the concern of immunosuppressive drugs and the effect on the fetus, which is commonly IUGR. Immunosuppressed women are also at risk of opportunistic infections.

During pregnancy the left ventricular function will be monitored as necessary. In labour, invasive monitoring may be necessary. Antibiotic cover is usually prescribed for Caesarean section or instrumental delivery. There is often involvement of a transplant physician, cardiologist and anaesthetist during labour and delivery. In the postnatal period, breastfeeding is usually not recommended as immunosuppressive drugs are mostly contraindicated, but this would need to be individually assessed.

ISCHAEMIC HEART DISEASE: CORONARY ARTERIAL DISEASE (CAD) AND MYOCARDIAL INFARCTIONS (MI)

Coronary arterial disease (or ischaemic heart disease) is a growing problem in women of child-bearing age, mainly as a result of changing lifestyles (*see* section *Blood supply to the heart*, Chapter 2). Risk factors for coronary arterial disease such as smoking, diabetes and stress are more frequently seen in pregnant women, and this is often combined with increased age, as older women are increasingly undertaking pregnancy. Risk factors in the younger population also include smoking, oral contraceptive use among smokers, hypercholesterolemia and thrombophilias or family hyperlipidaemia. As well as pre-pregnancy evaluation, effective counselling as to the specific risks is important. In addition, if medication is being used, it may need to be changed in order to protect the fetus from potential damage.

In pregnancy it is best to diagnose coronary arterial disease with a stress echo-cardiogram rather than using radionuclide perfusion agent. If imaging is positive, then cardiac catheterisation with abdominal shielding can be carried out. Angina can be treated as usual (there is little literature on its treatment in pregnancy as it has been such a rare condition), and surgery is possible during pregnancy for unstable angina or MI. When using nitrates in pregnancy, care should be taken not to cause hypotension, as this could compromise the fetus. Complications during pregnancy include congestive cardiac failure, arrhythmias, stroke and MI.

Myocardial infarctions can occur at any time throughout pregnancy but are most common in the third trimester. Signs and symptoms usually include crushing chest pain (*see* Box 3.1), but the chest pain is often mistakenly considered to be anything from heartburn to pulmonary embolism. As MI is rare in child-bearing women, it is often not considered; however, as it is becoming more common levels of suspicion need to rise. Cocaine may cause MI secondary to coronary artery spasm.

BOX 3.1: SIGNS AND SYMPTOMS OF MI

- Ischaemic chest pain
- Pain in arms (usually left), neck, back and/or lower jaw
- Nausea
- Sweating

To diagnose MI the clinical signs and symptoms (*see* Box 3.1) are evaluated and a 12-lead ECG and blood tests (primarily involving cardiac enzymes) will confirm the diagnosis.

The clot is usually on the anterior wall of the heart and mortality is reported as up to 21%. Treatment is as for the non-pregnant individual: thrombolytic agents, e.g., streptokinase or plasminogen, may be used. Low-dose aspirin is usually prescribed. Cardiac catheterisation with shielding can be carried out. Treatment following acute MI may also include open heart surgery (e.g., a cardio-pulmonary bypass). The mother is at the same risk as if she were not pregnant, but a high fetal loss has been reported (Roos-Hesselink, 2006). Following stabilisation, investigations are needed into thrombophilias.

In labour, extra oxygen may be required. Attention should be paid to pain control as pain leads to tachycardia, which leads to increased oxygen requirements by the myocardium that can result in ischaemia. Vaginal delivery is preferable, with a short second stage.

PERICARDITIS

Pericarditis (inflammation of the pericardium – the sac that surrounds the heart) is usually self-limiting. It may be idiopathic or arise from infection: viral (including mumps, infectious mononucleosis, Epstein-Barr virus, hepatitis B or HIV) or bacterial (including pneumococci, staphylococci, streptococci, gram-negative septicaemia, listeria). It also may be a complication of tuberculosis, SLE and rheumatoid arthritis.

Signs and symptoms include pleuritic chest pain, fever, cough, dyspnoea, fatigue and malaise. Diagnosis is made on clinical signs and examination, and ECG and echocardiogram results. Treatment is according to the underlying cause.

DRUGS COMMONLY USED IN CARDIAC DISEASE

This section gives an overview of the drugs used, how they work and possible side effects. Physicians prescribing medication need to consider fetal effects and balance these against indications for maternal well-being. Midwives should encourage women to discuss concerns with their physician or obstetrician.

ALPHA-ADRENOCEPTOR-BLOCKING DRUGS

Alpha blockers (e.g., prazosin, terazosin and doxazosin) reduce peripheral arterial resistance and thereby blood pressure without increasing heart rate or decreasing output. Side effects include dizziness, postural hypotension and headache. These drugs are not commonly used in pregnancy.

ANGIOTENSIN-CONVERTING ENZYME (ACE) INHIBITORS

ACE inhibitors (e.g., captopril and enalapril) control blood pressure and treat heart failure. They work by inhibiting the conversion of angiotensin I to angiotensin II, resulting in the dilation of arterioles, which reduces preload. These drugs influence sodium and water retention. Side effects include a dry cough, hypotension and acute renal failure (and are contraindicated in renal disease). They may not cause damage to the fetus in the first trimester (Tomlinson, 2006) but many fetal risks occur in the second and third trimester.

ANGIOTENSIN-II RECEPTOR (ATR) ANTAGONISTS

ATR antagonists (e.g., losartan, valsartan and eprosartan) influence vasoconstriction, aldosterone release and sodium retention. Limited information is available on their effect in pregnancy but they are thought to have the same fetal effects in the second and third trimester as ACE inhibitors (Saji, *et al.*, 2001). Side effects (not common) are hypotension, dizziness and hyperkalaemia.

ANTI-ARRHYTHMICS

Anti-arrhythmia drugs are generally used to correct cardiac arrhythmias such as atrial fibrillation and ventricular tachycardia. They are divided into five classes, and most commonly used in pregnancy are class II: beta blockers (*see* section following) and class IV: calcium channel blockers (*see* section following). Their side effects vary and depend on the specific drug. Although some anti-arrhythmics have teratogenic effects and/or may cause IUGR, most of the widely used anti-arrhythmics appear safe in pregnancy, although there is very limited data of the effects of many of the new drugs.

Beta blockers

Beta blockers (e.g., atenolol, labetalol and propranolol) inhibit the effects of adrenaline on beta receptor cells, decreasing the heart rate and the strength of the cardiac contraction. This therefore reduces the workload of the heart and also reduces the oxygen requirements of the myocardial cells. Gradual withdrawal from these drugs is needed. Side effects include fatigue, cold extremities, bronchoconstriction (therefore contraindicated in asthma), hypotension, bradycardia and heart block. All these drugs cross the placenta and although there is not considered to be a significant fetal risk in using them (Khalil and O'Brien, 2006). IUGR has been identified (Magee and Duley, 2003).

Calcium channel blockers

Calcium channel blockers (e.g., nifedipine and verapamil) have an anti-arrhythmic effect. Calcium entry induces contraction in the smooth muscle and in cardiac cells this causes vasoconstriction. Blocking the calcium channels will promote relaxation, allowing vasodilation and reduced cardiac contraction strength. Side effects – flushing, headache, dizziness, peripheral oedema and fall in blood pressure – may lead to tachycardia and palpitations. These drugs appear to have no adverse fetal effects.

ANTIHYPERTENSIVES

Hydralazine is a vasodilator taken orally or IV. It is usually used IV to manage acute hypertension. Side effects include headache, nausea, flushing and vomiting (note: these are the same signs as fulminating pre-eclampsia). It can cause rapid decrease in blood pressure, resulting in fetal heart rate abnormalities.

CENTRALLY ACTING ANTIHYPERTENSIVE DRUGS

Methyldopa stimulates alpha-adrenergic receptors, which results in the decreased activity of the sympathetic system, reducing vascular peripheral tone and vasoconstriction. Side effects include depression, drowsiness and fluid retention.

INOTROPIC DRUGS

This group includes digoxin, dopamine, adrenaline (epinephrine) and noradrenaline. Digoxin is commonly used to slow and strengthen arterial impulses. It is used in atrial flutter and fibrillation and in congestive heart failure. It is rarely administered IV, and is taken mainly orally (by a tablet or liquid). It crosses the placenta (Tikanoja, *et al.*, 1998). Levels need to be monitored in pregnancy to prevent toxicity (Downie, *et al.*, 2003).

Dopamine is used in cardiogenic shock. It increases the force of contractions and dilates coronary, intracerebral and renal vessels.

Adrenaline is primarily used in cardiac arrest. It enhances ventricular contraction but also causes a rise in the heart rate and vasoconstriction.

Noradrenaline increases contractibility and causes systemic vasoconstriction.

DIURETICS

Hydrochlorothiazide and furosemide promote excretion of fluid but can cause electrolyte imbalance. They are used in pulmonary oedema, congestive heart failure and hypertension. When used during pregnancy, regular electrolyte assessment and regular ultrasound to assess for IUGR or oligohydramnios is usual. The neonate may be at risk of an electrolyte imbalance.

ANTICOAGULANTS

(*See also* section on *Anticoagulation treatment of DVT and PE* in Chapter 4.)

Warfarin, heparin and low molecular weight heparin (LMWH) inhibit fibrin clot formation.

Unfractionated heparin does not cross the placenta and can be given IV or subcutaneously. However, long-term use can lead to osteoporosis and is associated with thrombocytopenia. To reverse the effect of heparin, protamine sulphate is used.

LMWH similarly does not cross the placenta, but it has a greater bioavailability and a longer half life, permitting once-daily subcutaneous injections. Further benefits over unfractionated heparin include a reduced incidence of heparin-induced thrombocytopenia and osteoporosis. LMWH is now considered the preferred anticoagulant to prevent and treat venous thromboembolism in pregnancy (Greer and Nelson-Piercy, 2005). However, for those women with prosthetic heart valves the data is more limited and the management more complex. For those women who are receiving long-term warfarin treatment, a plan is needed before pregnancy on how best to maintain effective anticoagulation balanced against risk to the fetus.

Warfarin is taken orally and in contrast to heparin crosses the placenta, with particular risk of damage to the embryo if taken between six and 12 weeks gestation. It is also associated with central nervous system malformations when taken at any time during pregnancy. In addition, if taken at the time of delivery it can lead to bleeding in the neonate and it increases the risk of post-partum haemorrhage in the mother (Jilma, *et al.*, 2003). Warfarin is a vitamin K antagonist and as such impairs the synthesis of several coagulation factors. Vitamin K can be given to reverse its effect. If it is used in the second trimester, it should be stopped at 35 weeks and heparin commenced (Warnes, 2007).

OXYTOCICS

Special care is needed when using oxytocin for women with cardiac disease. Oxytocin affects the vascular smooth muscle and can cause hypotension and compensating tachycardia; therefore rapid IV bolus doses should be avoided. Oxytocin also has an antidiuretic hormone effect, and large doses, especially when infused with a large volume of electrolyte-free fluid, can lead to water intoxication and pulmonary oedema.

UTEROTONICS

Ergometrine causes sustained hypertension, so it should be avoided in any woman with cardiac complications.

There is limited data on the use of misoprostol in women with heart disease.

METHODS OF ASSESSING, MONITORING AND DIAGNOSING CARDIAC CONDITIONS

ARTERIAL CATHETER

An arterial catheter is a specialised cannula inserted into the artery and when connected to special equipment it can continuously monitor the blood pressure (Woodrow, 2004) and usually also give a mean arterial pressure (MAP) reading. However, it is a good practice for the blood pressure to also be checked manually about once a shift (Garretson, 2005). Bloods can be taken for arterial blood gas estimation. To do this blood needs to be withdrawn and discarded first to avoid contamination with saline or heparin. Medications should never be given through an arterial line. Particular care of the site is necessary as dislodging the cannula will result in arterial bleeding. The cannula needs to be attached to an infusion (usually normal saline with or without heparin) under pressure.

MEAN ARTERIAL PRESSURE (MAP)

MAP represents the average pressure through the cardiac cycle and represents the perfusion pressure for body organs. It is determined by cardiac output and systemic vascular resistance and can be calculated from blood pressure readings.

$$MAP = diastolic + (systolic - diastolic) \text{ divided by } 3$$

It is shown on arterial line monitors or some electronic blood pressure machines. MAP readings can be used to underpin treatment.

CENTRAL VENOUS PRESSURE (CVP)

The CVP cannula is positioned in the superior or inferior vena cava. It directly reflects the right atrial pressure and indicates the preload of the right ventricle or right ventricle end-diastolic pressure. Recordings are influenced by peripheral resistance, the volume of the blood returning to the heart, the contractility of the heart and position (when standing, etc.). It measures the pressure of the blood filling the right atrium and is used to assess blood volume and guide fluid management. Medications can be given through the CVP line.

ARTERIAL BLOOD GASES (ABG)

Arterial blood gases are taken to evaluate the concentration of gases in the blood, most importantly oxygen, carbon dioxide and bicarbonate, together with assessing the pH. It can provide important information to underpin care of a woman with pulmonary or renal compromise.

PULSE OXIMETER

This correlates closely to arterial blood gases and so can give a continuous indication of respiratory status. It works by evaluating the colour of the blood and gives a continuous assessment of oxygen saturation (SaO_2) (normal 95–100%) and pulse rate. It is non-invasive and is normally positioned on the finger. Readings can be affected by dark nail polish. The probe needs to be moved regularly (about four hourly) in order to avoid pressure damage.

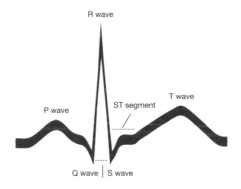

P wave – rapid spread of impulse as it sweeps over atria

QRS complex – rapid spread of impulse from AV node through the bundle of His and the Purkinje fibres. Represents electrical activity of ventricle muscle

T wave – represents relaxaton of ventricle muscle

FIGURE 3.10: Electrocardiogram waveform

ELECTROCARDIOGRAM (ECG)

The ECG is a record of the overall spread of electrical activity through the heart. By attaching electrodes to the surface of the skin, the pattern of electrical activity in the heart can be represented. The normal ECG shows five waves that have been named P, Q, R, S and T (*see* Figure 3.10). Variations can be significant and indicate diagnosis and/or treatment requirements.

Continuous ECG monitoring uses three or five electrodes clipped to adhesive patches on the woman's chest. A 12-lead ECG using leads on limbs and chest will give a more extensive view of the heart's activity and can pinpoint areas of concern, making it useful to diagnose arrhythmias and myocardial ischaemia.

Changes in the ECG occur in pregnancy as the position of the heart changes with the enlarging uterus and elevated diaphragm (Blackburn, 2007)

ECHOCARDIOGRAM (ECHO)

This is an ultrasound examination of the heart that can detect structural abnormalities of the chambers and valves. It can detect direction and magnitude of blood flow, thus making an assessment for conditions such as valvular regurgitation.

COMPUTED TOMOGRAPHY (CT) SCAN

CT scans use X-rays and an electronic detector, which results in cross-sectional images. For adequate assessment of blood vessels an IV contrast medium is needed, and this, plus the high radiation dose, makes it a rare investigation for pregnant women. It is most likely to be used to diagnose and assess aortic dissection.

MAGNETIC RESONANCE IMAGING (MRI)

MRIs use magnets and low-energy radio frequency signals to provide images of anatomy and function. It is non-invasive and does not use radiation. Movement must be avoided as this can cause artefacts. Its effect on the fetus has not been established (DeWilde, *et al.*, 2005) and therefore it should be used only when necessary and after the first trimester, if possible.

EXERCISE TESTING

Exercise testing usually consists of a treadmill where a woman can walk at various rates for variable times while attached to an ECG. There is no data of its safety in pregnancy but it may be useful preconception to establish functional capacity.

AMBULATORY ELECTROCARDIOGRAPHIC MONITORING (HOLTER)

This is a small ECG which is attached to the woman, usually for 24 hours, giving a picture of cardiac activity throughout the day, while she is undergoing various activities. Ambulatory monitoring can help clarify whether palpitations, which are frequent during pregnancy, are from common and benign causes or constitute a more potentially sinister arrhythmia.

REFERENCES

Armenti V, Moritz M, Davison JM. Pregnancy after transplantation. In: James DK, Weiner CP, Steer PJ, *et al.*, editors. *High Risk Pregnancy: management options.* 3rd ed. Philadelphia, PA: Elsevier Saunders; 2006. pp. 1174–86.

Bernstein P, Magriples U. Cardiomyopathy in pregnancy: a retrospective study. *Am J Perinatol.* 2001; **18**: 163–8.

Blackburn ST. *Maternal, Fetal and Neonatal Physiology.* 3rd ed. St Louis, MO: Saunders; 2007.

Bonnin M, Mercier F, Sitbon O, *et al.* Severe pulmonary hypertension during pregnancy. *Anesthesiology.* 2005; **102**: 1133–7.

Brochu M, Baril J, Dore A, *et al.* Improvement in exercise capacity in asymptomatic and mildly symptomatic adults after atrial septal defect percutaneous closure. *Circulation.* 2002; **106**: 1821–6.

Cabell C, Jollis J, Peterson G, *et al.* Changing patient characteristics and the effect on mortality in endocarditis. *Arch Intern Med.* 2002; **162**: 90–4.

Campuzano K, Roque H, Bolnick A, *et al.* Bacterial endocarditis complicating pregnancy: case report and systematic review of the literature. *Arch Gynecol Obstet.* 2003; **268**: 252–5.

Connolly H, Grogan M, Warnes C. Pregnancy among women with congenitally corrected transposition of great arteries. *J AM Coll Cardiol.* 1999; **33**: 1692–5.

Daliento L, Somerville J, Presbitero P, *et al.* Eisenmenger syndrome: factors relating to deterioration and death. *Eur Heart J.* 1998; **19**: 1845–55.

DeWilde J, Rivers A, Price D. A review of the current use of magnetic resonance imaging in pregnancy and safety implications for the fetus. *Prog Biophys Mol Biol.* 2005; **87**: 335–53.

Downie G, Mackenzie J, Williams A. *Pharmacology and Medicines: management for nurses.* 3rd ed. Edinburgh: Churchill Livingstone; 2003.

Drenthen W, Pieper P, Ploeg M, *et al.* Risk of complications during pregnancy after Senning or Mustard (atrial) repair of complete transposition of the great arteries. *Eur Heart J.* 2005; **26**: 2588–95.

Elkayam U. Pregnancy again after peripartum cardiomyopathy: to be or not to be? *Eur Heart J.* 2002; **23**: 753–6.

Elkayam U, Bitar F. Valvular heart disease and pregnancy: part 1: native values. *J Am Coll Cardiol.* 2005; **46**: 223–30.

Elkayam U, Akhter M, Singh H, *et al.* Pregnancy-associated cardiomyopathy: clinical characteristics and a comparison between early and late presentation. *Circulation.* 2005; **111**: 2050–5.

Freed L, Levy D, Levine R, *et al.* Prevalence and clinical outcome of mitral valve prolapse. *N Engl J Med.* 1999; **341**: 1–7.

Garretson S. Haemodynamic monitoring: arterial catheters. *Nurs Stand.* 2005; **19**(31): 55–64.

Gatzoulis M, Balaji S, Webber S, *et al.* Risk factors for arrhythmia and sudden cardiac death late after repair of tetralogy of Fallot: a multicentre study. *Lancet.* 2000; **356**: 975–81.

Ginsberg J, Chan W, Bates S, *et al.* Anticoagulation of pregnant women with mechanical heart valves. *Arch Intern Med.* 2003; **163**: 694–8.

Greer IA, Nelson-Piercy C. Low molecular-weight heparins for thromboprophylaxis and treatment of venous thromboembolism in pregnancy: a systematic review of safety and efficacy. *Blood. 2005;* **106**(2): 401–7.

Guedes A, Mercier L, Leduc L, *et al.* Impact of pregnancy on the systemic right ventricle after a Mustard operation for transposition of the great arteries. *J Am Coll Cardiol.* 2004; **44**: 433–7.

Head C, Thorne S. Congenital heart disease in pregnancy. *Postgrad Med J.* 2005; **81**: 292–8.

Hibbard J, Lindheimer M, Lang R. A modified definition for peripartum cardiomyopathy and prognosis based on echocardiography. *Am J Obstet Gynecol.* 1999; **94**: 311–16.

Horstkotte D, Follath F, Gutschik E, *et al.* Guidelines on prevention, diagnosis and treatment of infective endocarditis executive summary: The Task Force on Infective Endocarditis of the European Society of Cardiology. *Eur Heart J.* 2004; **25**: 267–76.

Immer F, Bansi A, Immer-Banoi A, *et al.* Aortic disease in pregnancy: an analysis of risk factors and outcome. *Ann Thorac Surg.* 2003; **76**: 309–14.

Jilma B, Kamath S, Lip YH. ABC of antithrombotic therapy: antithrombotic therapy in special circumstances – pregnancy and cancer. *BMJ.* 2003; **326**(7380): 37–40.

Joshipura K, Ritchie C, Douglass C. Strength of evidence linking oral conditions and systemic disease. *Compend Contin Educ Dent Suppl.* 2000; **30**: 12–23.

Khalil A, O'Brien P. Cardiac drugs in pregnancy. In: Steer P, Gatzoulis M, Baker P, editors. *Heart Disease and Pregnancy.* London: RCOG Press; 2006. pp. 79–94.

Kim KM, Sukhani R, Slogoff S, *et al.* Central hemodynamic changes associated with pregnancy in a long-term cardiac transplant recipient. *Am J Obstet Gynecol.* 1996; **174**: 1651–3.

Lewis G, editor. The Confidential Enquiry into Maternal and Child Health. *Why Mothers Die 2000–2002.* London: CEMACH; 2004.

Lewis G, editor. The Confidential Enquiry into Maternal and Child Health. *Saving Mothers' Lives: reviewing maternal deaths to make motherhood safer 2003–2005. The Seventh Report on Confidential Enquiries into Maternal Deaths in the UK.* London: CEMACH; 2007.

Magee L, Duley L. Oral beta-blockers for mild to moderate hypertension during pregnancy. *Cochrane Database Syst Rev.* 2003; **3**: CD002863.

Meijboom L, Mulder BJM. Management of pregnancy in Marfan syndrome, Ehlers-Danlos syndrome and other heritable connective tissue disorders. In: Oakley C, Warnes C, editors. *Heart Disease in Pregnancy.* 2nd ed. Oxford: Blackwell; 2007. pp. 122–35.

Mercer B, Arheart K. Antimicrobial therapy in expectant management of preterm premature rupture of the membranes. *Lancet.* 1995; **346**: 1271–9.

Montoya M, Karnath B, Ahmad M. Endocarditis during pregnancy. *South Med J.* 2003; **96**: 1156–7.

Moreillon P, Que Y. Infective endocarditis. *Lancet.* 2004; **363**: 139–49.

Murali S, Baldisseri M. Peripartum cardiomyopathy. *Crit Care Med.* 2005; **33**(Suppl. 10): S340–6.

Myerson SG, Mitchell AR, Ormerod OJ, *et al.* What is the role of balloon dilatation for severe aortic stenosis during pregnancy? *J Heart Valve Dis.* 2005; **14**(2): 147–50.

Parambil J, McGoon M. Pregnancy and pulmonary hypertension. In: Oakley C, Warnes C, editors. *Heart Disease in Pregnancy.* 2nd ed. Oxford: Blackwell; 2007. pp. 59–78.

Parry A, Westaby S. Cardiopulmonary bypass during pregnancy. *Ann Thorac Surg.* 1996; **61**: 1865–9.

Poppas A, Miller M. Peripartum cardiomyopathy. In: Rosene-Montella K, Keely E, Barbour L, *et al.*, editors. *Medical Care of the Pregnant Patient.* 2nd ed. Philadelphia, PA: ACP Press; 2008. pp. 340–3.

Pyeritz R. The Marfan syndrome. *Annu Rev Med.* 2000; **51**: 481–510.

Ray P, Murphy G, Shutt L. Recognition and management of maternal heart disease in pregnancy. *Br J Anaesth.* 2004; **93**: 428–39.

Roos-Hesselink J. Ischaemic heart disease. In: Steer P, Gatzoulis M, Baker P, editors. *Heart Disease and Pregnancy.* London: RCOG Press; 2006. pp. 243–50.

Saji H, Yamanaka M, Hagiwara A, *et al.* Losartan and fetal toxic effects. *Lancet.* 2001; **357**: 363.

Silverman D, Gray J, Roman M, *et al.* Family history of severe cardiovascular disease in Marfan syndrome is associated with increased aortic diameter and decreased survival. *J Am Coll Cardiol.* 1995; **26**: 1062–7.

Stuart G. Maternal endocarditis. In: Steer P, Gatzoulis M, Baker P, editors. *Heart Disease and Pregnancy.* London: RCOG Press; 2006. pp. 267–84.

Swan L. Aortopathies, including Marfan syndrome and coarctation. In: Steer P, Gatzoulis M, Baker P, editors. *Heart Disease and Pregnancy.* London: RCOG Press; 2006. pp. 169–82.

Tikanoja T, Kirkinen P, Nikolajev K, *et al.* Familial atrial fibrillation with fetal onset. *Heart.* 1998; **79**: 195–7.

Tomlinson M. Cardiac Disease. In: James DK, Weiner CP, Steer PJ, *et al.*, editors. *High Risk Pregnancy: management options.* 3rd ed. Philadelphia, PA: Elsevier Saunders; 2006. pp. 790–827.

Uebing A, Gatzoulis M. Right heart lesions. In: Steer P, Gatzoulis M, Baker P, editors. *Heart Disease and Pregnancy.* London: RCOG Press; 2006. pp. 191–210.

Veldtman G, Connolly H, Grogan M, *et al.* Outcomes of pregnancy in women with tetralogy of Fallot. *J Am Coll Cardiol.* 2004; **44**: 174–80.

Warnes C. Cyanotic congenital heart disease. In: Oakley C, Warnes C, editors. *Heart Disease in Pregnancy.* 2nd ed. Oxford: Blackwell; 2007. pp. 43–58.

Weiss B, Zemp L, Seifert B, *et al.* Outcome of pulmonary vascular disease in pregnancy: a systematic overview from 1978 through 1996. *J Am Coll Cardiol.* 1998; **31**: 1650–7.

Woodrow P. Arterial blood pressure monitoring. In: Moore T, Woodrow P, editors. *High Dependency Nursing Care: observation, intervention and support.* London: Routledge; 2004. pp. 301–8.

CHAPTER 4

Haematological disorders

CONTENTS

SUMMARY OF NORMAL HAEMATOLOGICAL CHANGES IN PREGNANCY

▶ Plasma volume increases by 50%.
▶ Red cell mass (total volume of red cells in circulation) increases by 20%.
▶ Physiological anaemia of pregnancy – as a result of the dilution effect of greater plasma increase in relation to increase in red blood cells (RBC).
▶ White blood cell increase.
▶ Hypercoagulable state – changes to coagulation and fibrinolysis.
▶ Venous stasis.
▶ Isolated mild thrombocytopenia – platelet count tends to fall progressively to lower threshold of normal or below near term. Needs to be distinguished from pathological causes such as pre-eclampsia.
▶ Increase in requirement for iron.
▶ Increase in folate requirement.

(Blackburn, 2007; Nelson-Piercy, 2006; Rodger, *et al.*, 2008)

RED BLOOD CELLS (RBCs)

Red blood cells (erythrocytes) contain significant amounts of haemoglobin (Hb) and their primary function is to transport oxygen in the blood. They are flat, disc-shaped cells. This shape gives them a large surface area for the diffusion of oxygen across the membrane and the thinness of the cell enables the oxygen to reach the inner part of the cell. RBCs are formed in the bone marrow, and their maturation is dependent on the presence of iron, vitamin B12 and folic acid, which are derived from the diet. They survive on average for just 120 days in the circulation. As the cell ages it becomes increasingly fragile and most red cells break down in the narrow vasculature of the spleen but some break down in the liver. The cells are recycled in the liver and spleen, which produces iron (reused) and bilirubin (which is changed by the liver to become water soluble and excreted). Hypoxia increases RBC production by stimulating the hormone erythropoietin.

Total RBC volume increases in pregnancy, reflecting the increased fetal and maternal demand for oxygen (Blackburn, 2007). Plasma volume expansion will alter usual reference ranges for red cell indices and these physiological changes are a challenge to the haematological status of a woman with haemoglobinopathies.

RBCs contain several hundred haemoglobin molecules that combine with oxygen, giving arterial blood its red colour and transporting oxygen around the body. Each haemoglobin molecule, as the name suggests, is composed of *haem* (derived from iron) and *globin*, which is the part that is inherited and determines the characteristics of the haemoglobin.

ANAEMIA

The WHO defines anaemia in pregnancy as an Hb level of less that 11 g/dL, although a level of less than 10.5 g/dL is more widely adopted in the second trimester, when physiological haemodilution is at its greatest (Strong, 2006). Iron deficiency is the most common cause (90%) of anaemia in pregnancy, followed by folate deficiency and they can occur together (Karovitch, 2008; Letsky, 2002; Strong, 2006). Vitamin B12 deficiency rarely causes anaemia in pregnancy (Strong, 2006). In HELLP syndrome a breakdown of RBCs results in haemolytic anaemia (Karovitch, 2008).

Anaemia is classified by examining differences in the RBC size (mean cell volume, MCV) and the amount of haemoglobin (mean cell haemoglobin, MCH). In iron deficiency anaemia the RBCs are smaller in size (microcytic) and lacking in haemoglobin, which makes them appear pale (hypochromic) (Bain, 2004). Box 4.1 summarises the causes of anaemia in pregnancy. Discussion will concentrate on the more common causes of anaemia in pregnancy.

BOX 4.1: CAUSES OF ANAEMIA

- Decreased RBC production
  — lack of required substrate such as iron, folate, vitamin B12
  — problems in bone marrow production
- Increased RBC loss
  — bleeding – menstrual loss, during childbirth, trauma
- Increased RBC destruction (haemolytic anaemia)
  — sickle cell anaemia
  — HELLP syndrome
  — Hereditary spherocytosis

(Karovitch, 2008)

IRON DEFICIENCY ANAEMIA

Iron stores in women entering pregnancy can be low due to menstrual loss and poor diet (Blackburn, 2007; Strong, 2006). *See* Box 4.2 for risk factors for anaemia in pregnancy. Pregnancy increases the demand for iron twofold to threefold (Nelson-Piercy, 2006). Iron is needed for extra RBC production, for certain enzymes required for the function of tissues, for the fetus and placenta and to replace the increased normal daily loss (Karovitch, 2008; Letsky, 2002). Fetal requirements, which are greatest in the last four weeks of pregnancy, will be met preferentially at a cost to the mother (Blackburn, 2007). The demand for iron in pregnancy is met partly by the absence of menses and increased absorption of dietary iron by the intestinal mucosa, but it does also rely on maternal iron stores. Absorption of iron is less than 10% of that contained in the diet and the average diet cannot meet this demand.

Iron deficiency not only impairs RBC production but also affects cellular function, resulting in impaired muscular and neurotransmitter function, changes to epithelial cells and alteration in gastrointestinal function (Strong, 2006). Complications of severe iron deficiency anaemia for mother and fetus/neonate are summarised in Box 4.3.

BOX 4.2: RISK FACTORS FOR IRON/FOLATE DEFICIENCY ANAEMIA IN PREGNANCY

- Eating disorders and/or dieting
- Malabsorption conditions such as coeliac disease
- Poor diet – poverty, convenience foods, substance abuse
- Previous heavy menstrual periods
- Childbirth-related – multiparity, recent pregnancy, twin pregnancies, hyperemesis
- Anti-epileptic drugs – increased risk of folate deficiency
- Hookworm infestation (commonest cause of iron deficiency worldwide)

(Coggins, 2001; Harrison, 2001; Karovitch, 2008; Nelson-Piercy, 2006)

Diagnosis of iron deficiency anaemia

Diagnosis of anaemia is usually made through blood investigations (*see* Box 4.4 for normal values). Initially suspicion is raised from a routine full blood count showing a low Hb. If the mean corpuscular volume (MCV) is also reduced, the most likely cause is iron deficiency, and serum ferritin levels are the most useful test for this (McGhee, 2000; McKay, 2000).

If both iron and folate or B12 are deficient, the MCV, which is an average of many measurements, may be normal, with a low Hb. A blood film will show two types of red cells, large and small, that explain the anaemia. Reduced ferritin levels, together with reduced folate and vitamin B12 levels, could indicate malabsorption. An elevated MCV needs further investigation for a variety of causes, such as high intake of alcohol, thyroid or liver anomalies or vitamin B12 or folate deficiencies. A woman with unusual abnormal haematological findings should be referred to a haematologist for an expert opinion.

Midwives working without an easy access to laboratories may find the haemoglobin colour scale a useful tool, and information can be accessed through the World Health Organization's website.

BOX 4.3: COMPLICATIONS OF IRON DEFICIENCY ANAEMIA

Maternal complications
- Fatigue
- Headaches
- Shortness of breath
- Chest pain
- Tachycardia
- Decreased resistance to infection
- Impaired muscle function
- Increased blood loss at delivery secondary to impaired uterine muscle function
- Lower tolerance to blood loss

Fetal/neonatal complications
- Low amniotic fluid volume
- Preterm delivery
- Low birth weight
- Poor iron stores – stores are important in first year of life when iron intake is low
- Poor cognitive performance

(Coggins, 2001; Karovitch, 2008; Strong, 2006)

BOX 4.4: NORMAL BLOOD VALUES IN PREGNANCY FOR USE IN DIAGNOSING ANAEMIA

- Haemoglobin (g/dL): 10.5–14
- Haematocrit (venous) or packed cell volume (PCV): 35–40%
- MCV (fl): 80–103
- Mean cell haemoglobin (MCH) (pg): 27–33
- Mean corpuscular haemoglobin concentration MCHC (g/dL): 32–36
- serum ferritin: 30–100 mg/L
- serum folate: 6–9 μg/L

Management of iron deficiency anaemia

Routine screening for anaemia for all women should take place at booking and 28 weeks gestation. NICE (2008) recommends that if the Hb is < 11 g/dL in early pregnancy, or <10.5 g/dL at 28 weeks, iron supplementation should be considered.

Many authors suggest that ferritin levels are low at the end of pregnancy and that stores cannot be built up through diet alone. They argue that routine supplementation with oral iron is the best way to prevent iron deficiency (Karovitch, 2008; Letsky, 2002; Nelson-Piercy, 2006). However, NICE (2008) advise that routine iron supplementation does not benefit maternal or fetal health and may have unpleasant side effects, such as heartburn, nausea and constipation. Unnecessary iron may also interfere with the absorption of other minerals (Boyle, 2006).

There is also a suggestion that it may be possible to predict those who will need supplements, by testing serum ferritin concentration in the first trimester. Serum ferritin levels in early pregnancy below 50–80 mg/L would benefit from iron supplementation (Letsky, 2002; Nelson-Piercy, 2006).

Iron deficiency anaemia is common in pregnancy, and many women are prescribed an iron supplement, usually in combination with folate, as there is some evidence this is more beneficial than iron alone when treating iron deficiency anaemia (Juarez-Vazquez, et al., 2002). Advice should be given to the woman (see Box 4.5) concerning the most effective way to take these tablets and, since non-compliance is common, it should be emphasised that if she feels unable to continue taking iron, she needs to let the midwife know so that a different formulation can perhaps be prescribed.

BOX 4.5: ADVICE FOR WOMEN WITH IRON DEFICIENCY ANAEMIA

- Absorption of iron from food depends on the type of iron. Iron from animal sources is more effectively absorbed, therefore those with a vegetarian or vegan diet need to be aware of possible deficiencies in their diet.
- Vitamin C increases absorption, whereas tea, coffee, chocolate and antacids inhibit it.
- Side effects are common with iron supplements (e.g., constipation or diarrhoea, nausea, black stools). Gradually introducing these supplements may reduce the side effects, as may taking medication with meals, although this may reduce absorption.

The inability in some women to take oral iron may necessitate intramuscular injections or IV infusions of iron. The effect on the anaemia, however, will not be any more rapid than oral medication (Nelson-Piercy, 2006) and Hb usually rises about 0.8 g/dL per week with treatment. For women with severe anaemia close to term, and in particular if they are at high risk of haemorrhage (for example, with a placenta praevia), a blood transfusion may be advised before delivery.

FOLATE DEFICIENCY

Folic acid is a B-complex vitamin found in green leafy vegetables, fruit, nuts and liver (Walker, 2007). Folate deficiency is the most usual cause of megaloblastic anaemia in pregnancy (Karovitch, 2008), although this condition is now uncommon in the UK (Letsky, 2002). In megaloblastic anaemia there is delayed maturation of the red cell nucleus in the bone marrow (Hoffbrand and Provan, 2007). RBCs that are larger, misshapen and have reduced survival time enter the bloodstream. There is a raised MCV, indicative of a macrocytic anaemia (Nelson-Piercy, 2006).

Folate requirements increase threefold in pregnancy due to the requirements of fetal growth, increased RBC production and increased urinary loss of folate (Karovitch, 2008). Folate deficiency may arise due to poor diet or from malabsorption in conditions like coeliac disease (Hoffbrand and Provan, 2007). Folic acid is essential for DNA synthesis and cell duplication, and folate deficiency increases the risk of neural tube defects and of cleft lip and palate (Goh, *et al.*, 2006). Deficiency in pregnancy increases the risk of having a low-birth-weight baby and without supplementation some women will develop a macrocytic anaemia in the puerperium as the demands of pregnancy may have depleted her stores.

Iron preparations for supplementation in pregnancy contain folate, and folate supplements should not be given without iron (Letsky, 2002).

HAEMOGLOBINOPATHIES (SICKLE CELL DISORDERS AND THALASSAEMIA)

Haemoglobinopathies is a broad term used to describe a range of disorders that affect the structure of haemoglobin, an essential component of RBCs. These include:

▶ alpha thalassaemia
▶ beta thalassaemia (also known as Cooley anaemia)
▶ sickle cell disease (SCD) – This is a general name for a disorder where the person has inherited two unusual haemoglobins, one of which is sickle haemoglobin. There are many haemoglobin variants but not all are significant. They are named after letters of the alphabet or the place they were identified. When one of these variants is inherited with the sickle variant they result in sickle cell disease (Oteng-Ntim, *et al.*, 2005). *See* Box 4.6 for some of these more common disorders.

BOX 4.6: COMMON DISORDERS GROUPED UNDER SICKLE CELL DISEASE

- HbSS – sickle cell anaemia*
- HbSC – haemoglobin SC disease
- HbSβ thal – sickle beta thalassaemia
- HbSD Punjab – haemoglobin SD Punjab disease
- HbSO Arab – haemoglobin SO Arab disease
- HbSE – haemoglobin SE disease
- HbS Lepore – haemoglobin S Lepore disease

NB: The carrier state, sickle cell trait HbAS, is not considered sickle cell disease, because it does not cause illness, although it is inevitably included in discussion.

(Okpala, 2004a; Oteng-Ntim, *et al.*, 2005; Strong, 2006; UK National Screening Committee, 2005; Zack-Williams, 2007)

* Sickle cell anaemia is frequently misnamed as sickle cell disease as confusingly it is also known as homozygous haemoglobin SS sickle cell disease. As it is the most common of the sickle cell disorders it is not surprising this confusion arises. In this text the authors will use the terms interchangeably in line with modern convention, making clear any reference to variant sickle disorders as those listed in Box 4.6.

NORMAL HAEMOGLOBIN

The *globin* part of haemoglobin is the part that is inherited and determines the characteristics of the haemoglobin. Globin is a protein consisting of two pairs of polypeptide chains and its structure influences how easily the RBCs store and release oxygen. Globin can contain several different types of polypeptide chains, termed alpha, beta, gamma and delta (American College of Obstetrics and Gynaecology (ACOG) 2007; Oteng-Ntim, *et al.*, 2005). *See* Figures 4.1 and 4.2.

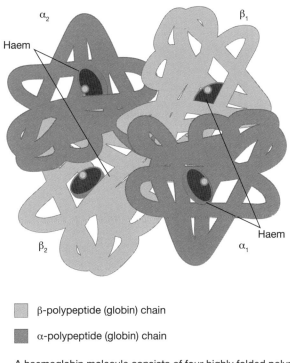

β-polypeptide (globin) chain

α-polypeptide (globin) chain

A haemoglobin molecule consists of four highly folded polypeptide chains (2 alpha and 2 beta) and four iron–containing haem groups

FIGURE 4.1: Haemoglobin molecule

Sickle cell disease is due to mutations in the beta chains of adult haemoglobin and in thalassaemia there is an imbalance in the globin chains.

Most of the haemoglobin found in healthy adults is termed HbA and contains two alpha chains and two beta chains, but there are other types. Fetal haemoglobin (HbF) contains a pair of alpha chains, but in place of the beta chains, it contains a pair of gamma chains. Fetal haemoglobin has enhanced oxygen-trapping capabilities useful for intra-uterine life and levels decrease to a minimum by six months of age. There is also HbA2, a minority adult haemoglobin (*see* Box 4.7).

PATHOPHYSIOLOGY IN SICKLE CELL DISEASE

SCDs are abnormalities of the quality of the haemoglobin. A genetically inherited amino acid substitution results in the production of an abnormal haemoglobin that can sickle. More than 300 variant (abnormal) haemoglobins have been identified,

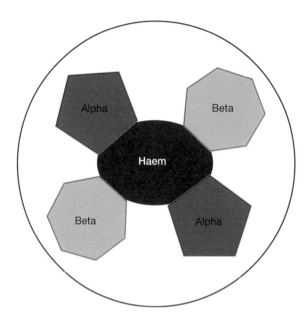

Alpha$_2$ + Beta$_2$ + Haem = Haemoglobin A

FIGURE 4.2: Schematic representation of haemoglobin structure
Source: UK National Screening Committee (2005)

although not all are clinically significant (Strong, 2006). Box 4.6 gives an overview of some of the significant variant combinations, the most common of which is sickle cell anaemia (HBSS).

BOX 4.7: TYPES OF HAEMOGLOBIN

An adult usually has:
- HbA (2 alpha and 2 beta chains)   95–8%
- HbF (2 alpha chains and 2 gamma chains)   1%
- HbA2 (2 alpha and 2 delta chains)   1.8–3.4%

Features of sickle cell disease

When a person with SCD experiences dehydration, infection or low oxygen supply, their fragile RBCs form crystals and assume the characteristic pointed and elongated sickle shape. This causes a breakdown of RBCs, increased viscosity of the blood and vasoocclusion, which further decreases oxygenation (Roberts, 2007). The average lifespan of RBCs in SCD is 17 days, compared to 120 days for normal RBCs (Okpala, 2004b; Oteng-Ntim, *et al.*, 2006). This results in *chronic anaemia* (average Hb 6.5–9 g/dL). Enlarged spleen and gallstone formation may occur secondary to excessive RBC destruction (Oteng-Ntim, *et al.*, 2006).

A sickle cell crisis is defined as an acute onset of severe pain, vital-organ involvement and the requirement for medical attention. It is a broad term used to describe a group of acute events that occur in response to triggers (*see* Box 4.8), but the most common is the vasoocclusive crisis. The abnormal cells clump and block the passage of blood through capillaries. The lack of oxygen and subsequent ischaemia is very painful. The decreased amount of oxygen in the blood damages local tissues and will cause permanent damage to the organs if it lasts long enough (ACOG, 2007) (*see* section following). This may occur at any time, and pregnancy, labour and the puerperium all have great potential to precipitate a crisis. Previous crises may have left residual organ or system damage, which may also compromise a successful pregnancy.

BOX 4.8: PRECIPITATING FACTORS FOR A CRISIS

- Infection
- Pyrexia
- Hypoxia
- Cold/hot (sudden change in temperature)
- Dehydration
- Physical exertion
- Acidosis
- Injury
- Anaesthetics
- Psychological stress
- Unknown

Possible complications of sickle cell crisis

Acute chest syndrome is a serious and often fatal complication due to sickling with vasoocclusion in the lungs. Acute chest syndrome can complicate 7–20% of pregnancies (Serjeant, *et al.*, 2004). Symptoms include fever, coughing, chest pain and shortness of breath with audible crackles. Infection may be involved (Oteng-Ntim, *et al.*, 2005) but recent findings also suggest embolus of bone marrow (Duffy, 2004). Treatment is difficult and may include mechanical ventilation, exchange blood transfusion, heparin and antibiotics (Oteng-Ntim, *et al.*, 2005).

Other potential complications of a vasoocclusive crisis include:

- impaired function of the spleen
- avascular necrosis of the head of the femur
- renal damage
- enlarged liver
- ventricular enlargement and pulmonary hypertension
- cerebrovascular accidents
- leg ulcers
- propensity to infection and sepsis.

(Roberts, 2007)

To summarise, in sickle cell disease:

◗ the RBCs become crescent shaped
◗ the lifespan of the RBC is shortened
◗ the fall in Hb leads to chronic anaemia
◗ blood vessel occlusion occurs
◗ painful sickling crisis and multisystem organ damage is possible
◗ there is susceptibility to infection, probably as a result of the reduced function of the spleen
◗ jaundice appears due to excess breakdown of RBCs.

(ACOG, 2007; Okpala, 2004b; Oteng-Ntim, *et al.*, 2005, 2006)

The physiological changes that occur in pregnancy, along with other features of childbirth, prove challenging to the management of a woman with SCD in pregnancy Box 4.9 summarises those features.

BOX 4.9: PHYSIOLOGICAL CHANGES AND OTHER FEATURES OF PREGNANCY RELEVANT TO SCD

- Increased plasma volume and red cell mass
- Increased requirement for folic acid and iron
- Increased risk of thromboembolism
- Increased vulnerability to infection – urinary tract infection, chrorioamnionitis, endometritis, mastitis
- Labour complications – dehydration, haemorrhage
- Surgical complications – infection, dehydration, immobility

(Blackburn, 2007; Khare and Bewley, 2004)

Subsequently, pregnancy-specific complications include:

- increased risk of vascular complications
- maternal anaemia, resulting in poor oxygen delivery to the fetus
- sickling in arterioles of the uterine placental decidua leading to hypoperfusion and hypoxia in the placental circulation
- higher incidence of placental abruption and placenta praevia
- increased incidence of IUGR
- pre-eclampsia more common
- premature labour more common.

(Walker, 2007)

PATHOPHYSIOLOGY IN THALASSAEMIA

Thalassaemias are usually quantitative abnormalities of globin chain synthesis. There is an impaired production and imbalance of the globin chains.

Alpha thalassaemia

The alpha chain is essential, as it is present in all types of haemoglobin and if this chain is omitted the condition known as *alpha thalassaemia major* is incompatible with life, with fetal demise occurring due to severe anaemia and hydrops, unless – rarely – intra-uterine blood transfusion is carried out. There are normally two pairs (i.e., four) of alpha globin genes and if one or two of these genes are missing the result is the *alpha thalassaemia* trait. A chronic haemolytic anaemia with normal life expectancy called haemoglobin H, or *alpha thalassaemia intermedia*, is where there is deletion of three alpha globin chains. Antenatal screening includes detecting those with carrier status for a number of alpha thalassaemia traits.

Beta thalassaemia

In simple terms beta thalassaemia is a quantitative deficiency of functional beta globin chains which results in the premature destruction of RBCs, causing anaemia (Thein, 2004).

Beta thalassaemia carrier (trait)

Figure 4.3 is a schematic representation of the impact of one defective beta globin chain. As the individual has another functional gene, they will make RBCs, but they will be smaller. A full blood count (FBC) will reveal reduced MCV (size of cell) and reduced MCH (the amount of haemoglobin in the cell). This finding is indicative

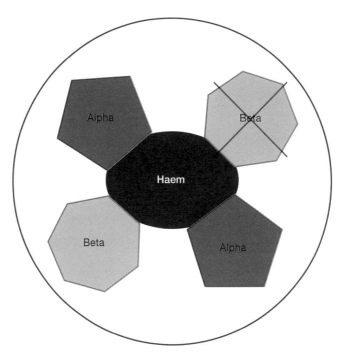

FIGURE 4.3: Beta thalassaemia carrier (trait)

Source: UK National Screening Committee (2005)

of iron deficiency anaemia and misdiagnosis will occur if serum ferritin levels (an indicator of body iron stores) are not checked. The establishment of carrier status for beta thalassaemia is important, as certain carrier combinations result in significant disease, including beta thalassaemia major.

The overall carrier rate in the UK is low compared to the one in seven rate identified in Cyprus (Strong, 2006). However, as a result of population integration, thalassaemia can occur in any racial group

Beta thalassaemia major

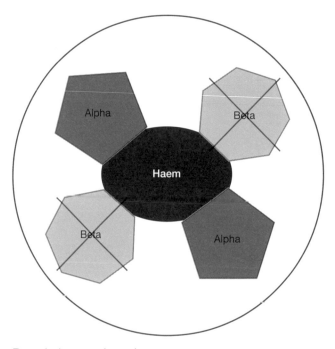

FIGURE 4.4: Beta thalassaemia major
Source: UK National Screening Committee (2005)

Figure 4.4 is a schematic representation to explain the impact of two defective beta globin chains. With no beta globin working, effective RBCs cannot be made. Children born with beta thalassaemia major are well at birth because they are making fetal haemoglobin (HbF), which uses gamma chains instead of beta chains. They gradually develop problems associated with severe anaemia by the time they are two years old (Strong, 2006). Routine frequent blood transfusions (often monthly) are required throughout their life. This results in an excess of iron, which eventually accumulates in their organs, such as the heart muscle, causing damage. Chelation therapy is therefore necessary to remove this excess iron.

The symptoms of beta thalassaemia major are related to anaemia and the features of this disease are:

▶ an enlarged liver and spleen because the excess amounts of empty RBCs block up the liver and spleen

▶ insufficient circulating RBCs. A message is sent to the bone marrow to make more red cells. In response the bone marrow expands. This expansion alters the bone structure, causing a decrease in bone density (therefore the potential for osteoporosis to develop) and an increase in bone prominence evident in the face (UK National Screening Committee, 2005)

▶ problems related to iron overload: excessive iron causes organ damage

▶ problems related to repeat blood transfusion: infections and red cell alloimmunisation

▶ women with beta thalassaemia major can be small in stature and have small pelvic bones, increasing the need for a Caesarian section

▶ transfusion requirements alter as blood requirements increase in pregnancy.

(Aessopos, *et al.*, 1999; UK National Screening Committee, 2005; Weatherall, 2007)

GENETIC INHERITANCE IN SICKLE CELL DISEASE AND THALASSAEMIA

The structural changes that cause haemoglobinopathies are inherited in an autosomal recessive fashion, meaning that two of the variants (one from each parent) must be inherited in order to be affected by the disease. Carriers for the defective haemoglobin structure have one normal and one abnormal allele. Examples given in this section are for sickle cell disease, although it should be noted that thalassaemia follows a similar pattern of inheritance.

When considering genetic inheritance for sickle cell, an abnormal allele is denoted S (sickle haemoglobin) and the healthy allele is denoted A (adult haemoglobin). Box 4.10 gives the different possible combinations.

BOX 4.10: POSSIBLE GENETIC COMBINATIONS OF HAEMOGLOBIN WITH REFERENCE TO SICKLE CELL

HbAA   Normal adult haemoglobin
HbAS*   Sickle cell trait – a carrier of the sickle cell haemoglobin gene. They have HbA from one parent and HbS from the other
HbSS   Sickle cell anaemia– symptoms of pain and anaemia. They have inherited HbS from both parents

* The sickle cell trait provides some protection against malaria.

Antenatal screening seeks to identify previously unknown carrier status and offer partner testing. The risk to a woman with sickle cell anaemia, or any of the other homozygous disorders of haemoglobin, of having a child with the disease is increased, although only if her partner has carrier status or in the rare event that he, too, has homozygous disease. Figure 4.5 shows the possible outcomes for the offspring of a mother with sickle cell anaemia if her partner has usual haemoglobin (HbAA) and Figure 4.6 shows the possible outcomes if her partner is found to have a haemoglobin

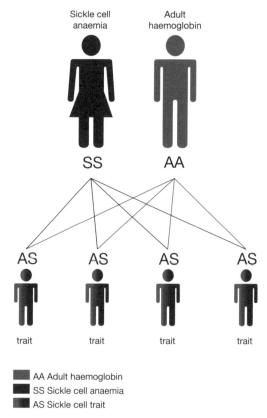

FIGURE 4.5: Possible outcome if one parent has sickle cell anaemia and the other has the usual adult haemoglobin

variant. In the second option parents need to understand that for each pregnancy there is a new risk.

CARE AROUND CHILDBIRTH FOR WOMEN WITH SICKLE CELL DISEASE OR BETA THALASSAEMIA

In the past, pregnancy put women with SCD and thalassaemia major at extreme risk; in fact, those with thalassaemia major rarely survived to child-bearing age; but new technology and advances in identification and care have lead to much improved outcomes for both mothers and babies, and today many women with haemoglobinopathies contemplate pregnancy.

However, pregnancy in women with SCD can increase morbidity and mortality, especially if underlying anaemia and multi-organ damage is present (ACOG, 2007). Pregnancy in women with beta thalassaemia major is far less common than in those with SCD. However, it is suggested that if women with beta thalassaemia major have minimal organ damage (in particular, normal cardiac function) and receive specialised pregnancy care, a successful outcome is possible (Aessopos, *et al.*, 1999; Tuck, 2005). It must be remembered that these are high-risk pregnancies and should

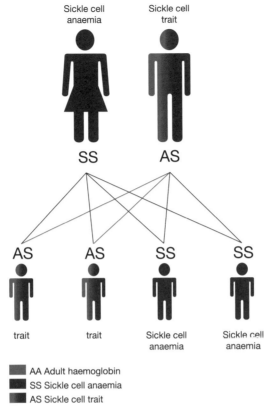

Sickle cell anaemia

Sickle cell trait

SS

AS

AS — trait

AS — trait

SS — Sickle cell anaemia

SS — Sickle cell anaemia

■ AA Adult haemoglobin
■ SS Sickle cell anaemia
■ AS Sickle cell trait

FIGURE 4.6: Possible outcome if the mother has sickle cell anaemia and her partner is a carrier

have all the resources necessary to achieve a good outcome. Care for women with SCD and thalassaemia should be undertaken by an experienced multidisciplinary team, including a haematologist.

Preconception care

Preconception care is concentrated on ensuring that a woman with SCD or thalassaemia is as healthy as possible to start the pregnancy. This includes a full assessment of all organs and body systems, as these are vulnerable to damage in both conditions (Hassell, 2008).

The ideal at this stage is testing partners and counselling the couple about the potential risk of producing an affected child, as well as providing information about antenatal fetal testing. This ensures that when pregnancy does occur the potential parents will have had time to consider all options and will have all the information for making an informed choice. Partner testing may produce a result in which the couple choose to have IVF and selected implantation to ensure a disease-free fetus (Xu, *et al.*, 1999).

Beta thalassaemia major

The role of iron chelation agents in teratogenicity is not known, and it has been recommended that those women undertaking regular iron chelation therapy should stop one month before contraception stops, then restart (with contraception) if there is no pregnancy in three cycles (Aessopos, *et al.*, 1999). If the pregnancy is unplanned then chelation should be discontinued when the pregnancy is confirmed. However, this woman needs to work closely with her doctors to ensure that her health is not compromised at this vulnerable time.

Beta thalassaemia major is associated with cholelithiasis – a preconception gall bladder and biliary tract assessment should be offered (Aessopos, *et al.*, 1999).

Sickle cell disease

As there is a faster turnover of RBCs in those with SCD, an increased dose of folic acid (5 mg daily) is recommended (ACOG, 2007; Khare and Bewley, 2004).

If the woman with SCD is taking hydroxycarbamide (hydroxyurea), it is recommended she stop 3–4 months before discontinuing contraception as it is thought to be teratogenic (Walker, 2007). Some women with SCD take regular pain medication, and this may also need to be reviewed.

Pregnancy care

It is extremely unlikely that those with SCD or beta thalassaemia major will reach child-bearing age with no knowledge of their condition. However, those with carrier status may have no obvious signs and symptoms, and their first diagnosis may be at a routine antenatal test. Screening on the basis of country of origin (Africa, Asia, Mediterranean, Middle and Far East) however, with current-day migration and inter-marriage, has proved ineffective in the UK. For example, in the North West Thames Health Region several white English women have been identified with haemoglobinopathies (Oni, *et al.*, 2002). Currently, in areas deemed to be high prevalence areas, all women are automatically screened by hospital laboratories, using electrophoresis on booking bloods. In areas considered to have a low prevalence, the family origin questionnaire (Department of Health, 2007) should be used by midwives to identify who to test.

Information for those newly diagnosed, as well as those who had not received preconception counselling, includes the offer to test partners and receive counselling regarding the risk of having an affected child. Information on antenatal diagnostic tests available is also given. Prenatal diagnosis can be done by chorionic villus sampling (CVS) at about 10–12 weeks or by amniocentesis (or more rarely, by fetal blood sampling). There is also a suggestion that ultrasound markers may be useful in predicting a fetus at risk of alpha thalassaemia major (Leung, *et al.*, 2006).

Parents' views on having an affected child will be influenced by their own experiences. Many with sickle cell trait will know someone with SCD and this may be mild or severe. Those with thalassaemia trait may not know anyone with thalassaemia major. It is estimated that in the UK approximately 50% of those diagnosed with beta thalassaemia major die before 35 years of age, and it is suggested that this is because of the difficulty in adhering to the arduous treatment (Modell, *et al.*, 2000) of repeated transfusion and frequent, painful infusions to remove excess iron (Ahmed, *et al.*, 2005).

Compliance with these regimes may not be optimal, resulting in increased medical problems. However, there are new advances in bone marrow transplant (La Nasa, *et al.*, 2002) and stem cell treatment, which may hold out hope for a cure in the future.

Research has shown about 50% of women choose to terminate a pregnancy following results showing an affected fetus (Khare and Bewley, 2004). Many countries have seen a decrease in births of those with beta thalassaemia major as a result of prenatal diagnosis (Ahmed, *et al.*, 2006). However, the number of births in the UK has not reduced and most of these are to parents of Pakistani origin (Hickman, *et al.*, 1999).

In a study of Pakistani women in England, most said they would accept antenatal diagnosis because they wanted to know but would not accept termination, although some did not know of the associated risk of a miscarriage in antenatal testing (Ahmed, *et al.*, 2006). This underlines the need to treat all women as individuals and ensure they have all the information possible to make an informed choice, although their decisions will be ultimately based on individual values and beliefs. Midwives need to ensure that all women are making informed choices at every stage of the decision-making path.

It has been suggested that routine maternity care does not enable fetal diagnosis and termination (if chosen) in early pregnancy (Dormandy, *et al.*, 2008). There is an argument for preconception screening for carrier status, or at least early pregnancy screening by GPs (Thomas, *et al.*, 2005; Wright, *et al.*, 2003).

Women with HbSC or HbSβ thal (*see* Box 4.6) may have only received their diagnosis during pregnancy. They, however, often have splenomegaly and splenic sequestration, and this may manifest as abdominal pain in pregnancy (Walker, 2007). Pregnancy may also precipitate a crisis for the first time in these women.

As there is a risk of IUGR for the fetus in most haemoglobinopathies, regular fetal surveillance for growth and well-being is recommended (Hassell, 2008).

Thalassaemia

In pregnancy, those with alpha thalassaemia trait can be offered normal management, whereas those with beta thalassaemia trait may need extra iron supplementation if they are iron deficient (Walker, 2007) and are at increased risk of IUGR and oligohydramnios (Sheiner, *et al.*, 2004). A pregnant woman with thalassaemia intermedia (HbH) may develop severe anaemia during pregnancy (Nassar, *et al.*, 2006). Women with beta thalassaemia major may need transfusions to maintain their Hb levels, although chelation treatment is discontinued as there is no knowledge of its safety in pregnancy (ACOG, 2007). In beta thalassaemia major the ideal is to maintain an Hb of 10 g/dl, and FBC and ferritin concentration should be monitored closely.

Although there is little literature concerning pregnancy in women with beta thalassaemia major, there is evidence that stillbirth, IUGR and premature labour are common (Hassell, 2008). Therefore, for most women with thalassaemia, frequent antenatal checks assessing the fetal growth and well-being as well as the maternal condition are necessary (Aessopos, *et al.*, 1999).

In those with beta thalassaemia minor (thalassaemia trait) there has been a demonstrated increased rate of IUGR, so it is advisable to offer these women increased fetal surveillance (Sheiner, *et al.*, 2004).

Sickle cell disease

Those with SCD generally continue their initial higher dose of folic acid throughout pregnancy, but iron is given only if specifically indicated (Oteng-Ntim, *et al.*, 2006).

The type and rate of complications in pregnancy depends on the specific SCD, but the most common disorder is sickle cell anaemia (HbSS) and this is the one in which the most information is available.

Women with HbSS are at risk of an increased early fetal loss and maternal morbidity (Serjeant, *et al.*, 2004). However, compared with women without SCD, there appears to be no difference in their increased blood pressure rates or late miscarriages (Mou Sun, *et al.*, 2001). Nevertheless, it is important to establish a BP baseline early in pregnancy, as women with HbSS often have a low normal rate and therefore the threshold for diagnosing pregnancy-induced hypertension should also be reduced – one authority has suggested as low as 125/75 (Hassell, 2008).

Research has shown that women with HbSS are more likely to be hospitalised in pregnancy, mainly for crises, infections, anaemia, premature rupture of membranes, preterm labour and postnatal infections. Other serious complications, such as left ventricular dysfunction or splenic sequestration, are not uncommon in women with SCD (Walker, 2007). However, there appears to be no increase in their rate of antepartum (APH) or post-partum (PPH) haemorrhage (Serjeant, *et al.*, 2004).

Crises are common in pregnancy and probably occur more in those with HbSS than in those with HbSC (Khare and Bewley, 2004). In general it is considered that those who suffered complications from their status pre-pregnancy are more at risk of complications during pregnancy (Walker, 2007). The signs and symptoms of a crisis can overlap with those of common serious pregnancy complications such as the pre-eclampsia/HELLP syndrome, pulmonary embolism or abruption. Pregnant women with SCD should have this information so they can seek medical help perhaps sooner than they normally would, as many of them are often used to coping with crises on their own. Box 4.11 provides a summary of care required during crisis.

A blood transfusion (either a top-up or an exchange) is used only when absolutely necessary, as women with SCD develop red cell antibodies more frequently than those without the disease (Davies and Olatunji, 1995). Other disadvantages to transfusion include exposure to infection, transfusion reaction, alloimmunisation, fluid volume fluctuation and, in those who have had frequent transfusions, iron overload. A delayed transfusion reaction can be seen many days afterwards and can be life-threatening (Proudfit, *et al.*, 2007).

Dehydration can be a trigger for a crisis, and care must be taken if the woman with SCD has nausea and vomiting in early pregnancy.

Minor infections are common in pregnancy, especially urinary tract infections. As infection is the most common cause of crises in SCD, these infections must be effectively screened for and treated. Women with a mild infection may even need to be hospitalised early to avoid dehydration and to allow increased levels of antibiotics to ensure that a severe crisis does not occur. Some women with SCD are on long-term prophylactic antibiotics and these are usually continued in pregnancy. In others, prophylactic antibiotics are started in pregnancy, but the decision to do so is taken on an individual basis.

Normal Hb readings in women with SCD are often low (7–9 g/dl) (Okpala, 2004c).

There does not appear to be an association between the baby's birth weight and the degree of anaemia in women with SCD (Hassell, 2008). However, chronic anaemia in these women predisposes them to pulmonary embolism, and therefore antenatal anticoagulation with the appropriate drug (usually LMWH) is often considered necessary (Khare and Bewley, 2004; Oni, *et al.*, 2002).

Women with SCD will have at least monthly Hb estimations, but iron supplementation is appropriate only if the ferritin levels decrease (Oteng-Ntim, *et al.*, 2006). Although a routine prophylactic blood transfusion is controversial, either a top-up or an exchange transfusion may be necessary for individual women. Transfusion may be necessary if anaemia increases, for haemorrhage, crises, septicaemia or acute chest syndrome (Walker, 2007). Routine renal function tests are also carried out for women with SCD where there is any indication of renal damage.

Perinatal mortality rates are approximately 4–5 times higher in some women with SCD than in unaffected pregnancies (Khare and Bewley, 2004). Miscarriage may also be more common in those with SCD (ACOG, 2007). For those with SCD an increased rate of placenta praevia and abruption has been reported, and the fetus is at risk of a premature rupture of the membranes, premature delivery (both spontaneous and iatrogenic), IUGR and stillbirth (ACOG, 2007; Serjeant, *et al.*, 2004; Walker, 2007). IUGR is more common in HbSS than in HbSC or HbS β thal. Increased fetal surveillance is therefore essential, and regular ultrasound estimations of growth, as well as a Doppler assessment, if necessary, are usually routine.

BOX 4.11: SUMMARY OF CARE DURING A CRISIS

- Analgesia. Ideally a patient-controlled analgesia pump is made available and diamorphine is usually effective.
- Hydration. It is usually necessary to maintain optimum hydration by means of IV infusion.
- Treatment of the cause. Infection is common, therefore all normal sites of infection must be assessed and appropriate antibiotics commenced, often IV
- Administration of oxygen. Saturation monitoring must be undertaken and if saturation levels are < 95%, oxygen is usually necessary and should be humidified.
- Maintenance of a comfortable temperature and stress-free environment, as far as possible.
- CTG monitoring when appropriate. If opiates are taken, this must be taken into account when analysing the trace.
- Monitoring pain, respirations and level of consciousness.
- Exchange transfusion if the condition is not responsive.
- If the woman is in the third trimester, delivery may be necessary to resolve the crisis.

Labour care

The antenatal care for all women with haemoglobinopathies is multidisciplinary, and a plan for these high-risk women should have been made by the team and the woman during pregnancy. It is likely that the haematologist would want to be informed when she is admitted in labour.

Induction of labour may be recommended for women with haemoglobinopathies, but this decision should be made on an individual basis. Blood should be grouped and cross-matched early in labour as the time necessary for cross-matching is increased when atypical antibodies are present, and these are common in women who have received many previous transfusions.

In both SCD and beta thalassaemia major the fetus is likely to be IUGR, so continuous electronic fetal monitoring is usual during labour.

Active management of the third stage is also normal practice for women with both thalassaemia and SCD to decrease the amount of blood lost. Cord blood is usually taken to screen the newborn.

Thalassaemia
Women with beta thalassaemia major who have had an uneventful pregnancy should be allowed to labour spontaneously and have a normal delivery (Aessopos, *et al.*, 1999). If complications have occurred, the care will be underpinned by individual circumstances. Elective Caesarean section may be the mode of delivery of choice for those with beta thalassaemia major if there is an indication such as subclinical impairment of cardiac function. If necessary, this woman could be transfused the day before to ensure optimum Hb levels.

Sickle cell disease
In labour women with SCD are vulnerable to dehydration, hypoxia, acidosis and sepsis, so care must be taken with monitoring them. Women with SCD may have chronic anaemia and hypoxaemia, which affects cardiac function, and labour may add to this (Walker, 2007). Oxygen therapy may be necessary in labour and the evaluation of this woman's oxygenation with pulse oximetry monitoring is recommended. Prophylactic antibiotics may be prescribed for labour and the immediate postnatal period (Oni, *et al.*, 2002). Temperature control of the environment is also important, as the woman must be kept warm but not overheated. Crises are common in labour and the first 24 hours postnatal, so care must be taken to avoid predisposing factors (*see* Box 4.8).

If a general anaesthetic is required for a Caesarean section, it is usual to admit the woman to the ICU for assisted ventilation for the first 24 hours.

Pethidine is not well cleared from the body in those with poor renal function (such as many women with SCD), so frequent doses may lead to maternal complications (Oni, *et al.*, 2002). Women with SCD may have increased tolerance to pain medication, and this may need to be considered during labour. If an epidural is used, care must be taken to avoid hypotension. However, an epidural can reduce catecholamine concentration in the circulation, reducing the risk of sickling (Walker, 2007). Dehydration is possible during labour, whatever analgesia is chosen, and the midwife must monitor fluids carefully to avoid this – IV fluids are usual.

For women with SCD, because of the increased risk of cerebral vascular accident (CVA) due to subarachnoid haemorrhage, pushing time may be limited.

Postnatal care

Antibiotics may be continued or commenced in the postnatal period, as the chance of infection is high for all women in the puerperium (Boyle, 2006), and these women may be deficient in iron and zinc, compromising wound healing.

Contraception advice is part of postnatal care, and for women with haemoglobinopathies, where planned pregnancies can contribute to their success, this is vital and can be seen as preconception care for the next pregnancy.

Babies born to women with SCD and beta thalassaemia major will probably have the cord blood sent for analysis at delivery to determine their status (or confirm it, if an antenatal diagnosis was carried out). All newborns in the UK are screened for SCD via the newborn blood spot screening programme (formerly Guthrie Test) at 5–8 days of age.

Sickle cell disease

For women with SCD, pain and hypovolaemia from blood loss are both potential triggers of a vasoocclusive crisis (*see* Box 4.8). As there also continues to be an increased risk of thrombosis, thromboprophylaxis and thromboembolic deterrent (TED) stockings are usual, and early ambulation is encouraged.

Thalassaemia

For women dependent on regular transfusions, chelation therapy is restarted at about 20 days, with regular follow-ups.

THROMBOEMBOLIC DISEASE

Since the Confidential Enquiries into Maternal Deaths began, thromboembolic disease has been known to be a leading cause of maternal mortality in the UK (Nelson-Piercy, 2006). Pregnancy is known to increase the risk of deep vein thrombosis (DVT) and pulmonary embolism (PE). Studies differ on when a child-bearing woman is at highest risk of thromboembolism, but it can occur at any time in pregnancy, including the first trimester, and in the postnatal period (Rodger, *et al.*, 2008).

PATHOPHYSIOLOGY

The risk of venous thromboembolism is up to 10 times higher in a pregnant woman compared to a non-pregnant woman of similar age (RCOG, 2007). Rudolf Virchow (1821–1902) first described the triad of factors that are associated with venous thrombosis, all of which are present during pregnancy.

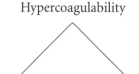

Hypercoagulability

Vascular damage   Venous stasis

Hypercoagulability: A normal pregnancy is associated with alterations in the proteins of the coagulation and fibrinolytic systems, resulting in a relative state of hypercoagulability.

These changes are thought to minimise bleeding in the third stage of labour and help maintain the placenta–uterine interface.

Venous stasis: Sluggish venous return from the lower limbs occurs when the pregnant uterus compresses the inferior vena cava, compounded by the reduction in the muscle tone of veins during pregnancy caused by progesterone. Blood flow in the veins depends on the action of the voluntary muscles and periods of inactivity further slow blood flow. The anatomy of the venous drainage from the lower limb, where the left iliac vein is crossed by the right iliac artery, means that DVTs are more common in the left leg, although this is not unique to pregnancy (Bothamley, 2002; Greer, 1999).

Vascular damage: Damage to the vessel walls sets off a series of chemical reactions that promote platelet aggregation and fibrin formation at the site of injury, resulting in clot formation. Endothelial damage to the pelvic vessels can occur during vaginal or operative delivery (Bothamley, 2002; Greer, 1999).

PREVENTION OF THROMBOEMBOLISM
Prevention, detection and appropriate treatment of DVT is crucial in limiting deaths from PE. In consideration of the increased risk of venous thromboembolism (VTE) that pregnancy poses, all pregnant women should be assessed at the earliest possible time for any additional risk factors, with an ongoing reassessment of pregnancy-related risks, particularly if they are admitted to hospital (Lewis, 2007). *See section Risk factors for DVT and PE* below. Midwives should be familiar with risk assessment guidance produced by the RCOG: Risk assessment profile for thromboembolism in Caesarean section (RCOG, 1995) and *Thromboprophylaxis during Pregnancy, Labour and after Vaginal Delivery* (RCOG, 2004). An antenatal risk assessment tool has been proposed to aid midwives and other clinicians to identify and provide prophylaxis to women at increased risk (Whapshott, 2007). There are a number of medical and midwifery measures that can be introduced to help prevent VTE, with the midwife playing an important role in educating women, administering medication, fitting TED stockings and detecting signs and symptoms of DVT. Box 4.12 lists common prophylactic measures to prevent DVT.

RISK FACTORS FOR DVT AND PE
General conditions
▶ Personal or family history of DVT, PE or thrombophilia.
▶ Obesity (BMI > 30).
▶ Prolonged immobilisation.
▶ Surgery.
▶ Major current illness, e.g., heart, lung, bowel disease, malignancy.
▶ Anti-cardiolipin antibodies (antiphospholipid syndrome or as part of systemic lupus erythematosis).
▶ Inherited thrombophilias – e.g., Factor V Leiden.
▶ Sickle-cell disease.
▶ Long-distance air travel.
▶ Gross varicose veins.
▶ Smoking.
▶ Combined oral contraceptive pill.

Pregnancy-related factors

◗ Caesarean section.
◗ Maternal age over 35.
◗ Parity > four (RCOG, 2007)/ parity > one (Knight, 2008).
◗ Multiple pregnancies.
◗ Severe infection.
◗ Pre-eclampsia.
◗ Immobility (including bed rest).
◗ Surgical procedures in pregnancy.
◗ Dehydration, hyperemesis.
◗ Excessive blood loss.

(Bothamley, 2002; Knight, 2008; Lim, *et al.*, 2007; RCOG, 2004; Whapshott, 2007)

BOX 4.12: PROPHYLACTIC MEASURES THAT MAY BE USED TO PREVENT THROMBOEMBOLISM

For those at higher risk
● Thromboprophylaxis with prescribed LMWH
● Prescribed low-dose aspirin

Following instrumental or surgical delivery
● Avoiding long period of immobilisation
● Wearing correctly fitting TED stockings
● Deep-breathing exercises to encourage venous return
● Effective post-partum pain relief to enable mobility

General measures for all pregnant women
● Doing leg exercises to encourage venous return
● Avoiding dehydration
● Avoiding tight-fitting garments, such as garters around the legs
● Avoiding sitting with legs crossed
● Taking regular breaks on long car journeys
● Seeking specific advice about air travel in pregnancy

DEEP VEIN THROMBOSIS
Diagnosis of DVT

Signs and symptoms (*see* Box 4.13) can create suspicion of a DVT but in up to 50% of cases this will not be confirmed (Nelson-Piercy, 2006). As there is also evidence that most women who die from PE showed no clinical signs and symptoms of DVT (Hamilton-Fairley, 2004), this underlines the difficulty in identifying this potentially serious occurrence.

BOX 4.13: SIGNS AND SYMPTOMS OF DVT

- Redness or discoloration of the affected leg
- Swelling (at least 2 cm difference between the two legs)
- Leg pain or discomfort
- Calf tenderness
- Change in limb colour or temperature
- Homan's sign (pain on dorsiflexion of the foot) (unreliable)
- Low-grade pyrexia (< 37.5°C)
- Tachycardia (pulse > 100/min)
- Lower abdominal pain

(Bothamley, 2002)

Diagnostic tools for DVT

Ultrasonography is the primary diagnostic test for detecting DVT in pregnancy. However, when results are equivocal or when iliac vein or higher-level thrombosis is suspected, MRI or venography (injection of contrast medium) may be used. Measuring blood levels of fibrin degradation products (using the D-dimer test) is a common test for DVT outside pregnancy. However, these are known to be unreliable in pregnancy and the postnatal period, but a low level can suggest there is no thrombus (RCOG, 2007).

Management of DVT

Anticoagulation treatment (*see* p. 102) is the main treatment for DVT, but other interventions will aid recovery and are aimed at promoting good venous return, thereby preventing further clot formation. Leg elevation is recommended when sitting, but in pregnancy inguinal congestion may occur, so the leg should not be raised at too acute an angle and pressure behind the knee should be avoided. Once anticoagulants have been commenced and compression stockings fitted, mobility is encouraged, and standing still should be avoided. Graduated compression TED stockings minimise the risk of clot formation by providing external compression, which increases the velocity of blood flow in the veins, reducing venous stasis (Agu, *et al.*, 1999; RCOG, 2007). TED stockings must be accurately fitted.

PULMONARY EMBOLISM

Signs and symptoms of PE (*see* Box 4.14) are largely dependent on the size of the clot obstructing the pulmonary circulation. A major PE will cause collapse with hypotension and may even be fatal, with cardiac or respiratory arrest. However, a minor PE may be non-specific and diagnosis may be difficult.

Diagnostic tools for PE

Assessment of the woman's condition will be undertaken with a chest X-ray, an ECG and tests of oxygen levels (saturation and blood gases) and although this will not lead to a diagnosis, the findings may identify other aetiologies and underpin treatment.

A *ventilation/perfusion (V/Q) scan* is the most common diagnostic test for PE and consists of assessment of the pulmonary blood flow following an intravenous injection of albumin labelled with radioactive technetium (a low radiation dose is not believed to be associated with a substantial increased risk for the fetus) (RCOG, 2007).

A *CT pulmonary angiogram* (CTPA) can be used, in which the chest is assessed using CT following the injection of a dye into the bloodstream; however, the RCOG Guidelines (2007) suggest there is a high radiation dose to the breasts.

BOX 4.14: SIGNS AND SYMPTOMS OF PE

Most common signs and symptoms
- Breathlessness
- Pleuritic chest pain
- Cough
- Peripheral oedema
- Chest sounds: crackles

Associated signs and symptoms
- Haemoptysis
- Tachypnoea
- Tachycardia
- Hypertension
- Distended neck veins
- Cyanosis
- Tricuspid flow murmur
- Pyrexia
- Anxiety

Treatment of pulmonary embolism

Early diagnosis and treatment is vital when PE is suspected, as deaths caused by PE can occur very quickly following an embolic event.

Immediate treatment should include standard assessment, with the commencement of continuous vital-sign measurement as well as ECG, intravenous access and oxygen therapy. Cardiac arrest procedures, including intubation, may be necessary and it is vital the entire emergency team, including a senior anaesthetist, is summoned. An echocardiogram or CTPA should be undertaken within one hour (RCOG, 2007). The midwife's responsibilities are summarised in Box 4.15.

Although anticoagulation treatment (*see* following section) will be used in most cases, other medical or surgical interventions may be necessary in life-threatening pulmonary embolism. *Thrombolytic therapy* ('clot busting' drugs such as streptokinase) may be used, but this has not previously been common in pregnancy except in a life-threatening situation, due to the risk of major haemorrhage (Ahearn, *et al.*, 2002). In cases where recurring clots are developing, *inferior vena cava filters*, which work by intercepting emboli travelling to the pulmonary vasculature, have been used safely in pregnancy (Kawamata, *et al.*, 2005). *Pulmonary embolectomy* is rarely used, but *pulmonary angiography*, with the use of a guideline wire via a cardiac catheter, may be successful in breaking up the clot (Manganaro, *et al.*, 2000) although there is a high radiation exposure (RCOG, 2007).

BOX 4.15: MIDWIFE'S RESPONSIBILITIES IN PULMONARY EMBOLISM EMERGENCY

- Summon the emergency response team or arrange emergency transfer to hospital if at home.
- Administer CPR if necessary.
- Assist with endotracheal intubation as necessary.
- Give oxygen.
- If appropriate, sit the woman up to maximise the respiratory effort.
- Initiate IV access.
- Assess and record cardiovascular and respiratory vital signs.
- Attach oximeter and record ECG.
- Give heparin and other drugs according to medical orders.
- Maintain accurate fluid balance.
- Monitor fetal well-being as appropriate.
- Support the woman and her family.

Following any thromboembolic event, anticoagulation maintenance is used and continued for several weeks through pregnancy and the puerperium. This may involve regular monitoring. All anticoagulants commonly used are not contraindicated in breastfeeding. Midwives may be involved in teaching women to give their daily injections, advise about side effects such as bleeding from gums and bruising and generally provide ongoing support following what may have been a very frightening experience.

ANTICOAGULATION TREATMENT OF DVT AND PE

The aims of treatment include preventing an extension of the thrombosis, restoring venous patency and reducing the risk of a PE recurrence. In the acute phase this is undertaken by producing as high an anticoagulation as possible without putting the woman at risk of spontaneous bleeding (de Swiet, 2002).

Unfractionated (standard) heparin (UH) is administered via the IV or subcutaneous route. Different regimens will be used depending on the individual condition of the woman and local guidelines; however, all regimes need to be supported by appropriate monitoring (*see* Table 4.1) to quickly establish and maintain therapeutic levels. Potential side effects include thrombocytopenia and osteoporosis (with long-term use).

Low molecular weight heparin (LMWH) is administered by subcutaneous injection. It has several advantages over UH, including a longer half-life (therefore enabling once-daily injections), less incidence of heparin-induced thrombocytopenia and osteopaenia (Aguilar and Goldhaber, 1999; Greer and Nelson-Piercy, 2005) and less need for laboratory monitoring. LMWH is commonly used for prophylaxis or in the chronic phase of treatment, but authorities now say that LMWH is also safe and effective for treatment of acute thromboembolism in pregnancy (Greer and Nelson-Piercy, 2005; Quinlan, *et al.*, 2004).

Women taking LMWH maintenance therapy should discontinue its use when labour begins – and if delivery is planned, it should be discontinued 24 hours before the planned delivery (RCOG, 2007). Women receiving heparin therapy prior to a regional block should have their coagulation screen checked before the insertion of an epidural catheter, to prevent potential spinal haematoma. Midwives also need to be aware of anaesthetist's instructions and local policies regarding the timing of removal of an epidural catheter.

Warfarin is an oral anticoagulant and, unlike heparin, is able to cross the placenta. It is not recommended for use in pregnancy except as an alternative to LMWH in the post-partum period. Regular assessment of the international normalised ratio (INR) is necessary, particularly in the first 10 days of treatment, which can prove inconvenient for the newly delivered mother.

TABLE 4.1: Laboratory tests for monitoring heparin therapy

Assay	Nature of the test	Comments
Activated partial thromboplastin time	Measures time to clot formation after adding an activating agent	Can be difficult to measure and unpredictable in pregnancy
Protamine titration	Determines the plasma level of heparin	
Prothrombin time, also called international normalised ratio (INR)	Thrombin is added to the plasma and time to clot recorded	Used to monitor blood clotting in people who take warfarin
Anti-factor Xa assay	Measures the rate of factor-Xa inhibition by optical density determination	Expensive; LMWH-specific; not widely available

Source: Toglia and Nolan (1997)

RESOURCE
NHS Sickle Cell and Thalassaemia Screening Programme. Available at: www.kcl-phs.org.uk/ haemscreening/publications.htm#InfoStrategy

REFERENCES

Aessopos A, Karabatsos F, Farmakis D, *et al.* Pregnancy in patients with well-treated beta-thalassaemia: outcome for mothers and newborn infants. *Am J Obstet Gynecol.* 1999; **180**: 360–5.

Agu O, Hamilton G, Baker D. Graduated compression stockings in the prevention of venous thromboembolism. *Br J Surg.* 1999; **86**: 992–1004.

Aguilar D, Goldhaber S. Clinical uses of low molecular weight heparins. *Chest.* 1999; **115**: 1418–23.

Ahearn G, Hadjiliadis M, Govert J, *et al.* Massive pulmonary embolism during pregnancy successfully treated with recombinant tissue plasminogen activator. *Arch Intern Med.* 2002; **162**: 1221–7.

Ahmed S, Green J, Hewison J. Antenatal thalassaemia carrier testing: women's perceptions of 'information' and 'consent'. *J Med Screen.* 2005; **12**(2): 69–77.

Ahmed S, Green J, Hewison J. Attitudes towards prenatal diagnosis and termination of pregnancy for thalassaemia in pregnant Pakistani women in the North of England. *Prenat Diag.* 2006; **26**(3): 248–57.

American College of Obstetricians and Gynaecologists (ACOG). ACOG practice bulletin no. 78, January: hemoglobinopathies in pregnancy. *Obstet Gynecol.* 2007; **109**(1): 229–36.

Bain BJ. *A Beginner's Guide to Blood Cells.* 2nd ed. Oxford: Blackwell; 2004.

Blackburn ST. *Maternal, Fetal and Neonatal Physiology: A Clinical Perspective.* 3rd ed. Philadelphia, PA: Saunders Elsevier; 2007.

Bothamley J. Thromboembolism in pregnancy. In: Boyle M, editor. *Emergencies Around Childbirth.* Oxford: Radcliffe Publishing; 2002. pp. 21–39.

Boyle M. *Wound Healing in Midwifery.* Oxford: Radcliffe Publishing; 2006.

Coggins J. Iron deficiency anaemia: a complication of pregnancy or a foregone conclusion? A midwife's view. *MIDIRS.* 2001; **11**(4): 469–74.

Davies S, Olatunji P. Blood transfusion in sickle cell disease. *Vox Sang.* 1995; **68**: 145–51.

Department of Health. Family origin questionnaire, NHS antenatal and newborn screening programmes. London: Department of Health; 2007. Available at: www.sickleandthal.org.uk/Documents/F_Origin_Questionnaire.pdf (accessed 5 December 2008).

de Swiet M. Thromboembolism. In: de Swiet M, editor. *Medical Disorders in Obstetric Practice.* Oxford: Blackwell; 2002.

Dormandy E, Gulliford M, Reid E, *et al.* Delay between pregnancy confirmation and sickle cell thalassaemia screening: a population-based cohort study. *Br J Gen Pract.* 2008; **58**(548): 154–9.

Duffy TP. Hematologic aspects of pregnancy. In: Burrow GN, Duffy TP, Copel JA, editors. *Medical Complications during Pregnancy.* 6th ed. Philadelphia, PA: Elsevier Saunders; 2004. pp. 69–86.

Goh YI, Bollano E, Einarson TR, *et al.* Prenatal multivitamin supplementation and rates of congenital anomalies: a meta-analysis. *J Obstet Gynaecol Can.* 2006; **28**(8): 680–9.

Greer IA. Thrombosis in pregnancy: maternal and fetal issues. *Lancet.* 1999; **353**: 1258–65.

Greer IA, Nelson-Piercy C. Low molecular-weight heparins for thromboprophylaxis and treatment of venous thromboembolism in pregnancy: a systematic review of safety and efficacy. *Blood.* 2005; **106**(2): 401–7.

Hamilton-Fairley D. *Lecture Notes on Obstetrics and Gynaecology.* 2nd ed. Oxford: Blackwell; 2004.

Harrison K. Anaemia in pregnancy. In: Lawson J, Harrison K, Bergstrom S, editors. *Maternity Care in Developing Countries.* London: RCOG Press; 2001. pp. 112–28.

Hassell K. Hemoglobinopathies and thalassemias. In: Rosene-Montella K, Keely E, Barbour L, *et al.*, editors. *Medical Care of the Pregnant Patient.* 2nd ed. Philadelphia, PA: ACP Press; 2008. pp. 486–96.

Hickman M, Modell B, Greengross P, *et al.* Mapping the prevalence of sickle cell and beta-thalassaemia in England: estimating and validating ethnic-specific risks. *Br J Haematol.* 1999; **104**: 860–7.

Hoffbrand AV, Provan D. Macrocytic anaemias. In: Provan D, editor. *ABC of Clinical Haematology.* 3rd ed. Oxford: Blackwell; 2007. pp. 6–10.

Juarez-Vazquez J, Bonizzoni E, Scotti A. Iron plus folate is more effective than iron alone in the treatment of iron deficiency anaemia in pregnancy: a randomised, double blind clinical trial *BJOG.* 2002; **109**(9): 1009–14.

Karovitch A. Hemoglobinopathies, thalassemias, and anemia part 11: anaemia. In: Rosene-Montella K, Keely E, Barbour LA, *et al.*, editors. *Medical Care of the Pregnant Patient.* 2nd ed. Philadelphia, PA: ACP Press; 2008. pp. 497–508.

Kawamata K, Chiba Y, Tanaka R, *et al.* Experience of temporary inferior vena cava filters inserted in the perinatal period to prevent pulmonary embolism in pregnant women with deep vein thrombosis. *J Vasc Surg.* 2005; **41**: 652–6.

Khare M, Bewley S. Management of pregnancy in sickle cell disease. In: Okpala IE, editor. *Practical Management of Haemoglobinopathies.* London: Blackwell; 2004. pp. 107–19.

Knight M, on behalf of UKOSS. Antenatal pulmonary embolism: risk factors, management and outcomes. *Br J Obstet Gynaecol.* 2008; **115**: 453–61.

La Nasa G, Giardini C, Argiolu F, *et al.* Unrelated donor bone marrow transfusion for thalassaemia: the effect of extended haplotypes. *Blood.* 2002; **99**(12): 4350–6.

Letsky EA. Blood volume, haematinics, anaemia. In: de Swiet M, editor. *Medical Disorders in Obstetric Practice.* 4th ed. Oxford: Blackwell; 2002. pp. 29–60.

Leung K, Liao C, Li Q. A new strategy for prenatal diagnosis of homozygous alpha-thalassemia. *Ultrasound Obstet Gynecol.* 2006; **28**(2): 173–7.

Lewis G, editor. The Confidential Enquiry into Maternal and Child Health (CEMACH). *Saving Mothers' Lives: reviewing maternal deaths to make motherhood safer 2003–2005. The Seventh Report on Confidential Enquiries into Maternal Deaths in the UK.* London: CEMACH; 2007.

Lim W, Elkelboom JW, Ginsberg JS. Inherited thrombophilia and pregnancy associated venous thromboembolism. *BMJ.* 2007; **334**: 1053–4.

McGhee M. *A Guide to Laboratory Investigations.* 3rd ed. Oxford: Radcliffe Medical Press; 2000.

McKay K. Blood tests in pregnancy (2): iron deficiency anaemia. *Pract Midwife.* 2000; **3**(4): 25–7.

Manganaro A, Buda D, Calabro D, *et al.* Physical treatment of deep vein thrombosis. *Minerva Cardioangiol.* 2000; **48**: 53–6.

Modell B, Khan M, Darlison M. Survival in beta-thalassaemia major and UK data from the UK Thalassaemia Register. *Lancet.* 2000; **355**(9220): 2051–2.

Mou Sun P, Winburn W, Raynor D, *et al.* Sickle cell disease in pregnancy: twenty years of experience at Grady Memorial Hospital, Atlanta, Georgia. *Am J Obstet Gynecol.* 2001; **184**(6): 1127–30.

Nassar A, Usta I, Rechdan J. Pregnancy in patients with beta-thalassemia intermedia: outcome of mothers and newborns. *Am J Hematol.* 2006; **81**(7): 499–502.

National Institute for Health and Clinical Excellence (NICE). *Antenatal Care: routine care for the healthy pregnant woman NICE guideline 62.* London: NICE; 2008. www.nice.org.uk/guidance/CG62

Nelson-Piercy C. *Handbook of Obstetric Medicine.* 3rd ed. Abingdon: Informa Healthcare; 2006.

NHS. Sickle Cell and Thalassaemia Screening Programme. Available at: www.kcl-phs.org.uk/haemscreening/publications.htm#InfoStrategy (accessed 8 December 2008).

Okpala IE. The concept of comprehensive care of sickle cell disease. In: Okpala IE, editor. *Practical Management of Haemoglobinopathies.* Oxford: Blackwell; 2004a. pp. 1–9.

Okpala IE. Epidemiology, genetics and pathophysiology of sickle cell. In: Okpala IE, editor. *Practical Management of Haemoglobinopathies.* Oxford: Blackwell; 2004b. pp. 20–5.

Okpala IE. Sickle cell crisis. In: Okpala IE, editor. *Practical Management of Haemoglobinopathies.* Oxford: Blackwell; 2004c. pp. 63–71.

Oni L, Okuyiga E, Sweeney M. *Care and Management of Women with Sickle Cell Disease in Maternity Care Settings.* London: Brent Sickle Cell & Thalassaemia Centre; 2002.

Oteng-Ntim E, Cottee C, Bewley S, *et al.* Sickle cell disease in pregnancy. *Curr Obstet Gynecol.* 2006; **16**(6): 353–60.

Oteng-Ntim E, Lupton M, Mensah S, *et al.* Sickle cell disease and pregnancy. In: Studd J, editor. *Progress in Obstetrics and Gynaecology.* Vol 16. London: Elsevier; 2005. pp. 73–82.

Proudfit C, Atta E, Doyle N. Hemolytic transfusion reaction after preoperative prophylactic blood transfusion for sickle cell disease in pregnancy. *Obstet Gynecol.* 2007; **110**(2 Pt. 2): 471–4.

Quinlan D, McQuillan A, Eikelboom J. Low-molecular-weight heparin compared with intravenous unfractionated heparin for treatment of pulmonary embolism: a meta-analysis of randomized, controlled trials. *Ann Intern Med.* 2004; **140**: 175–83.

Roberts S. Sickle cell disease. In: Queenan JT, Spong CY, Lockwood CJ, editors. *Management of High-Risk Pregnancy: an evidenced-based approach.* 5th ed. Oxford: Blackwell; 2007. pp. 109–12.

Rodger M, Rosene-Montella K, Barbour L. Acute thromboembolic disease. In: Rosene-Montella K, Keely E, Barbour L, *et al.*, editors. *Medical Care of the Pregnant Patient.* 2nd ed. Philadelphia, PA: ACP Press, 2008. pp. 426–44.

Royal College of Obstetricians and Gynaecologists (RCOG). *RCOG Working Party on Prophylaxis against Thromboembolism in Gynaecology and Obstetrics.* London: RCOG; 1995.

Royal College of Obstetricians and Gynaecologists (RCOG). *Green-top Guideline No. 37: Thromboprophylaxis during Pregnancy, Labour and after Vaginal Delivery.* London: RCOG; 2004.

Royal College of Obstetricians and Gynaecologists (RCOG). *Green-top Guideline No. 28: Thromboembolic Disease in Pregnancy and the Puerperium: acute management.* London: RCOG; 2007.

Serjeant G, Loy L, Crowther M, *et al.* Outcome of pregnancy in homozygous sickle cell disease. *Obstet Gynecol.* 2004; **103**(6): 1278–85.

Sheiner E, Levy A, Yerushalmi R, *et al.* Beta-thalassemia minor during pregnancy. *Obstet Gynecol.* 2004; **103**: 1273–7.

Strong J. Anemia and white blood cell disorders. In: James DK, Gonik, Steer P, editors. *High Risk Pregnancy: management options.* 3rd ed. Philadelphia, PA: Saunders Elsevier; 2006. pp. 865–88.

Thein SL. The genetics and multiple phenotypes of beta thalassaemia. In: Okpala IE, editor. *Practical Management of Haemoglobinopathies.* Oxford: Blackwell; 2004. pp. 26–39.

Thomas P, Oni L, Alli M, *et al.* Antenatal screening for haemoglobinopathies – a whole system participatory action research project. *Br J Gen Pract.* 2005; **55**: 424–8.

Toglia MR, Nolan TE. Venous thromboembolism during pregnancy: a current review of diagnosis and management. *Obstet Gynecol Surv.* 1997; **52**: 60–72.

Tuck S. Fertility and pregnancy in thalassemia major. *Ann N Y Acad Sci.* 2005; **1054**: 300–7.

UK National Screening Committee. *The Sickle Cell, Thalassaemia Training CD.* Version 2. 2005. Available at: www.screening.nhs.uk/cpd/fasttrack/main.htm (accessed 5 December 2008).

Walker I. Hematological disorders. In: Greer A, Nelson-Piercy C, Walters B, editors. *Maternal Medicine: medical problems in pregnancy.* Edinburgh: Churchill Livingstone Elsevier; 2007. pp. 134–45.

Weatherall DJ. The hereditary anaemias. In: Provan D, editor. *ABC of Clinical Haematology.* 3rd ed. Oxford: Blackwell; 2007. pp. 11–16.

Whapshott HC. Antenatal assessment for risk of venous thromboembolism. *Br J Midwifery.* 2007; **15**(9): 545–9.

World Health Organization. Available at: http://search.who.int/search?ie=utf8&site=default_co llection&client=WHO&proxystylesheet=WHO&output=xml_no_dtd&oe=utf8&q=haemo globin+colour+scale+&Search=Search&sitesearch= (accessed 8 December 2008).

Wright J, Rati N, Kennefick A, *et al*. A pilot study of 'fast track' antenatal screening for haemoglobinopathies. *J Med Screen*. 2003; **10**(4): 169–71.

Xu K, Shi Z, Veeck L, *et al*. First unaffected pregnancy using preimplantation genetic diagnosis for sickle cell anaemia. *JAMA*. 1999; **281**(18): 1701–6.

Zack-Williams D. Sickle cell anaemia in pregnancy and the neonate: ethical issues. *Br J Midwifery*. 2007; **15**(4): 205–9.

CHAPTER 5

The renal system, hypertension and pre-eclampsia

CONTENTS

[Note: Diabetic nephropathy is in Chapter 1 and lupus nephritis is in Chapter 9]

PHYSIOLOGY OF THE RENAL SYSTEM AND PREGNANCY CHANGES

Marked changes to the physiology and anatomy of the renal system are required to support the physiological changes of pregnancy (Box 5.1). Successful pregnancy for women with renal disease will depend on pre-pregnancy renal function. Figure 5.1 illustrates the main components of the renal system.

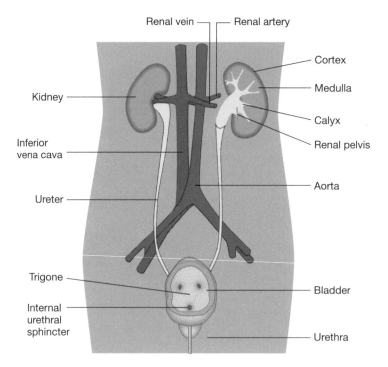

FIGURE 5.1: The renal system

KIDNEY

The kidney filters plasma to produce urine, retaining substances required by the body and eliminating waste. Pregnancy creates an increase in plasma volume with increased metabolic wastes. The kidney acts as an excretory organ for fetal waste as well. In pregnancy renal blood flow increases 50–80% over non-pregnant levels, although this reduces a little by the late third trimester (Gibson and Rosene-Montella, 2008). This rise in renal blood flow causes the kidney to swell, increasing its length by 1 cm (Williams, 2006). In addition to the formation of urine, the kidney also has an endocrine function, playing an important part in the control of blood pressure. Box 5.2 lists the functions of the kidney.

NEPHRONS AND THE FORMATION OF URINE

The kidney is made up of approximately 1.2 million nephrons, which are the functional units of the kidney and consist of a tubule that is closed at one end and opens into the collecting tubule at the other. Through the production of urine by the kidneys, waste products of metabolism are excreted, electrolyte balance is regulated and the pH balance is maintained. Urine is formed through a process of filtration, selective reabsorption and tubular secretion in the nephrons (*see* Figures 5.2 and 5.3).

Glomerular filtration

The *Bowman's capsule* is a cup-like structure forming the closed end of the tubule. It surrounds a network of capillaries known as the *glomerulus*. The wall of the glomerular

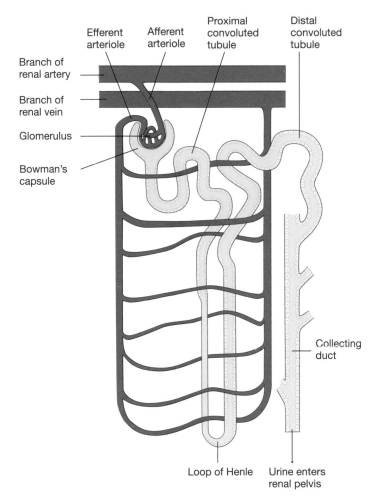

FIGURE 5.2: Nephron and associated blood vessels

capillary serves as a filtration membrane, allowing all the components of the blood to filter through except blood cells and certain plasma proteins. The fluid (termed filtrate, which ultimately becomes the urine) passes from the glomerular capillaries, collects in the Bowman's capsule and filters into the *proximal tubule*.

Selective reabsorption and tubular secretion
Selective reabsorption, as the term implies, allows those filtered constituents that are needed to maintain fluid and electrolyte balance to be reabsorbed into the bloodstream. In the proximal tubule, solutes, nutrients, electrolytes and proteins are reabsorbed, followed by the *loop of Henle*, where a concentration of the urine occurs as water is reabsorbed.

In the *distal convoluted tubule* more solutes are reabsorbed but some substances, such as drugs, are also secreted into the filtrate at this point. The filtrate (urine) drains into *collecting ducts* and then passes into the calyces of the kidney (*see* Figure 5.3).

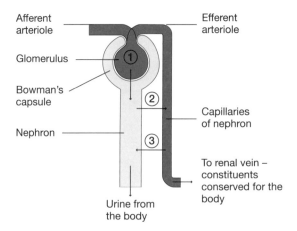

1 Glomerular filtration: Filtration of blood into
  Bowman's capsule
2 Tubular reabsorbtion: Selective movement of
  filtered substances from filtrate back into blood
3 Tubular secretion: Selective movement of some
  non-filtered substances from blood to nephron

Anything from the blood that is filtered or secreted but
not reabsorbed remains in the filtrate and is excreted
as urine

FIGURE 5.3: Summary of the processes that form urine

Selective reabsorption is controlled by various mechanisms and varies according to body need and in some cases it is regulated by hormones. The hormones regulating the formation of urine include the *parathyroid hormone* (regulating calcium and phosphorus), the *antidiuretic hormone (ADH)* (regulating water) and *aldosterone* (regulating sodium and potassium). Atrial natriuretic peptide secreted by the atria of the heart in response to stretching of the walls of the atria decreases the reabsorption of sodium and water in the proximal convoluting tubules and collecting ducts (Sherwood, 1994).

Box 5.3 lists components of urine, which is mostly water, electrolytes and waste products of metabolism.

GLOMERULAR FILTRATION AND TUBULAR FUNCTION IN PREGNANCY

The glomerular filtration rate (GFR) is the volume of fluid filtered by the kidneys per unit of time. In an average person the kidneys filter 180 L/day. This increases in pregnancy by about 40–60%, mediated by increased renal blood flow (Williams, 2006). Women pass urine more often during pregnancy and more urine is produced (Blackburn, 2007; Gibson and Rosene-Montella, 2008; Thorp, *et al.*, 1999). Changes associated with increased GFR in pregnancy are summarised in Box 5.4.

BOX 5.1: SUMMARY OF CHANGES RELATED TO THE URINARY SYSTEM IN PREGNANCY

- Increase in kidney volume, weight and size
- Marked dilation of ureters and renal calyces, which is more pronounced on the right side
- Pressure from enlarging uterus and displacement of bladder
- Increased renal blood flow (50–80%) with an accompanying increase in glomerular filtration rate (GFR) (50%)
- Changes to tubular handling of certain substances
- Accumulation of sodium
- Oedema in 35–85% of healthy pregnant women
- Decreased tone and increased capacity of bladder
- Increased potential for bladder damage and urinary tract infection
- Changes to parameters of renal function
- Decrease in the half-life of drugs cleared by the kidney

(Blackburn, 2007; Gibson and Rosene-Montella, 2008)

BOX 5.2: FUNCTIONS OF THE KIDNEY

- Regulates water and electrolyte balance
- Excretes metabolic waste products and foreign substances
- Conserves nutrients
- Secretes erythropoietin for the production of red blood cells
- Has a role in the control of blood pressure through renin–angiotensin–aldosterone system with regulation of sodium and water balance
- Converts vitamin D into an active form
- Regulates the acid–base balance by the urinary output of hydrogen and bicarbonate

BOX 5.3: COMPONENTS OF URINE

- Water 96%
- Urea 2%
- Uric acid
- Creatinine
- Ammonia
- Sodium
- Potassium
- Chlorides
- Phosphates
- Sulphates
- Oxalates

BOX 5.4: CHANGES ASSOCIATED WITH INCREASED GFR AND TUBULAR FUNCTION IN PREGNANCY

- Increased excretion of solutes including glucose, amino acids, protein, electrolytes and water-soluble vitamins, although tubular reabsorption increases to prevent the depletion of essential electrolytes.
- Decreased tubular glucose reabsorption means glycosuria is a common finding in pregnancy.
- Sodium filtration is increased but reabsorption increases also and results in a net retention of sodium in pregnancy.
- Excretion of water-soluble vitamins increases, so maternal diet needs to include vitamins B12, B2, B6 and C, folate and niacin.
- Urinary calcium excretion is increased but this is balanced by increased intestinal absorption of calcium.
- Increased secretion of urea, creatinine, uric acid and nitrogen in urine.
- Decrease in serum levels of urea, blood urea nitrogen, creatinine and uric acid.
- Alteration in renal excretion of drugs.
- Renal acid–base balance is altered to compensate for the respiratory alkalosis caused by increased alveolar ventilation with increased renal loss of bicarbonate.

(Blackburn, 2007; Thorsen and Poole, 2002; Williams, 2006)

Proteinuria

The filtrate in the Bowman's capsule contains all the substances in the plasma component of blood, except protein and some substances that are bound to plasma proteins. In reality, some protein leaks through as the glomerular membranes are not perfect barriers, but usually it is reabsorbed back by the tubules. In diseased kidneys the glomerular membrane becomes damaged and therefore allows protein through more readily and the tubules lose their ability to reabsorb protein from the filtrate (Challinor, 1998). Proteinuria occurs more frequently during pregnancy and a finding of 1+ protein on the dipstick is not necessarily indicative of pathology (Waugh, *et al.*, 2004). However, proteinuria is an important sign in the diagnosis of pre-eclampsia and should therefore never be ignored.

RENAL ENDOCRINE FUNCTION

The kidney also acts as an endocrine organ. *Erythropoietin* produced by the kidney is responsible for stimulating the bone marrow to produce red blood cells in response to tissue hypoxia.

Vitamin D can be obtained in the diet or by the action of UV radiation on the skin. These forms of vitamin D are inactive and require activation by a process in the liver and kidney. This active form of vitamin D is thus made in the body, making it technically a hormone, not a vitamin. Vitamin D is responsible for the absorption of calcium and phosphorus by the small intestine, from where the minerals are used in forming or remoulding bone.

Renin is formed and stored in the cells of the arterioles of the juxtaglomerular apparatus. These specialised cells are located around the afferent arterioles which control renal blood flow and the GFR. If blood pressure drops, renin is excreted into the circulation. Renin acts on angiotensinogen (a plasma protein) to convert it to angiotensin I. Enzymes further convert this to angiotensin II, which is a powerful vasoconstrictor and increases blood pressure. Renin and raised potassium levels also stimulate the adrenal gland to secrete aldosterone, which causes retention of sodium (and water), thus increasing blood volume.

In pregnancy there is an increase in all the components of the renin–angiotensin–aldosterone mechanism which maintain homeostasis with expanded extra cellular volume of pregnancy. The production of vitamin D and erythropoietin similarly increases during pregnancy in a healthy woman, although their effects are masked by other haemodynamic changes (Williams, 2006).

THE URETERS

The ureters are 25 cm-long tubes with a diameter of about 3 mm that convey urine from the kidney to the urinary bladder. The ureters penetrate the posterior walls of the bladder obliquely, passing through the wall for several centimetres before opening into the bladder cavity. This anatomical arrangement means that when urine volume increases, pressure in the bladder rises, the ureters are compressed and backflow (reflux) of urine is prevented (Sherwood, 1994). Urine does not flow through the ureters by gravity alone, as peristaltic contractions of the smooth muscle in the walls of the ureters propel the urine forward.

In pregnancy there is marked dilation of the calyces, the renal pelvis and the ureters that is referred to as *physiological hydronephrosis of pregnancy*. This occurs as a result of smooth-muscle relaxation mediated by the action of progesterone and prostaglandins (Davison and Baylis, 2002; Faúndes, *et al.*, 1998: Gibson and Rosene-Montella, 2008). There is also some compression of the ureters at the pelvic brim by the growing uterus. The portions of the ureters below the pelvic brim are not usually enlarged. The dilation is more prominent on the right-hand side, where the right ureter makes a more acute angle turn at the pelvic brim because of the location of the iliac and ovarian veins, slowing the passage of urine and increasing urinary stasis (Faúndes, *et al.*, 1998). There can also be some vesicouteric reflux (reflux of urine from the bladder into the ureters) as the enlarging uterus displaces the ureters laterally, flattening the angle of insertion into the bladder (Baylis and Davison, 1998). The ureters may contain as much as 300 mL by the third trimester (Blackburn, 2007). This can influence the accuracy of timed urine collections as well as increase risk of urinary tract infection. Dilation may persist for up to three months post-partum (Thorsen and Poole, 2002).

URINARY BLADDER AND URETHRA

The bladder is distensible, being able to accommodate large fluctuations in urine volume and, when full, it rises above the pelvic brim. Pressure from the growing fetus may impede bladder capacity in the third trimester (Blackburn, 2007).

The three openings into the bladder wall form a triangle area called the trigone. The two upper openings are the ureters and the lower one the urethra. The female urethra is 4 cm long and has two separate sphincters. The internal sphincter at the base of the bladder is composed of smooth muscle, like the bladder, and is under involuntary control. When the bladder is relaxed the internal sphincter closes the outlet of the bladder. The external urethral sphincter is composed of skeletal muscle and is reinforced by the muscle layers of the pelvic floor. This sphincter is under voluntary control (Waugh and Grant, 2006).

In pregnancy there is a reduction in bladder tone as a result of the relaxing effect of progesterone on the smooth muscle layer of the bladder. The bladder is displaced upwards and backwards. Under the influence of oestrogen there is hyperplasia and an increased blood supply to the bladder mucosa, making it more oedematous and vulnerable to trauma and infection (Blackburn, 2007).

The pregnancy changes of decreased tone, oedema and mucosal hyperplasia can be aggravated by prolonged labour, forceps delivery, analgesia and anaesthesia. The pressure of the fetal head on the bladder during labour can result in trauma and a transient loss of bladder sensation, which can lead to over-distension of the bladder with incomplete emptying. The post-partum period is characterised by a rapid and sustained diuresis (Blackburn, 2007).

GENERAL PRINCIPLES OF CARE
RENAL DISEASE IN PREGNANCY

Pregnancy, for women with renal disease, may be detrimental to their health, causing an acceleration in decline of their renal function with poor pregnancy outcome (*see* Box 5.5 for risks associated with renal disease). Factors associated with poor maternal and fetal outcome in pregnancy include:

▶ a declining level of renal function (defined by serum creatinine levels)
▶ pre-existing hypertension
▶ proteinuria
▶ recurrent urinary tract infection
▶ poor glycaemic control in women with diabetic nephropathy.

(Williams, 2006, 2007)

Although there are many pre-existing conditions that may affect the renal system and compromise maternal and fetal well-being in pregnancy, most – especially the more severe – are rare. Therefore, general principles for care will be included, and these will be relevant, depending on the individual woman's condition, for all women with renal disease.

PRECONCEPTION CARE

As with all chronic conditions, preconception care should be available to ensure these women have their condition assessed, medications reviewed and health optimised before becoming pregnant.

The presence of abnormal serum values and/or proteinuria representing compromised renal function, and/or hypertension will contribute to the risk of a poor pregnancy outcome for the woman or baby (Williams, 2008). However, it has been shown that maximising health, such as effective treatment of chronic hypertension in the preconception period, may reduce the risks (Williams, 2008).

BOX 5.5: RISKS ASSOCIATED WITH RENAL DISEASE IN PREGNANCY

- Deterioration of renal function
- Increased thrombosis
- Increased risk of ascending urinary tract infection (UTI)
- Hypertension
- Pre-eclampsia
- Preterm delivery
- IUGR
- Increased Caesarean section rate

PREGNANCY CARE

During pregnancy, renal function should be closely monitored with regular blood testing and 24-hour urine collections. Women may be taught to test their own urine in between antenatal visits. Careful regular screening for, and treatment of, urinary tract infection will be carried out and prophylactic antibiotics may also be used for those with recurrent renal system infections.

There is an increased risk of hypertension developing or worsening for all women with renal disease, and this must also be assessed regularly and treated as appropriate. Superimposed pre-eclampsia may occur, and screening for this in a woman with possible pre-existing proteinuria and hypertension is challenging. Some renal disease is complicated with hyperuricaemia and causes IUGR, but if hepatic transaminases are raised and thrombocytopenia is present, this is likely to represent pre-eclampsia (Williams and de Swiet, 1997). The midwife can give information to the woman about recognising pre-eclampsia and signs of early labour, including who to contact if concerns arise.

As the renal system is responsible for production of erythropoietin (necessary for haemoglobin), anaemia is screened for regularly. Some authorities prescribe prophylactic low-dose aspirin to women with renal disease, as they believe this may prevent glomerular capillary thrombosis (RCOG, 2007; Williams, 2008).

Increased fetal surveillance, in particular regular growth scans, is normal to ensure fetal well-being. In addition to the fetus being at risk from uteroplacental insufficiency, a reduced maternal glomerular filtration may produce higher levels of toxic materials or drugs in the maternal circulation, and these may cross to the fetus (Thorsen and Poole, 2002). Fetal compromise may be the first sign of a deteriorating maternal condition (Thorsen and Poole, 2002).

It has been suggested that renal biopsy is not contraindicated during pregnancy (Chen, et al., 2001) if considered necessary, but this is controversial. If renal function declines to the stage where dialysis is required, the woman may be offered the choice of terminating the pregnancy, but her renal function may continue to decline even after the pregnancy is stopped. It may be possible for pregnancy to continue successfully while on dialysis (Williams, 2008), but it is a very high-risk situation.

LABOUR CARE

Due to a compromised renal function, fluid overload can occur at any time for a woman with renal disease; however, this is much more likely in labour, when intravenous fluids are commonly used. This may increase hypertension and ultimately lead to pulmonary oedema. Pulmonary oedema may also result from progressive renal damage, and observation for respiratory signs and symptoms (shortness of breath, rising respiratory rate, decreased oxygen saturation levels, frothy sputum and crackles heard during lung auscultation) is necessary. A strict fluid balance must be observed and documented clearly.

Cardiac monitoring may be undertaken during labour, depending on the woman's condition, and abnormalities may represent increasing serum potassium, which will need to be speedily reversed. Arterial blood gas analysis may indicate metabolic acidosis, and this will also need rapid treatment.

POSTNATAL CARE

As with all medical conditions, breastfeeding is encouraged, but a review of any medication being taken must be undertaken first and this should be done during pregnancy to enable feeding to commence immediately after birth. Renal assessment continues as necessary, and the midwife should ensure that appropriate follow-up is organised.

SUMMARY OF MIDWIFERY CARE

◗ Ensure women have information about symptoms of pre-eclampsia and signs of premature labour and who to contact if there are any concerns.
◗ Provide information on how to collect an accurate mid-stream specimen of urine (MSU) and 24-hour urine collection, and enable the woman to make home assessments of proteinuria, if appropriate.
◗ Provide information on a healthy diet and lifestyle to improve immunity, avoid infections and prevent anaemia.
◗ Give advice about preventing thromboembolism.
◗ Avoid catheterisation and ensure impeccable technique if necessary.
◗ Maintain accurate fluid balance records in appropriate situations.

SPECIFIC RENAL CONDITIONS

This section gives an overview of some of the renal conditions that may affect pregnant women. The list is not exhaustive and the reader is directed to more specialist renal texts as required.

URINARY TRACT INFECTION (UTI)

UTI occurs more frequently in pregnant women because of the anatomical and physiological changes that take place in the renal system in pregnancy. They include:
◗ increased glucose excretion with glycosuria (which is not necessarily indicative of diabetes, but is a good medium in which bacteria can grow)
◗ elongation and dilation of the ureters and physiological hydronephrosis
◗ decreased bladder tone as pregnancy advances, leading to urinary stasis
◗ change in the angle at which the ureters enter the bladder, causing urine reflux.

Symptoms suggestive of UTI in pregnancy are dysuria (pain and difficulty in passing urine) and offensive smelling urine. Urinary frequency, urgency and nocturia are signs of UTI but are frequent symptoms in healthy pregnant women, making the diagnosis less straightforward (Blackburn, 2007; Williams, 2006). Diagnosis is by urine microscopy and culture of a freshly obtained MSU. This will enable quantification of pyuria (leukocytes in the urine) and detection of urinary pathogens. More than 100 000 bacteria/mL of a single organism (usually *Escherichia coli*) is diagnostic.

Asymptomatic bacteriuria (ASB)
The prevalence of ASB is estimated at between 2–10% of pregnant women (Thorsen and Poole, 2002). ASB has been associated with adverse conditions such as premature labour, a reduction in fetal/infant weight, maternal anaemia, hypertension and pre-eclampsia (Thorsen and Poole, 2002). Since this condition is, by definition, asymptomatic, ASB is routinely screened for during antenatal care, and it is diagnosed by a laboratory finding of > 100 000 bacteria/mL. Untreated ASB can lead to a symptomatic urinary tract infection and/or pyelonephritis. It has been estimated that about 25% of women with untreated ASB will develop pyelonephritis (Vazquez and Villar, 2003).

Pyelonephritis
Pyelonephritis is an acute bacterial infection of the renal pelvis which can spread into the tissue of the kidney. It occurs in approximately 1–2% of all pregnancies and is most commonly the result of an ascending urinary tract infection (Thorsen and Poole, 2002). Screening and treatment for ASB reduces the incidence of pyelonephritis, thus reducing maternal and fetal morbidity (Williams, 2006).

Common symptoms of pyelonephritis include lower UTI symptoms, backache, tenderness, high fever, rigors and nausea and vomiting. The right side is more commonly affected (Thorsen and Poole, 2002). There is usually a raised serum CRP (C-reactive protein) and high leukocytes, and screening with blood cultures for septicaemia is also carried out. Urine cultures are positive and pyuria is found – and often seen. Women with pyelonephritis are usually hospitalised, closely monitored and treated with intravenous antibiotics. Acute pyelonephritis can trigger uterine contractions and is a cause of preterm labour (Williams, 2006). Acute respiratory distress syndrome (ARDS) can occur, especially in women who have received tocolysis for threatened premature labour (Gilstrap and Ramin, 2001), so monitoring of the respiratory system should take place. Other complications for the woman include septic shock with an increased risk of pulmonary oedema due to fluid shift.

REFLUX NEPHROPATHY
Reflux nephropathy is one of the most common complications of the renal system for young women, and they are at particular risk in pregnancy of both superimposed complications such as pre-eclampsia and a decline in the general renal function. Reflux nephropathy involves reflux of urine from the bladder to the ureters (vesicoureteric reflux: VUR), which causes the development of infection in the kidneys and progressive loss of functioning nephrons and is one of the most frequent causes of renal disease in women of child-bearing age (Williams, 2006). Up to 30% of women who develop end-stage renal failure have reflux nephropathy (Davison and Baylis, 2002).

Reflux nephropathy is characterised by moderate to severe renal damage, reduced GFR, proteinuria, recurrent urinary tract infection and concurrent hypertension. This combination of features gives rise to a poor pregnancy outcome. There can be a sudden escalation of blood pressure with superimposed pre-eclampsia and irreversible progression of renal damage during pregnancy. Severe intra-uterine growth restriction may occur (Davison and Baylis, 2002).

Women who had VUR in childhood, even if surgically corrected, are at increased risk of reflux nephropathy and should be screened for ASB every 4–6 weeks during pregnancy (Williams, 2006). Those whose nephropathy stems from VUR in childhood may be offered fetal or neonatal screening by ultrasound, as this condition is familial (Davison and Baylis, 2002).

NEPHROTIC SYNDROME

Nephrotic syndrome is itself not a disease but is a feature of several renal disorders. Features of the syndrome include:

- marked proteinuria (non-pregnant value of > 0.35 g per day)
- hypoalbuminaemia
- generalised oedema
- hyperlipidaemia.

(Waugh and Grant, 2006)

When glomeruli are damaged, plasma proteins pass through into the filtrate (they are normally too big to do so). Albumin is the most common plasma protein and it is a relatively small molecule. When there is significant loss in the urine, plasma oncotic pressure changes result in a shift of fluid out of the vascular space, resulting in oedema and a reduction in plasma volume. The juxtaglomerular apparatus detects the fall in blood flow to the kidneys, which stimulates the renin–angiotensin–aldosterone system to conserve water and sodium, setting up a vicious cycle of fluid retention and worsening oedema (Huether, 2006). Nephrotic syndrome occurs with *glomerulonephritis, diabetic nephropathy* or *lupus nephritis,* with the most common cause in pregnancy being *pre-eclampsia.* A low dietary intake of protein with anorexia or malnutrition may contribute to low levels of plasma albumin (Davison and Baylis, 2002).

The outcome for pregnancy depends on renal function, level of hypertension and extent of proteinuria. The physiological changes of pregnancy exacerbate symptoms, with increased protein excretion, increased fluid retention and worsening oedema (Davison and Baylis, 2002).

GLOMERULONEPHRITIS

Glomerulonephritis involves a reduction in urine output, the presence of proteinuria, and haematuria. Inflammation of the endothelial lining of the glomerular capillaries leads to diminished blood flow and there is a reduction in the amount of urine produced. The damage to the endothelium also alters its permeability, allowing more protein to leak through. Further damage allows blood cells to escape, resulting in haematuria. Oedema, renal impairment and hypertension commonly accompany glomerulonephritis (Huether, 2006). There are numerous types of glomerulonephritis.

The classification of the disorder is complex and can be described according to cause, pathological lesion seen on biopsy tissue, disease progress (acute/chronic) or on clinical presentation (Macfarlane, *et al.*, 2000). Overall, the type of glomerulonephritis does not affect the pregnancy as much as the impact of co-existing hypertension, proteinuria, the degree of renal impairment and urinary tract infection (Williams, 2007).

RENAL CALCULI (NEPHROLITHIASIS, RENAL STONES)

Stones can form in the kidney and bladder when urinary constituents such as oxalates, phosphates and calcium crystallise. Most originate in the collecting tubules and pass into the renal pelvis, where they may increase in size. Dehydration, stasis and, in particular, infection, which alters the pH of the urine, predisposes to the development of calculi (Macfarlane, *et al.*, 2000).

The incidence of renal stone disease is the same in pregnancy as it is outside pregnancy and is estimated at one in 244 pregnancies (Lewis, *et al.*, 2003). It is more common in the Caucasian population, more likely to present in the second or third trimester and affects multiparous women more than women having their first baby (Williams, 2007). Pregnancy creates optimum conditions for the development of calculi, including renal tract dilation, urinary stasis and an increase in calcium in the urine. However, inhibitors of stone formation such as magnesium and citrate are excreted in larger amounts in pregnancy as well (Davison and Baylis, 2002).

The necessity for treating renal calculi (stones) is rare in pregnancy, but some operations are safe. However, most pregnant women with renal colic spontaneously pass the stones and treatment is restricted to hydration, analgesia and antibiotics. Signs and symptoms of renal colic include pain (often spasmodic), pyrexia, UTI and haematuria. Diagnosis can be by ultrasound (about 50%), abdominal radiograph or magnetic resonance urography (Williams, 2008). UTI associated with renal stones is associated with an increased risk of premature rupture of the membranes (Lewis, *et al.*, 2003).

SINGLE KIDNEY

A single kidney can be associated with other urological abnormalities as well as abnormalities of the uterus and genital tract. A single kidney may be present congenitally or because of the surgical removal of one kidney for disease or, occasionally, because the woman has been a living donor. These women are vulnerable to obstruction of their one kidney in pregnancy. They can have an incomplete obstruction that can cause renal damage despite seemingly normal urine output. High back pressure can compress and damage the renal medulla (Williams, 2006).

ACUTE RENAL FAILURE (ARF)

Acute renal failure is an abrupt reduction in renal function and is usually associated with diminished urine output of less than 30 mL per hour and less than 400 mL per day. It can occur in those with known renal compromise, in conjunction with another pregnancy complication (for example, pre-eclampsia, haemorrhage) or due to trauma (*see* Box 5.6). Often changes in blood urea nitrogen and serum creatinine levels are the earliest signs of acute renal failure.

The complication of ARF should be considered when caring for a woman with any of the possible causes, and monitoring urinary output is part of routine care. When suspected, serum screening (electrolytes and renal function tests – *see* Appendix at the end of this chapter for normal values) and possibly renal ultrasound if obstruction is suspected, will establish the diagnosis. Management is focused on identifying and treating the cause plus fluid replacement, ideally guided by CVP levels to prevent fluid overload. It is a very serious condition but full recovery is possible with treatment. In pregnancy, however, the physiological changes make permanent renal damage more common (Williams, 2006). Dialysis may be necessary in the short term or, rarely, in the long term.

BOX 5.6: POSSIBLE CAUSES OF ACUTE RENAL FAILURE

- Haemorrhage
- Obstruction; for example, from the uterus (in particular in multiple pregnancies), broad ligament/pelvic haematoma, damage to ureters, renal calculi
- Reaction to blood transfusion or drugs
- Pre-eclampsia
- Acute fatty liver disease of pregnancy
- Amniotic fluid embolism
- Pyelonephritis or other sepsis
- Hyperemesis gravidarum

CHRONIC RENAL FAILURE

Chronic renal failure is progressive and irreversible damage to about 75% of nephrons. The kidneys exhibit remarkable adaptive abilities and so the onset of symptoms is slow. The main causes are glomerulonephritis, diabetes, reflux nephropathy and hypertension. There is reduced glomerular filtration, which leads to a build up of urea and creatinine in the blood. A large quantity of urine is produced as reabsorption of water is impaired. Acidosis occurs as the kidney buffer system that normally maintains pH fails. An imbalance of sodium and potassium occurs. Hypertension can be a cause and a result of renal failure (Huether, 2006; Macfarlane, *et al.*, 2000; Waugh and Grant, 2006).

The woman with chronic renal failure is likely to have a degree of hypertension and be taking antihypertensive medication. She may be prescribed diuretics as she has the potential for systemic oedema, and she may be anaemic due to the suppression of erythropoietin. The outcome of her pregnancy depends on the severity of her condition, and careful monitoring, as described in the general care section earlier in this chapter, is necessary.

ORGAN TRANSPLANT: GENERAL INFORMATION

There are similarities in the preconception, antenatal, labour and postnatal care of women who have had organ transplants. These principles of care are given below. Most experience in pregnancy following transplant is in relation to renal transplant (Expert Group on Renal Transplantation, 2002). Details concerning each particular organ are given in the relevant chapter.

PRECONCEPTION CARE

Fertility is usually reduced with worsening disease, but it can return within weeks of a transplant, so contraception information is vital. The usual advice to a woman following organ transplant is to wait 1–2 years, using good contraception, before becoming pregnant. This is to allow the graft function to stabilise and necessary immunosuppressant medication to be reduced to maintenance level. Many drugs can be altered to divided doses to avoid peaks that may affect the fetus.

Since most transplant procedures result in an underlying chronic hypertension, cardiac screening for baseline information should be undertaken prior to pregnancy (Armenti, *et al.*, 2006). Any antihypertensive medication should also be reviewed. General health should be assessed, paying particular attention to nutrition, obesity, anaemia, proteinuria, smoking and alcohol intake, to ensure optimum well-being.

PREGNANCY CARE

BOX 5.7: COMMON ADVERSE EFFECTS FOR WOMEN (AND FETUS) WITH ORGAN TRANSPLANT

- Hypertension/pre-eclampsia
- Anaemia
- Infection
- Gestational diabetes
- Increased Caesarean sections
- Miscarriage
- Prematurity*
- IUGR*

* Some report that up to 50% of births to women following transplant are premature, but do not divide them into spontaneous or planned early delivery due to the mother's condition. Also many of the studies use a birth weight of < 2500 g as an indication of prematurity, but do not give the gestation, so information as to whether the baby is premature or IUGR is not available.

Care should be guided by a multidisciplinary team, including a representative from the transplant team. Mild rejection may occur and be largely asymptomatic, so the graft should be monitored regularly and, depending on the organ, this is done through blood/urine analysis or ultrasound/MRI examination (Armenti, *et al.*, 2006). Rarely, an organ biopsy may be necessary. A severe graft rejection may present with pyrexia and pain over organ site.

Medication taken following a transplant may need regular monitoring of serum levels as the haemodilution effect of pregnancy may adversely affect them. As steroids are often used routinely by women following an organ transplant, particular care needs to be taken to avoid infection.

Pre-eclampsia screening may be a challenge, as not only do many women have chronic hypertension and proteinuria, but many markers used in routine PET screening (see Appendix at the end of this chapter) are normal for those who have had a transplant.

Fetal surveillance is vital, considering the large amount of low-birth-weight babies born to women following an organ transplant (*see* Box 5.7). Depending on individual situations, all women may be offered regular growth ultrasound evaluation, and many will also have liquor volume estimation and Doppler assessments.

LABOUR CARE

Glucocorticoids are usual maintenance medication for women following transplant. Depending on the dosage given, stress dose steroids may be given during labour. There is a high Caesarean section rate for women who have undergone organ transplantation, and it is vital that an accurate assessment of where the donor organ is situated, and whether the original organ remains, is undertaken before any procedure is carried out. The midwife needs to ensure these records are available for every woman, as even planned vaginal deliveries may turn into Caesarean sections. Transplant surgeons often attend Caesarean sections to offer obstetricians specialist advice.

POSTNATAL CARE

Immunosuppressive drugs make the woman more susceptible to infection, and as the puerperium is a high-risk time for all women (Boyle, 2006), special care needs to be taken with infection prevention. Any medication dosage increase during pregnancy should be assessed and perhaps reduced as the haemodilution effect of pregnancy is lost. Breastfeeding needs to be considered according to the drugs the woman is taking, but if they are safe, then it should be encouraged.

RENAL TRANSPLANT

(*See also Organ transplant: general information* earlier in this chapter.)

Spontaneous pregnancy in those receiving dialysis has been reported (Hou, 1999) but it carries a high complication rate for the mother and baby; therefore waiting to become pregnant until after a transplant is recommended. There are no reports of pregnancy affecting the rate of transplant rejection (Williams, 2008).

Screening for pre-eclampsia may be problematic as many women may have degrees of hypertension and proteinuria, together with abnormal renal function tests, including a raised uric acid. As symptoms of organ rejection may not be obvious, monitoring serum creatinine is usual, and since these levels normally decrease in pregnancy, any rise should trigger further investigations (Fuchs, *et al.*, 2007).

Assessment of children born to mothers following a renal transplant has been made. One study involved 48 children aged from nine months to 18 years, and it found that 56% were premature and 44% IUGR, but 98% demonstrated a normal development (Willis, *et al.*, 2000).

The UK Obstetric Surveillance System (UKOSS) (2008) is currently undertaking a study of pregnancy in renal transplant recipients, and these findings may change the estimation of risk and underpin care in the future.

HYPERTENSION

Hypertension is the most common medical condition affecting women of child-bearing age (Powrie and Miller, 2008). There is a close relationship between the kidney and high blood pressure. Many renal diseases cause hypertension and hypertension can cause renal damage. Renal disorders with concurrent hypertension have a poorer outcome for mother and infant (Blackburn, 2007; Williams, 2007). Hypertensive disorders in pregnancy include:

 ▶ chronic hypertension
 ▶ transient hypertension of pregnancy
 ▶ pre-eclampsia.

Chronic hypertension currently complicates 3–5% of pregnancies, although with the increase in obesity and the tendency to delay child-bearing the incidence is likely to rise (Powrie and Miller, 2008). A woman with chronic hypertension has greater risk (20–40%) of developing pre-eclampsia (Powrie and Miller, 2008).

Changes to blood pressure in pregnancy are discussed in Chapter 2. In summary, blood pressure decreases in the second trimester, with a greater decrease in the diastolic blood pressure. Towards term the blood pressure rises to the pre-pregnancy baseline. The onset of a blood pressure greater than 140/90 mmHg after 20 weeks' gestation should prompt investigation for pre-eclampsia (Milne, *et al.*, 2005). Chronic severe hypertension (with a high risk of superimposed pre-eclampsia) is associated with:

 ▶ preterm delivery
 ▶ increased risk of a low-birth-weight baby
 ▶ IUGR
 ▶ placental abruption
 ▶ increased perinatal mortality.

(Powrie and Miller, 2008)

PRE-ECLAMPSIA
PATHOPHYSIOLOGY

Pre-eclampsia is a multisystem disorder with a complex aetiology that is unique to pregnancy. It is usually defined as raised blood pressure and proteinuria that develop after 20 weeks' gestation (Milne, *et al.*, 2005). However, pre-eclampsia may affect different body systems, as well as complicate pregnancies in women with other pre-existing pathologies, leading to varied presentations of pre-eclampsia that do not fit classical definitions (Roberts and Cooper, 2001). Sibai *et al.* (2005) even describe two syndromes of pre-eclampsia: the maternal syndrome (hypertension and proteinuria with or without multisystem abnormalities) and the fetal syndrome (fetal growth restriction, reduced amniotic fluid and poor fetal oxygen perfusion). Pre-eclampsia remains a disease of theories and is the subject of much research to understand its aetiology and improve its detection and management.

The changes seen in pre-eclampsia appear to be caused by a complex interplay of abnormal genetic, immunological and placental factors. Early changes in the way the placenta embeds in the uterus are a strong predisposing factor in the development of the systemic disease (Sibai, *et al.*, 2005). The establishment of normal placental implantation requires the trophoblast cells to invade the uterine decidua and myometrium, modifying and enlarging the uterine spiral arteries. This modification involves breaking down the elastic walls of the vessels, which lowers resistance and ensures a good blood supply to the placenta and fetus. Inflammatory agents of the innate immune system such as natural killer (NK) cells and cytokines have more recently been identified in this process (Sibai, *et al.*, 2005). In pre-eclampsia there is a defective invasion by the trophoblast cells; the spiral arteries retain their tone and dilate to only 40% of that seen in normal pregnancies. This results in under-perfusion of the placenta and chronic fetal hypoxia. Figure 5.4 depicts normal trophoblast invasion. In pregnancies complicated by pre-eclampsia this invasion is halted at 14–15 weeks (Morley, 2004).

BOX 5.8: RISK FACTORS FOR PRE-ECLAMPSIA

- Primigravida or > 10 years since last baby
- First pregnancy with a new partner
- Previous history of pre-eclampsia
- A family history of pre-eclampsia, in particular in the mother or sister (of both the woman and her partner)
- Multiple pregnancy
- Certain medical conditions such as essential hypertension, renal disease, diabetes
- Booking proteinuria (> 1+ on more than one occasion or > 0.3 g/24 h)
- Age ≥ 40 years
- Obesity (BMI > 35)
- IVF

As a consequence of poor placentation (and possible fetal compromise), generalised endothelial dysfunction occurs, leading to multi-organ involvement and the development of the classic features of pre-eclampsia, such as raised blood pressure and proteinuria, along with symptoms such as headaches, visual disturbances and epigastric pain. The endothelial cells that line the maternal blood vessels mediate immune and inflammatory responses, maintain the integrity of the vascular compartment, prevent intravascular coagulation and modify the contractile response of the underlying smooth muscle (Vander, *et al.*, 2001). Endothelial dysfunction in pre-eclampsia causes increased cell permeability, increased platelet aggregation, increased thrombosis, decreased production of nitric oxide (a powerful vasodilator) and an imbalance of the ratio of thromboxane A2 to prostacyclin (Powrie and Rosene-Montella, 2008; Walfisch and Hallak, 2006). The result is profound vasoconstriction leading to hypoperfusion of organs, 'leaky' vessels and raised blood pressure.

The mechanism for endothelial dysfunction is poorly understood. Antioxidant treatment (vitamins C and E) aimed at controlling the oxidative stress that may cause endothelial dysfunction has been disappointing in large clinical trials (Poston, *et al.*, 2006). Similarly, anti-platelet treatment aimed at restoring the prostacyclin–thromboxane imbalance has shown limited benefit (Duley, *et al.*, 2001). The role of nitric oxide and inflammatory responses are two areas of current research focus (Sibai, *et al.*, 2005). *See* Figure 5.5 for summary of the pathophysiology.

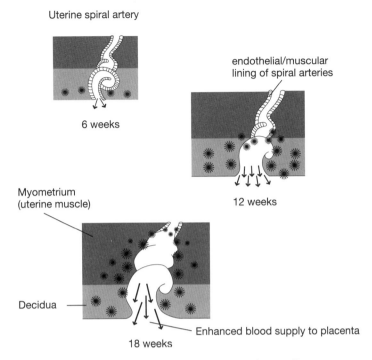

FIGURE 5.4: Invasion of the spiral arteries by trophoblast cells

PRECONCEPTION CARE

Although ensuring the best possible health before pregnancy is always advisable, since a full understanding of the aetiology of pre-eclampsia is not available, it is difficult to suggest specific measures. However, it would be sensible to change lifestyle issues that are known to predispose to pre-eclampsia, such as reducing weight to a normal level, stopping smoking and treating existing hypertension.

PREGNANCY CARE

By reviewing the risk factors (*see* Box 5.8), women can be identified as high risk for pre-eclampsia at booking. However, many women who have risk factors do not develop pre-eclampsia, and it is impossible at present to specifically target a group of women in whom pre-eclampsia will be anticipated. Of course women who have several risk factors and, in particular, those with a history of severe pre-eclampsia in previous pregnancies are more likely to develop the disease.

Since even women with no risk factors can develop pre-eclampsia, the midwife should ensure that all women receive information concerning symptoms and know how to self-refer when appropriate.

Routine antenatal screening for pre-eclampsia should be done at every antenatal visit, and this consists of measuring blood pressure (*see* Box 5.9), assessments for proteinuria (*see* Box 5.10) and discussion of possible symptoms (*see* Box 5.11). If there is a cause for concern, then blood tests (*see* Appendix) should be taken and, if appropriate, an ultrasound arranged to assess fetal well-being.

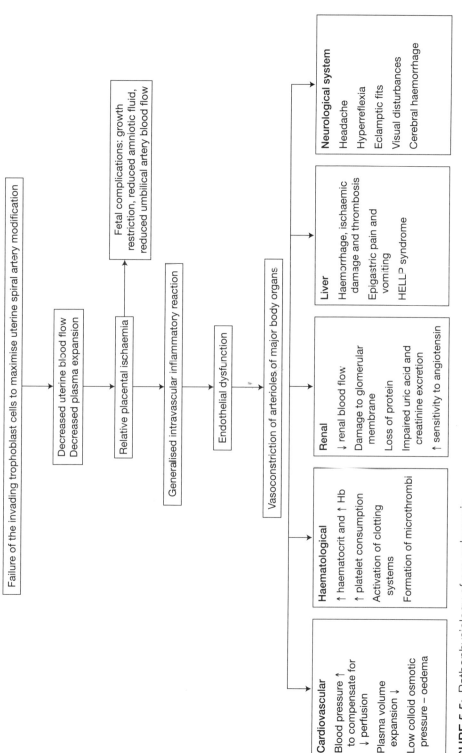

FIGURE 5.5: Pathophysiology of pre-eclampsia
Source: adapted from Roberts and Cooper (2001)

If a woman is diagnosed with pre-eclampsia, monitoring of blood pressure, proteinuria and presence or development of symptoms, as well as blood results (PET screening – *see* Appendix) and fetal assessment form the basic underpinning for care.

BOX 5.9: MEASURING BLOOD PRESSURE

Blood pressure readings that may indicate the need for further investigation are usually considered higher than 140/90 mmHg or an increase of 15–20 mmHg over booking. Although traditionally the diastolic was considered the most important component when assessing pre-eclampsia, it is now clear that equal attention should be paid to the systolic reading. Measurement of blood pressure is a vital screening tool and midwives should ensure their practice is optimum. Recommended best practice to ensure errors are not made includes:

- using an appropriate device and understanding the limitations of automated machines
- ensuring that the woman is relaxed and both the woman and equipment are positioned appropriately
- using the correct size of cuff
- slowly deflating the cuff
- measuring to the nearest 2 mmHg and avoiding digit preference where findings are rounded off
- using Korotkoff V (disappearance) for the diastolic reading
- using mean arterial pressure readings.

(Bothamley and Boyle, 2008a, 2008b; PRECOG, 2004; RCOG, 2006)

BOX 5.10: ASSESSMENT OF PROTEINURIA

Although proteinuria is often caused by a urinary tract infection, it is also possible that it may be the first sign of pre-eclampsia in a woman with normal blood pressure. There are many areas where the assessment of proteinuria may be variable and the midwife should ensure there is as little margin for error as possible. Common methods of assessment are:

- dipsticks: 1+ of protein needs further attention. Manufacturer's recommendations must be followed when caring for and using dipsticks (e.g., dating when they are opened and replacing lids) to ensure the most accurate results. Using automated dipstick readers may help to avoid observer error
- urinary spot protein: creatinine ratios can be used to assess whether a 24-hour urinary collection is necessary
- 24-hour urinary collection: a primary test to quantify excreted protein and > 0.3 g/24 hours is considered significant.

(Cote, *et al.*, 2008; PRECOG, 2004)

When pre-eclampsia is diagnosed, it is usually classified as mild, moderate or severe. Care pathways have been devised (Perez-Cuevas, *et al.*, 2003) and all maternity units provide guidelines and protocols for care of these women, but it is vital to remember that the unpredictability of pre-eclampsia means women classified as mild will not always stay within these defined boundaries. Equally, while it is usual that the earlier the signs and symptoms appear, the more severe the disease manifestation is, women have developed severe pre-eclampsia at term or even postnatally. Therefore, when caring for any woman with pre-eclampsia the midwife must be constantly alert for changes in her condition (*see* Box 5.12 for features of worsening pre-eclampsia).

BOX 5.11: POSSIBLE SIGNS AND SYMPTOMS OF PRE-ECLAMPSIA

- Headache
- Visual disturbances
- Epigastric pain
- Vomiting
- Reduced fetal movements
- Small for gestational age fetus

(McDonald, 2002; PRECOG, 2004)

BOX 5.12: FEATURES OF WORSENING (FULMINATING) PRE-ECLAMPSIA

- Rising blood pressure
- Increasing proteinuria
- Increasing severity of symptoms and signs listed in Box 5.11
- Signs of clonus
- Papilloedema
- Liver tenderness
- Platelet count falling
- Abnormal liver enzymes
- HELLP syndrome

(McDonald, 2002; RCOG, 2006)

Drugs (*see* Box 5.13) are an important part of the management of pre-eclampsia, and they are usually given to reduce blood pressure (antihypertensives) or to prevent or treat eclampsia (anticonvulsives). Antihypertensive drugs are given to reduce blood pressure, largely in order to prevent a cerebral vascular accident (stroke), and are considered vital when the blood pressure is > 160/110 (RCOG, 2006), although medication can be started with lower levels of hypertension. However, lowering the blood pressure does not mean that the woman has recovered from pre-eclampsia, as the disease process can continue. Careful observation of blood results should enable a more accurate assessment of her condition to be made.

Fluid management is vital to the successful management of pre-eclampsia. In the past, Confidential Enquiries into Maternal Deaths frequently reported an overload of fluid as a contributing factor to maternal mortality from pre-eclampsia. A careful assessment of fluid balance is integral to the care of a woman with moderate or severe pre-eclampsia. An indwelling urinary catheter, with hourly urine measurement and fluid restriction, may be necessary, and a CVP line may be useful to underpin fluid administration in severe cases. Continuous oxygen saturation monitoring may give an early warning of the onset of pulmonary oedema.

BOX 5.13: DRUGS COMMONLY GIVEN IN PRE-ECLAMPSIA

- *Methyldopa:* commonly used as first-line management in pregnancy, usually for mild or moderate pre-eclampsia, as lowering blood pressure is slow. It is a centrally acting hypotensive, reducing the blood pressure without adverse changes in the heart rate, cardiac output, renal perfusion or uteroplacental blood flow.
- *Nifedipine:* generally used when methyldopa has not been effective or if a more rapid response is required. This is a calcium channel blocker and works by preventing the transfer of calcium ions from extracellular space and inhibiting its uptake by the smooth muscle cells, therefore contractility is reduced and peripheral resistance is lowered. Although available in a sublingual preparation, this route is not used in pregnancy. Grapefruit can increase the potency of the drug, so should not be taken when it is used.
- *Labetalol:* given orally if methyldopa and nifedipine are ineffective, but more commonly used as an intravenous infusion in severe pre-eclampsia. As a combined alpha and beta antagonist, it works by reducing peripheral resistance and cardiac output.
- *Hydralazine:* mainly used as an intravenous infusion in severe pre-eclampsia. It acts directly on the smooth muscles of the arterial wall, causing vasodilation. Care must be taken to avoid sudden hypotension.
- *Magnesium sulphate:* recommended as a first-line treatment of eclampsia and to prevent eclampsia in those at high risk. It is usually given as a bolus IV injection, followed by an IV infusion. Although its primary function is as an anti-convulsive, it also has a strong hypotensive effect, and further antihypertensive medication may not be necessary for the pre-eclamptic woman. Careful monitoring of the woman's respiratory/neurological state is necessary as high serum levels (usually $> 7\,mmol/L$) are associated with respiratory depression and eventually cardiac arrest. Since the drug is cleared through the kidneys and women with pre-eclampsia often have renal impairment, without regular assessment and observation, a toxic serum level could easily be reached. Calcium gluconate can be given to treat respiratory depression and should be readily available.

Since IUGR of the fetus is a common component of pre-eclampsia, and in fact may sometimes be evident even before maternal signs and symptoms, fetal surveillance is necessary. Growth scans are usually carried out every two weeks, and other tests for fetal well-being, such as CTG, liquor volume estimation and umbilical artery Doppler assessment, are done as frequently as necessary, depending on the individual case. If the woman is preterm, since it is possible that delivery could take place imminently, steroids are routinely administered to her to aid in the maturation of the baby's lungs and help prevent complications after birth.

LABOUR CARE

Since delivery of the baby is necessary before the woman can start to recover from pre-eclampsia, this may take place at any gestation, dependent on the woman's condition. Induction of labour or, more commonly if preterm, a Caesarean section may be carried out. With mild pre-eclampsia at term, labour may start spontaneously, but regardless of the gestation or planned mode of delivery, the woman with pre-eclampsia will need a continuation of the monitoring that she was receiving antenatally. It is salutary to remember that one in five cases of eclampsia occur in labour, so vigilance should not be relaxed.

Syntometrine should not be given for management of the third stage as the ergometrine component is associated with increasing the blood pressure.

POSTNATAL CARE

Following delivery, it is usual to care for women with pre-eclampsia in a high-dependency area, as it is during this time that eclampsia is most common. Carefully monitoring her condition, along with the appropriate medication and support, will reduce her risk of long-term complications.

It must also be remembered that pre-eclampsia can present for the first time in the puerperium (RCOG, 2006).

SUMMARY OF MIDWIFERY CARE IN PRE-ECLAMPSIA
▶ Assessment of risk at booking, with referral as necessary.
▶ Ensuring that all women appreciate the importance of routine antenatal checks and know the symptoms that should lead them to seek help.
▶ Midwives should ensure regular and accurate blood pressure and urine screening takes place, with referral and blood testing when appropriate.
▶ Close observation (by whatever means appropriate to her condition) of any woman hospitalised, to ensure that any deterioration of her condition is immediately noted and acted on.
▶ All medications given as prescribed, and their effects noted.
▶ A midwife is a valuable resource who can offer explanations and information to women and their families, who are probably confused and distressed by this unexpected and potentially serious condition.

ECLAMPSIA

Eclampsia is defined as the convulsions associated with the signs and symptoms of pre-eclampsia. Midwifery treatment is initially concerned with the safety of the woman (for example, protecting her from injury as far as possible during the fit and positioning her in the recovery position, maintaining a clear airway and administering oxygen when the convulsion is over) and calling for urgent help. This is a multidisciplinary emergency and assistance is required from other midwives, obstetricians and anaesthetists. Attention must then be paid to:

‣ obtaining IV access
‣ medication (e.g., magnesium sulphate +/– antihypertensives)
‣ monitoring vital signs and blood tests
‣ monitoring fluid balance
‣ assessing fetal well-being
‣ planning delivery once the maternal condition has been stabilised.

HELLP SYNDROME

HELLP (haemolysis, elevated liver enzymes, low platelets) syndrome is usually considered to be a complication or variant of pre-eclampsia. Signs and symptoms (*see* Box 5.14) vary from those of pre-eclampsia but there is a significant overlap. Potential complications, such as eclampsia, haemorrhage, stroke, renal failure and deterioration of the fetal condition, are also common to pre-eclampsia, although in HELLP syndrome specific liver damage or even rupture is possible. Monitoring of the condition is similar to that of pre-eclampsia, with an added emphasis on assessment of liver enzymes (*see* Appendix). Treatment is also similar to that of pre-eclampsia, and the 'cure' is the same: delivery of the baby. Following birth, as in pre-eclampsia, there is an initial period of continued risk, followed by stabilisation, and there is a possibility of recurrence in the next pregnancy.

BOX 5.14: SIGNS AND SYMPTOMS OF HELLP SYNDROME

- Right upper quadrant pain
- Epigastric pain
- Gastrointestinal bleed
- Nausea and vomiting
- Malaise, fatigue
- Headache
- Hypertension
- Proteinuria
- Oliguria

(McDonald, 2002)

PSYCHOSOCIAL ISSUES AND PRE-ECLAMPSIA

In some cases of pre-eclampsia the outcome is tragic, resulting in a dead or extremely premature baby. The woman may also be very ill and spend time in an ICU. Midwives caring for these families should be highly skilled in meeting their psychosocial needs as well as being competent and knowledgeable concerning the physical side of pre-eclampsia.

The unexpectedness and unpredictability of pre-eclampsia make this condition a very potent risk factor for post-traumatic stress disorder (Creedy, *et al.*, 2000; Lyons, 1998), which is often seen in women who feel an acute lack of control. A supportive, knowledgeable midwife with good communication skills providing continuity of care could go some way in preventing this. It might also be appropriate to offer more long-term support than the midwife is able to provide, and community support groups, 'befrienders' or expert impartial advice sources, in particular those organised by Action on Pre-eclampsia, may be invaluable (PRECOG, 2004).

REFERENCES

Armenti V, Moritz M, Davison J. Pregnancy after transplantation. In: James DK, Steer P, Weiner CP, *et al.*, editors. *High Risk Pregnancy: management options.* 3rd ed. Philadelphia, PA: Elsevier Saunders; 2006. pp. 1174–86.

Baylis C, Davison JM. The urinary system. In: Chamberlain G, Broughton Pipkin F, editors. *Clinical Physiology in Obstetrics.* 3rd ed. Oxford: Blackwell Science; 1998. pp. 263–307.

Blackburn ST. *Maternal, Fetal and Neonatal Physiology.* 3rd ed. St Louis, MO: Saunders; 2007.

Bothamley J, Boyle M. How to measure blood pressure. *Midwives.* Feb/Mar 2008a: 29.

Bothamley J, Boyle M. How to use automated blood pressure monitoring. *Midwives.* Apr/May 2008b: 19.

Boyle M. *Wound Healing in Midwifery.* Oxford: Radcliffe Publishing; 2006.

Challinor P. Renal physiology. In: Challinor P, Sedgewick J, editors. *Principles and Practice of Renal Nursing.* Cheltenham: Stanley Thornes; 1998. pp. 14–35.

Chen H, Lin H, Yehy J, *et al.* Renal biopsy in pregnancies complicated by undetermined renal disease. *Acta Obstet Gynecol Scand.* 2001; **80**(10): 888–93.

Cote A, Brown M, Lam E, *et al.* Diagnostic accuracy of urinary spot protein:creatinine ratio for proteinuria in hypertensive pregnant women: systematic review. *BMJ.* 2008; **335**(7651): 103–6.

Creedy DK, Shochet IM, Horsfall J. Childbirth and the development of acute trauma symptoms: incidence and contributing factors. *Birth.* 2000; **27**(2): 104–11.

Davison J, Baylis C. Renal disease. In: de Swiet M, editor. *Medical Disorders in Obstetric Practice.* 4th ed. Oxford: Blackwell; 2002. pp. 198–266.

Duley L, Hendreson-Smart D, Knight M, *et al.* Antiplatelet drugs for prevention of pre-eclampsia and its consequences: systematic review. *BMJ.* 2001; **332**: 329–3.

Expert Group on Renal Transplantation. European best practice guidelines for renal transplantation. Section IV: Long-term management of the transplant recipient. 10. Pregnancy in renal transplant recipients. *Nephrol Dial Transplant.* 2002; **17**(Suppl. 4): 50–5.

Faúndes A, Br'cola-Filho M, Pinto e Silva JL. Dilatation of the urinary tract during pregnancy: proposal of a curve of maximal caliceal diameter by gestational age. *Am J Obsete Gynecol.* 1998; **178**(5): 1082–6.

Fuchs K, Wu D, Ebcioglu Z. Pregnancy in renal transplant recipients. *Semin Perinatol.* 2007; **31**: 339–47.

Gibson P, Rosene-Montella K. Normal renal and vascular changes in pregnancy. In: Rosene-Montella K, Keely E, Barbour LA, *et al.*, editors. *Medical Care of the Pregnant Patient.* 2nd ed. Philadelphia, PA: ACP Press; 2008. pp. 149–52.

Gilstrap L, Ramin S. Urinary tract infections during pregnancy. *Obstet Gynecol Clin North Am.* 2001; **28**: 581–91.

Hou S. Pregnancy in chronic renal insufficiency and end stage renal disease. *Am J Kidney Dis.* 1999; **20**: 235–52.

Huether SE. Structure and function of the renal and urologic systems. In: McCance KL, Huether SE, editors. *Pathophysiology: the biological basis for diseases in adults and children.* 5th ed. St Louis, MO: Elsevier Mosby; 2006. pp. 1279–300.

Lewis D, Robichaux A, Jaekle R, *et al.* Urolithiasis in pregnancy: diagnosis, management and pregnancy outcome. *J Reprod Med.* 2003; **48**: 28–32.

Lyons S. Post-traumatic stress disorder following childbirth: causes, prevention and treatment. In: Clement S, editor. *Psychological Perspectives on Pregnancy and Childbirth*. Edinburgh: Churchill Livingstone; 1998. pp. 123–43.

McDonald S. Pre-eclampsia and eclampsia. In: Boyle M, editor. *Emergencies Around Childbirth*. Oxford: Radcliffe Publishing; 2002. pp. 83–8.

Macfarlane PS, Reid R, Callander R. *Pathology Illustrated*. 5th ed. Edinburgh: Churchill Livingstone; 2000.

McGhee MA. *Guide to Laboratory Investigations*. Oxford: Radcliffe Medical Press; 2000.

McKay K. Biochemical and blood tests in midwifery practice (1): pre-eclampsia. *Pract Midwife*. 1999; **2**(3): 28–31.

Milne F, Redman C, Walker J, *et al*. The pre-eclampsia community guideline (PRECOG): how to screen for and detect onset of pre-eclampsia in the community. *BMJ*. 2005; **330**(12): 567–80.

Morley A. Pre-eclampsia: pathophysiology and its management. *Br J Midwifery*. 2004; **12**(1): 30–7.

Perez-Cuevas R, Fraser W, Reyes H, *et al*. Critical pathways for the management of preeclampsia and severe preeclampsia in institutionalised health care settings. *BMC Pregnancy and Childbirth*. 2003; **3**(6). Available at: www.biomedcentral.com/1471–2393/3/6 (accessed 8 December 2008).

Poston L, Briley AL, Seed PT, *et al*. Vitamin C and vitamin E in pregnant women at risk for pre-eclampsia (VIP Trial): randomized placebo-controlled trial. *Obstet Gynecol Surv*. 2006. **61**: 560–6.

Powrie RO, Miller M. Hypertension. In: Rosene-Montella K, Keely E, Barbour LA, *et al*., editors. *Medical Care of the Pregnant Patient*. 2nd ed. Philadelphia, PA: ACP Press; 2008. pp. 153–62.

Powrie R, Rosene-Montella K. Pre-eclampsia. In: Rosene-Montella K, Keely E, Barbour LA, *et al*., editors. *Medical Care of the Pregnant Patient*. 2nd ed. Philadelphia, PA: ACP Press; 2008. pp. 163–81.

Pre-eclampsia Community Guideline Development Group (PRECOG). Pre-eclampsia community guideline. 2004. Available at: www.apec.org.uk/pdf/guidelinepublishedvers04.pdf (accessed 8 December 2008).

Roberts JM, Cooper DW. Pathogenesis and genetics of pre-eclampsia. *Lancet*. 2001; **357**: 53–6.

Royal College of Obstetricians and Gynaecologists (RCOG*). The Management of Severe Pre-eclampsia/Eclampsia. Guideline 10 (A) March*. London: RCOG; 2006.

Royal College of Obstetricians and Gynaecologists (RCOG). *Renal Disease in Pregnancy: consensus views arising from the 54th study group*. London: RCOG; 2007.

Sherwood L. *Fundamentals of Physiology*. 2nd ed. Minneapolis, MI: West; 1994.

Sibai B, Dekker G, Kupferminc M. Pre-eclampsia. *Lancet*. 2005; **364**(9461): 785–99.

Thorp JM Jr, Norton PA, Wall LL, *et al*. Urinary incontinence in pregnancy and the puerperium: a prospective study. *Am J Obstet Gynecol*. 1999; **181**(2): 266–73.

Thorsen MS, Poole JH. Renal disease in pregnancy. *J Perinat Neonatal Nurs*. 2002; **15**(4): 13–26.

UK Obstetric Surveillance System (UKOSS). *Pregnancy in Renal Transplant Recipients*. 2008. Available at: www.npeu.ox.ac.uk/ukoss/current-surveillance (accessed 8 December 2008).

Vander A, Sherman J, Luciano D. *Human Physiology: the mechanisms of body function*. 8th ed. Boston, MA: McGraw Hill; 2001.

Vazquez J, Villar J. Treatments for symptomatic urinary tract infections during pregnancy. *Cochrane Database Syst Rev*. 2003: CD002256.

Walfisch A, Hallak M. Hypertension. In: James DK, Weiner CP, Steer PJ, *et al.*, editors. *High Risk Pregnancy: management options.* 3rd ed. Philadelphia, PA: Elsevier Saunders; 2006. pp. 772–89.

Waugh JJ, Clark TJ, Divakaran TG, *et al.* Accuracy of urinalysis dipstick techniques in predicting significant proteinuria in pregnancy. *Obstet Gynaecol.* 2004; **103**(4): 769–7.

Waugh A, Grant A. *Ross and Wilson Anatomy and Physiology in Health and Illness.* 10th ed. Edinburgh: Elsevier Churchill Livingstone; 2006.

Williams D. Renal disorders. In: James DK, Steer P, Weiner CP, *et al.*, editors. *High Risk Pregnancy: management options.* 3rd ed. Philadelphia, PA: Elsevier Saunders; 2006. pp. 1098–124.

Williams D. Renal disease in pregnancy. *Obstet Gynaecol Reprod Med.* 2007; **17**(5): 147–53.

Williams D. Acute and chronic renal disease. In: Rosene-Montella K, Keely E, Barbour LA, *et al.*, editors. *Medical Care of the Pregnant Patient.* 2nd ed. Philadelphia, PA: ACP Press; 2008. pp. 182–99.

Williams D, de Swiet M. Pathophysiology of pre-eclampsia. *Intensive Care Med.* 1997; **23**: 620–9.

Willis F, Findlay C, Gorrie M, *et al.* Children of renal transplant recipient mothers. *J Paediatr Child Health.* 2000; **36**(3): 230–5.

APPENDIX
LABORATORY TESTS

Although the following values are generally accepted as normal for pregnant women, individual reference ranges may vary depending on the laboratory and analytical methods used. When interpreting findings it is also important to remember that serial tests are usually most valuable, as they will indicate a trend, which will give a much more accurate assessment of a woman's condition.

RENAL FUNCTION TESTS AND NORMAL RESULTS

▶ Urea
  — 2.8–4.2 mmol/L (first trimester)
  — 2.5–4.1 mmol/L (second trimester)
  — 2.5–3.8 mmol/L (third trimester)
▶ Electrolytes
  — Sodium: 133–144 mmol/L
  — Potassium: 3.3–4.1 mmol/L
▶ Serum creatinine
  — 52–68 µmol/L (first trimester)
  — 44–68 µmol/L (second trimester)
  — 55–73 µmol/L (third trimester)
▶ Serum uric acid (urates)
  — 0.14–0.23 µmol/L (first trimester)
  — 0.14–0.29 µmol/L (second trimester)
  — 0.21–0.38 µmol/L (third trimester)
▶ Serum GFR > 70 mL/min (should not be < 50 mL/min. Severe disease < 25 mL/min)
▶ Plasma proteins: total proteins 48–64 gL
▶ Urine proteinuria: < 0.33 g per 24 hours
▶ Urinary creatinine clearance

- — 140–162 mL/min (first trimester)
- — 139–169 mL/min (second trimester)
- — 119–139 mL/min (third trimester)

LIVER FUNCTION TESTS AND NORMAL RESULTS

- ◗ AST (aspartate transaminase)
  - — 10–28 IU/L (first trimester)
  - — 11–29 IU/L (second trimester)
  - — 11–30 IU/L (third trimester)
- ◗ ALT (alanine transaminase)
  - — 6–32 IU/L
- ◗ ALP (alkaline phosphate)
  - — 32–100 IU/L (first trimester)
  - — 43–135 IU/L (second trimester)
  - — 133–140 IU/L (third trimester)
- ◗ Total albumin: 28–37 gL
- ◗ Total bilirubin
  - — 4–16 μmol/L (first trimester)
  - — 3–13 μmol/L (second trimester)
  - — 3–14 μmol/L (third trimester)

BLOOD TESTS IN PRE-ECLAMPSIA ('PET PROFILE')

- ◗ Full blood count:
  - — haemoglobin: 10.5–13 g/dL
  - — platelets: 150–400 10^9/L
- ◗ Renal function tests: plasma creatinine, serum uric acid, urea, creatinine clearance, total urinary protein (*see* results above)
- ◗ Liver function tests: AST, ALT, alkaline phosphatase, total albumin, total bilirubin (*see* results above).
- ◗ Clotting studies may also be carried out

CHAPTER 6
Disorders of the respiratory system

CONTENTS
→ The respiratory system and changes in pregnancy
→ Routine assessment of respiratory function
→ Asthma
→ Cystic fibrosis

THE RESPIRATORY SYSTEM AND CHANGES IN PREGNANCY

Enhanced respiratory efficiency is required in pregnancy to meet the increased metabolic demands of the woman, fetus and placenta and yet by comparison to exercise pregnancy makes little demand on respiratory reserve function. Anatomical and functional changes occur to lung volume and ventilation. Figure 6.1 illustrates the anatomical features of the respiratory system and Box 6.1 presents a summary of the changes to the respiratory system in pregnancy.

BOX 6.1: SUMMARY OF CHANGES TO THE RESPIRATORY SYSTEM IN PREGNANCY

- 20% ↑ in oxygen consumption
- ↑ metabolic demand for oxygen by maternal body and fetoplacental unit
- Position of diaphragm rises
- ↑ transverse diameter of chest
- Capillary engorgement of respiratory tract with increased friability of mucous membranes
- 40–50% ↑ in resting minute ventilation mainly from a rise in tidal volume
- Mild respiratory alkalosis
- Respiratory rate remains unchanged at 12–15 breaths per minute at rest
- Subjective feelings of breathlessness are common

(Blackburn, 2007; de Swiet, 2002; Nelson-Piercy, 2001; Rankin, 2005)

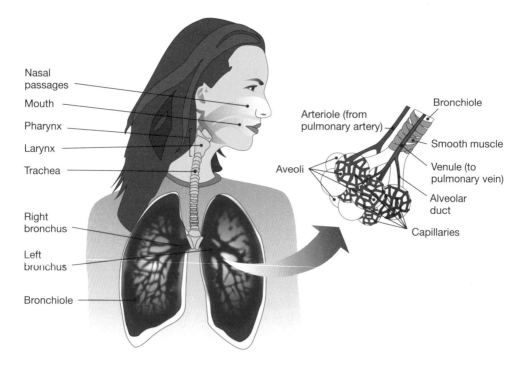

FIGURE 6.1: The respiratory system

Hormonal changes during pregnancy alter the vessels of the mucosal lining of the respiratory tract, leading to capillary engorgement and swelling of the lining in the nose, pharynx, larynx and trachea. Women may experience nasal congestion and notice a change to the tone of their voice. These symptoms can be exacerbated by oedema and fluid overload associated with pre-eclampsia, making endotracheal intubation more difficult (Ezri, *et al.*, 2001).

The inner lining of the *trachea* is a ciliated-lined mucus membrane which wafts mucus and particles upwards. Nerve endings in the larynx, trachea and bronchi are sensitive to irritation. A cough reflex is generated via the vagus nerve to expel mucus and/or foreign material. *Bronchioles* are made up of smooth muscle. This makes them responsive to autonomic nerve stimulation. The diameter of the air passages is therefore altered by the contraction or relaxation of these involuntary muscles.

LUNG VOLUMES AND CAPACITIES
The lungs during normal quiet breathing contain about 2.5 litres of air but their capacity is much greater, with the ability to expand to 4–5 litres. Air can be forced out, leaving a residual volume of around one litre. Lung volumes will be affected by the elasticity and compliance of the lungs and by the resistance created by narrowing or distension of the airways. There are a number of changes to lung volumes in pregnancy in response to an increased demand for oxygen and driven mainly by increased levels

of progesterone (*see* Table 6.1 for an explanation of lung volumes and changes in pregnancy).

TABLE 6.1: Lung volumes and changes in pregnancy

Name	Definition	Changes in pregnancy
Tidal volume	The amount of air passing in and out of the lungs during a single breath	Increases by 40% from 500 to 700 mL
Inspiratory capacity	The total amount of air that can be inspired with maximal effort	Increased by about 200–300 mL by late pregnancy
Residual volume	The minimum volume of air remaining in the lungs after maximal expiration. It cannot be directly measured	
Functional residual capacity	The volume of air in the lungs at the end of normal passive expiration	Decreases by about 500 mL
Vital capacity	The maximum volume of air that can be moved out of the lungs during a single breath following maximal inspiration	Studies are conflicting. Overall there is probably an increase in the order of 100–200 mL, although body size may impact vital capacity in pregnancy, with obese woman showing a reduction in vital capacity
Respiratory rate	12–15 breaths per minute at rest	No change in pregnancy
Minute ventilation	Tidal volume X respiratory rate	Increases in parallel with increases in tidal volume
Alveolar ventilation	Tidal volume less anatomical dead space	Increased by as much as 50%

Source: de Swiet (1998, 2002)

These alterations in lung volumes are due largely to anatomical changes which allow greater lung expansion. The lower ribs flare, increasing the transverse diameter of the chest by 2 cm and the subcostal angle increases. These changes begin before the enlarging uterus applies mechanical pressure (de Swiet, 1998). Relaxation of the soft tissues of the rib cage is caused by increasing levels of the hormones progesterone and relaxin, which contribute to increased rib cage elasticity (Blackburn, 2007). The enlarging uterus shifts the resting position of the diaphragm up by about 4 cm (Blackburn, 2007).

The pregnant woman at rest increases her ventilation by breathing more deeply rather than more frequently (de Swiet, 1998). This will help maintain normal oxygenation but can contribute to a sense of breathlessness, which is experienced by up to 75% of women during pregnancy. A reduced amount of CO_2 in arterial blood (owing to enhanced ventilation), with a consequent reduction in serum bicarbonate, results in a mild respiratory alkalosis, which is normal in pregnancy. This balance favours an optimal oxygen/carbon dioxide exchange.

During labour the strong contractions of the uterus increase metabolism and increase the demand for oxygen. Women tend to breathe more often and increase their depth of breathing. Pain and anxiety may further increase the hyperventilatory response. Contractions decrease blood flow in the intervillous space. Changes in acid–base status due to this hyperventilation and increased oxygen consumption are potentially hazardous to both mother and fetus. Sometimes mothers experience tingling and dizziness as a result of hyperventilation. The woman should be encouraged to slow down her rate of breathing, relax and breath more deeply between contractions in order to promote oxygenation (Blackburn, 2007).

Following delivery there is a rapid reversal of changes, with a reduction in progesterone and a decrease in intra-abdominal pressure. With delivery of the baby, blood gases return to pre-pregnant levels within 24 hours of delivery, with anatomical and ventilatory changes taking 1–3 weeks (Rankin, 2005).

ROUTINE ASSESSMENT OF RESPIRATORY FUNCTION

Assessment will include observing *respiratory rate*, depth and pattern and noting the presence of cough, wheeze or production of sputum. The respiratory rate at rest is 12–15 breaths per minute and breathing should seem relaxed. When breathing becomes difficult, such as during an asthmatic event, inspiratory accessory muscles in the neck and abdomen may be used, raising the sternum and ribs.

Peak expiratory flow rate (PEFR) is the maximum ability of exhalation during forced expiration, and it is measured by a peak flow meter. In normal pregnancy the peak flow is unaffected. This is probably because there is a balance between bronchodilating forces (PGE2 and progesterone) and bronchoconstricting (PGF2a) (Blackburn, 2007; de Swiet, 1998). However, if the airways are narrowed, such as occurs in asthma, air cannot be blown out from the lungs with as much force and velocity.

It is common for women with potentially compromised respiratory function to do home PEFR monitoring, and these findings can help them manage their condition, and records can guide medication prescription.

Forced expiratory volume in one second (FEV1) is the amount of air that can be forcibly expired after maximal inspiration in one second. It is measured by a spirometer and its normal values are also unaffected by pregnancy (Nelson-Piercy, 2006).

A *pulse oximeter* is an electronic machine used to measure pulse rate along with the level of oxygen saturation in the peripheral blood (SAO_2). It is non-invasive and usually positioned on the finger (*see* Chapter 3).

A *chest X-ray* will show the lungs, heart and major blood vessels and reveal any abnormalities of the chest. It is one of the single most helpful investigations in medicine. When having a chest X-ray the woman is asked to breathe in deeply and hold her breath while the X-ray is taken. This allows a picture of the lungs at full expansion. The exposure received is equivalent to 1–2 years' background radiation. When she is pregnant her uterus can be shielded.

ASTHMA

Asthma is a chronic inflammatory disorder of the airways. The inflammation causes recurrent episodes of wheezing, breathlessness, chest tightness and cough, and symptoms are more common at night or in the early morning (*see* Box 6.2). The cause is not completely understood but includes an allergic response to inhaled antigens such as house dust mites and pollen, with a role for environmental pollution and a genetic disposition. Inflammation makes the airways sensitive to stimuli such as chemical irritants, smoking, cold air or exercise. Stimuli that exacerbate the symptoms vary between women. When exposed to these stimuli the airways become swollen, constricted and filled with mucus. This narrowing of the airway is usually reversible either spontaneously or with treatment (British Thoracic Society, 2008; Global Initiative for Asthma, 2006).

The prevalence of asthma has increased substantially over the last 20 years, so that up to 12% of pregnant women now have asthma, making it the most common preexisting condition encountered in pregnancy (Rey and Boulet, 2007).

BOX 6.2: SIGNS AND SYMPTOMS IN ASTHMA

- Cough
- Increased respiration
- Breathlessness
- Tachycardia
- Wheezy breathing
- Use of accessory muscles
- Chest tightness
- Inability to complete sentence
- Worse at night and early morning

There are two mechanisms of airway obstruction: bronchial hyper-responsiveness and airway inflammation. Asthma involves an abnormal response of the airways, making them constrict easily in response to a wide range of possible stimuli (*see* Box 6.3 for a list of triggers to asthma). In addition, the bronchial mucosa of the airways is chronically thickened with inflammatory cells.

DRUGS

There are two main types of drugs used for the treatment of asthma. Corticosteroids aim to reduce the chronic inflammatory processes in the airways and bronchodilator drugs are used intermittently to relieve breakthrough symptoms of wheeze and shortness of breath. Anti-inflammatory drugs have been described as 'preventors' and bronchodilator drugs as 'reliever' drugs (Chung, 2002, p. 61).

Many women with asthma may have an intolerance or allergy to aspirin or NSAIDs, and if not already identified, this should be established, as these drugs are commonly used during the antenatal and postnatal periods.

BOX 6.3: TRIGGERS OF ASTHMA

- Upper respiratory tract viral infections
- House dust mites, pollens, animal dander
- Exercise
- Reduction or omission of regular medication
- Cold air
- Hyperventilation
- Drugs such as aspirin and non-steroidal anti-inflammatory drugs (NSAIDs)
- Food and drinks such as nuts, milk and egg allergies, preservatives or colouring agents
- Gastro-oesophageal reflux
- Environmental pollutants such as cigarette smoke and traffic fumes
- Stress and psychological factors (these may relate to hyperventilation)

(Chung, 2002)

IMPACT OF PREGNANCY ON ASTHMA

For about 20% of women with asthma their symptoms will deteriorate when pregnant, nearly 50% will stay the same and the remaining 30% will improve (Williamson and Nelson-Piercy, 2000). Improvement is attributed to progesterone-mediated broncho-dilators, which open up airways and an increase in free-cortisol levels, which minimise the inflammatory response. How an individual woman will be affected is unpredictable. However, those with mild asthma are more likely to have no problems and those with severe disease are at greatest risk of deterioration, particularly in late pregnancy (Murphy, *et al.*, 2005; Nelson-Piercy, 2001).

Murphy *et al.* (2005) found that winter, respiratory viral infections and non-adherence to medication were the most common causes of exacerbation of asthma during pregnancy. Obese women are also at higher risk of exacerbation of their asthma in pregnancy (Hendler, *et al.*, 2006). Urinary tract infections were implicated in another, smaller study (Minerbi-Codish, *et al.*, 1998).

PRECONCEPTION CARE

As with all medical conditions, preconception counselling is valuable for a woman with asthma. In particular, it is beneficial to ensure her medications are maintaining optimum health. Those who have been experiencing symptoms at least once a day may require more regular inhaled anti-inflammatory medication. If the condition is more severe, inhaled steroids combined with long-acting inhaled beta-agonists may be helpful.

Most importantly, women may also need education concerning the effects of drugs on pregnancy and the fetus. There are no known disadvantages to common medications taken for asthma (Nelson-Piercy, 2006), but women are often understandably anxious about taking drugs when trying to become pregnant or in pregnancy. However, reducing or omitting regularly prescribed drugs can put the woman at risk of an acute severe asthma attack.

Teaching and commencing home PEFR monitoring, if not already used, is important for pregnancy. It is worth noting that those with marked 'morning dips' are at increased risk of sudden severe attacks.

Identification and strategies to avoid triggers (*see* Box 6.3) can be valuable. Other subjects for preconception counselling include general health advice, especially concerning smoking cessation if appropriate.

PREGNANCY CARE
Impact of asthma on pregnancy

Mild and moderate asthma should pose no problems in pregnancy and outcomes should be good. However, poorly controlled severe asthma may compromise fetal outcome and contribute to maternal morbidity as a result of chronic or intermittent maternal hypoxaemia. Murphy *et al.* (2005) studied the rate of severe asthma attacks and their associated perinatal outcome in a prospective study of 146 women. They found an association between severe attacks, stillbirth, low birth weight and poor maternal weight gain. Despite a long list of potential complications of pregnancy and asthma (*see* Box 6.4), adverse perinatal outcomes are not common and are related to the degree of control of asthma. Midwives should reassure women appropriately about risks of asthma in pregnancy related to individual signs and symptoms and promote preventative care and prompt referral.

BOX 6.4: POSSIBLE COMPLICATIONS OF PREGNANCY ASSOCIATED WITH ASTHMA*

- Premature labour
- Low birth weight
- Stillbirth
- Low maternal weight gain
- Pregnancy-induced hypertension or pre-eclampsia
- Caesarean section
- Transient tachypnoea of the newborn
- Neonatal hypoglycaemia
- Neonatal seizure
- Admission to neonatal intensive care unit

* Note: studies have generally been inconclusive or conflicting in relation to risks of asthma in pregnancy and this list should therefore be viewed cautiously, noting that the complications listed are possible, not confirmed.

(Dombrowski, 2006; Nelson-Piercy, 2001; Powrie, 2006; Rey and Boulet, 2007; Rudra, *et al.*, 2006)

Most severe symptoms occur around 24–36 weeks' gestation, therefore, in moderate and severe asthma, an accurate dating scan, regular growth scans and regular assessment of fetal well-being may be appropriate (Dombrowski, 2006).

Respiratory function testing

Home testing of peak flow is encouraged and if a record is kept women can discuss these findings, perhaps identifying triggers to symptoms, at antenatal visits. However, findings may be influenced by the stage of pregnancy. According to a small recent study (Beckmann, 2006), peak flows differ according to trimester; the highest is in the second trimester, then it is lower in the third trimester. Women need this information to evaluate their readings.

Drug treatment

The aim of treatment is to prevent the exacerbation of asthma, thereby preventing maternal hypoxic episodes which could impact on the oxygenation of the fetus (Dombrowski, 2006). A US study showed that women decreased their use of asthma medication in early pregnancy (Enriquez, *et al.*, 2006). This has also been observed in the UK (Nelson-Piercy, 2006) and, as mentioned earlier in this chapter, women need to know that most asthma medication has no demonstrated adverse effects on the fetus, and there is far more danger from asthma exacerbations.

A check of inhaler techniques by a practitioner skilled in this should be offered to all women.

Regular oral steroids (which very few women find necessary as most can be maintained with inhaled medication) may cause an increased rate of gestational diabetes. Infrequently those taking high doses of steroids may feel agitated and find it difficult to sleep (Williamson and Nelson-Piercy, 2000). Oral prednisolone is often prescribed for emergency or rescue medication, and it is important for women to know that this subsequently needs to be tapered off with a gradual reduction of the dose.

SUMMARY OF SPECIFIC CARE IN PREGNANCY

▶ Ongoing monitoring of respiratory function, including home monitoring and clinical assessments.
▶ Identifying and developing avoidance strategies for triggers.
▶ Maintaining medication and adapting it only if it is necessary to treat or prevent exacerbations.
▶ Educating the woman to promote self-care, the correct use of inhalers and general health.
▶ Smoking cessation support if appropriate.

ACUTE SEVERE ASTHMA

An exacerbation (or acute severe asthma) is defined as symptoms severe enough to result in an admission to hospital (or attendance at A&E), or unscheduled attendance by a doctor, or additional oral corticosteroids to normal medication (Murphy, *et al.*, 2005). Acute severe asthma is considered to be the triad of usual signs and symptoms of asthma but to a more serious degree: wheezing, breathlessness and a cough. Acute severe asthma may occur rapidly or gradually build up over days. These attacks can rapidly become life-threatening, so the prompt attention of the multidisciplinary team and medication are necessary.

In life-threatening asthma, oxygen saturation will be < 92%, the woman may be cyanosed, hypotensive and making only a weak respiratory effort and heart monitoring may show arrhythmias and/or bradycardia. She may also appear confused and finally become comatose (Nelson-Piercy, 2006).

Initial treatment involves high-flow oxygen therapy, then nebulised bronchodilators (via an appliance which administers medication in the form of a mist) and intravenous or oral steroids, depending on her condition. In a particularly severe episode, or one that does not quickly respond to these treatments, intravenous aminophylline or intravenous beta-2 agonists may be necessary. Intravenous magnesium sulphate may also be used.

Obviously, depending on the woman's condition, one or two cannulas need to be sited and attention needs to be paid to rehydration if this is appropriate.

It is important to monitor potassium levels and replace if necessary. Continuous oxygen saturation monitoring is usual and frequent arterial blood gases assessment may be necessary.

A chest X-ray may be necessary, especially if there is chest pain. There may be signs of infection or a pneumothorax. The abdomen can be shielded during the X-ray.

As the severity of the signs and symptoms abate, the drug treatment with IV hydrocortisone can be changed to oral prednisolone and, as previously mentioned, it needs to be tapered off gradually.

LABOUR CARE

Acute attacks may be very rare in labour because of increased endogenous steroids that cause bronchodilatation that are present at this time (Williamson and Nelson-Piercy, 2000; de Swiet, 2002). However, others have suggested exacerbations of asthma symptoms occur in up to 20% (Rey and Boulet, 2007; Stenius-Aarniala, *et al.*, 1996).

Regular inhalers should be continued during labour – there is no evidence that inhaled asthma medication interferes with contractions (Nelson-Piercy, 2006). If oral steroids (> 7.5 mg daily prednisolone) have been taken for more than two weeks prior to labour, IV hydrocortisone should be given during labour until the oral medication can be restarted (Nelson-Piercy, 2006).

PEFR may be monitored during labour and frequent oxygen saturation monitoring is often a convenient way of assessing the woman's condition. It is important to maintain hydration throughout labour.

All analgesics offered during labour are safe, but in the unlikely event of acute severe asthma, opiates should be avoided (Nelson-Piercy, 2006). In the case of a post-partum haemorrhage, if Hemabate (carboprost/PGF2a) is used, it may cause bronchospasm (Williamson and Nelson-Piercy, 2000).

POSTNATAL CARE

There is a chance that a woman's condition may worsen in the postnatal period (Nelson-Piercy, 2006); therefore frequent PEFR monitoring should probably be continued for at least 12 hours postnatal and then progression made to her pre-pregnancy regime.

Most inhalants and oral medication used by women to treat asthma are safe in breastfeeding. Breastfeeding is particularly important as there is some evidence that prolonged breastfeeding may reduce the incidence of atopic disease in the infant (Williamson and Nelson-Piercy, 2000).

While most babies of asthmatic mothers have no problems, some rare conditions have been reported: transient tachypnoea of the newborn, hypoglycaemia, seizures and admission to the neonatal unit (Nelson-Piercy, 2006), but these are not common and are restricted in the main to those whose mother has had severe or uncontrolled asthma. There is some suggestion that baby boys are more at risk (Murphy, *et al.*, 2005).

CYSTIC FIBROSIS

Cystic fibrosis is the most common autosomal recessive condition in the Caucasian population, with an approximate incidence of 1:2000. About one in 20 people are thought to be carriers (Powrie, 2007). Although in the past most of those with cystic fibrosis died in childhood, with recent medical advances life expectancy has improved and the average age of survival is now 31 years (Cystic Fibrosis Trust, 2007). Transplant, either heart and lungs or including pancreas, is already taking place and may improve the outcome of those with cystic fibrosis in the future. A woman with cystic fibrosis may also have liver disease and/or diabetes.

Although most women with cystic fibrosis will have been diagnosed in childhood, the general incidence of late diagnosis is considered to be about 7.8% (Widerman, *et al.*, 2000). These are normally women with a milder form of the disease, although most will have a history of many respiratory infections. Diagnosis will be by sweat testing for raised chloride levels and/or DNA testing.

Cystic fibrosis is caused by a faulty gene on chromosome 7 called the cystic fibrosis transmembrane conductance regulator (CFTR) gene. This gene contains the information cells needed to make an important protein that regulates the transfer of sodium (salt) across cell membranes in certain glandular cells in the body. Those with cystic fibrosis have faulty copies of both the CFTR genes inherited from their parents and therefore cannot produce this vital protein. As a result, transport across the cell membrane is altered and secretions such as sweat and pancreatic juice are very salty and abnormally thick. Thickened mucus in the lungs causes respiratory difficulties and there is incomplete digestion of food and increased salt loss from sweat glands (Thibodeau and Patton, 2007). Table 6.2 summarises the impact of cystic fibrosis on body systems and the concerns these may cause in pregnancy. It is important to note that women will experience differing degrees of symptoms of cystic fibrosis due to variation in mutation and therapeutic interventions (Turner, *et al.*, 2005).

GENETICS OF CYSTIC FIBROSIS

Those who are carriers of cystic fibrosis have one faulty gene and one functioning gene and therefore they can produce the vital salt-transporting gene and do not suffer the symptoms of cystic fibrosis. Most people will be unaware that they carry the faulty gene, although they may seek genetic testing if they have a family history of cystic fibrosis. However, finding the faulty mutation is not entirely straightforward. The most common mutation (found in 75% of people) that affects the CFTR gene is called the delta F508 mutation. However, there are over 1200 places along the CFTR gene that have been identified as areas of change that can impact upon the function of the gene, making it difficult to test for all these changes. Testing is carried out on the 30 most common points, including delta F508 and yields approximately 90% of mutations.

TABLE 6.2: Features of cystic fibrosis and concerns for pregnancy

Body system	Impact of cystic fibrosis	Concerns for pregnancy
Fertility	• About 98% males infertile with obstructive azoospermia • Menstrual irregularities as women are underweight • Thick cervical mucus impedes the passage of sperm	• Pregnancy following assisted reproduction
Respiratory system	• Thick secretions clog air passages • Increased bacterial growth and respiratory infection • Lung disease, hypoxaemia • High-dose, long-term antibiotics • Nebulised drugs to improve respiratory function • Chest physiotherapy • Lung transplant	• Increased demands for pulmonary function in pregnancy can affect already compromised lungs • Increased risk of death from pulmonary hypertension • Increased risk of prematurity • Oxygen saturation and peak flow must be monitored • Postural drainage becomes more difficult in late pregnancy
Cardiac	• Women with pulmonary hypertension and right ventricular hypertrophy (cor pulmonale) are at increased risk during pregnancy • Digital clubbing	• Increased cardiac demands of pregnancy • Risk of cardiovascular collapse • Compromise of oxygen to fetus
Gastrointestinal tract	• Pancreatic insufficiency with malabsorption of fat and protein • Oral supplementation of pancreatic enzyme extracts • Nutrient and calorie depletion • Weight loss and difficulty in achieving weight gain. Extra calories consumed • Poor absorption of fat-soluble vitamins • Vitamin K deficiency affects blood clotting	• Pregnancy-related gastrointestinal tract symptoms pose additional challenge • Difficult to maintain a healthy weight gain in pregnancy • Anaemia and disordered clotting • Malnutrition may lead to IUGR
Hormonal	• Insulin production impaired with increasing pancreatic disease	• Diabetes-related problems of pregnancy • Pregnancy may unmask impaired glucose tolerance • Tight control of blood sugars required • Risk of gestational diabetes

(continued)

Body system	Impact of cystic fibrosis	Concerns for pregnancy
Fetus		• Teratogenicity of medical treatments must be balanced against the need to optimise maternal health • Fetal IUGR • Prematurity • Impact of malnutrition
Liver	• Impact on nutrition and clotting	
Bone	• Osteoporosis and joint disease due to nutritional deficits, inactivity and steroid use	• May affect mobility
Psychosocial	• Strive to maintain normal life with demands of daily treatment to control symptoms • Impact on life expectancy • Carry genetic fault	• Concerns over long-term parenting – health, life expectancy • Genetic counselling and decisions

Sources: Dack, *et al.* (2007); Connors and Ulles (2005); Powrie (2007)

Testing can be more accurate when the mutation has been identified in an index case (a relative of the person being tested with cystic fibrosis) (Turner, *et al.*, 2005).

Figure 6.2 shows how cystic fibrosis may be inherited from carrier parents. Where both parents carry the faulty gene, each child has a one in four chance of having cystic fibrosis, a two in four chance of being a carrier (like their parents) and a one in four chance of not inheriting any faulty cystic fibrosis genes. Figure 6.3 shows the impact for a woman with cystic fibrosis who is having a baby. She has two faulty recessive genes. If her partner is not a carrier, it is unlikely any of their offspring will be affected with cystic fibrosis, although they will be carriers. Figure 6.4 shows the possible outcome for an affected mother whose partner is a carrier. Antenatal screening for cystic fibrosis should be offered, but it will be an emotive issue that requires sensitive handling (Powrie, 2007). Options for couples affected by this genetic fault include carrier screening (preferably preconception, to inform the couple's reproductive choice), pre-implantation diagnosis (the chance of a live birth is currently low due to technical difficulties), antenatal testing and newborn screening. The development of a national newborn screening programme for cystic fibrosis began in 2004. Early diagnosis allows early access to specialist care with improved outcomes (Turner, *et al.*, 2005).

PRECONCEPTION CARE

As in most medical conditions, the outcome for both mother and baby following pregnancy largely depends on the severity of the disease. Preconception care should be targeted at assessment and maximising health, as well as optimising drug treatment.

Pulmonary function is considered to be the most important feature when planning pregnancy, and a full cardiac pulmonary assessment should be made. Women with

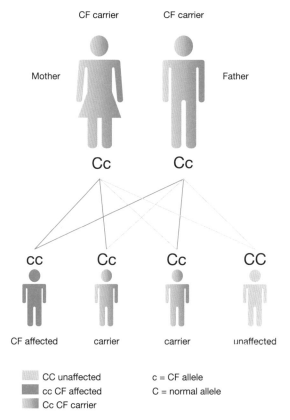

FIGURE 6.2 Genetic inheritance: both parents carriers of faulty gene for cystic fibrosis

pulmonary hypertension and cor pulmonale are counselled against pregnancy (Bourjeily, *et al.*, 2008).

Pancreatic insufficiency can be present in varying degrees, and assessment of a woman's nutritional status is a vital part of preconception care. Achieving a normal weight prior to pregnancy will help the woman keep up with the nutritional demands of pregnancy (Powrie, 2007). If the woman is also diabetic (*see* Chapter 1), careful blood sugar monitoring and attention to diet is necessary to enable conception and for the early embryonic stages to take place in the circumstances that are ideal for the health of the fetus.

As discussed in the previous section, genetic counselling and partner testing should be undertaken, and if the partner is a carrier, explanation of antenatal fetal testing and options if an affected fetus is diagnosed should be sensitively explored.

Burkholderia cepacia is an infection common to those with cystic fibrosis and its presence is a predictor of poor outcome of a pregnancy (Powrie, 2007).

PREGNANCY CARE

The pregnant woman with cystic fibrosis has a great need of a multidisciplinary approach to her care. Professionals involved along with the midwife and obstetrician will

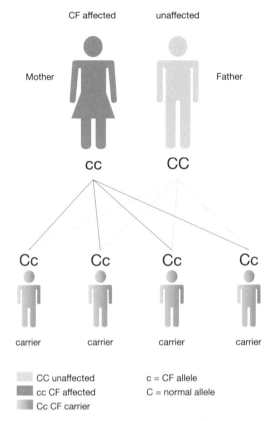

FIGURE 6.3 Genetic inheritance: mother with cystic fibrosis, partner not a carrier

include physicians, physiotherapists and dieticians with an expertise in cystic fibrosis management.

Women with cystic fibrosis usually give themselves chest physiotherapy at least daily. Physiotherapy, respiratory assessment and treatment may be increasingly necessary throughout the pregnancy (King, *et al.*, 2007). They also usually take bronchodilating medication, which may need to be modified during pregnancy. As pulmonary infections are common, it is likely that antibiotic therapy will be necessary. Stress incontinence is common in women with cystic fibrosis (Dodd and Langman, 2005), and physiotherapists also have a role in treatment of this condition.

Even when they are not pregnant, women with cystic fibrosis often need to eat 120–150% of normal requirements daily, and this can prove to be a challenge in pregnancy. They also often suffer from nutrient deficiencies from malabsorption, especially malabsorption of fat-soluble vitamins (Canny, 1993). This difficulty in managing her diet may be compounded if the woman is also diabetic, and help from a dietician may be particularly valuable in these circumstances. Osteoporosis can result from malabsorption, so women with cystic fibrosis are vulnerable to fractures.

Even if they are not diabetic before pregnancy, many women with cystic fibrosis have impaired glucose tolerance (Mackie, *et al.*, 2003), so early screening for gestational

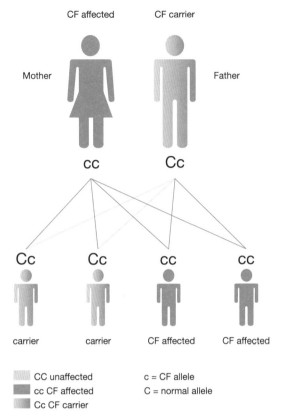

CF affected   CF carrier

Mother   Father

cc   Cc

Cc   Cc   cc   cc

carrier   carrier   CF affected   CF affected

CC unaffected   c = CF allele
cc CF affected   C = normal allele
Cc CF carrier

FIGURE 6.4 Genetic inheritance: mother with cystic fibrosis, partner is a carrier

diabetes should be done. It is common for these women to need insulin during pregnancy (Powrie, 2007).

Ideally the woman and her partner will already have a knowledge of the options available concerning antenatal fetal testing. The woman with cystic fibrosis and a partner who is a carrier (or parents who are both carriers) may choose to undertake antenatal testing for a fetal diagnosis. New maternal serum tests are being developed (Saker, *et al.*, 2006), and if these prove reliable and become widely available, they will avoid putting the pregnancy at risk. Regular fetal assessment is usually offered, as IUGR is common (Bourjeily, *et al.*, 2008). There appears to be an increased perinatal mortality rate (Hilman, *et al.*, 1996) and the risk is directly related to the severity of the cystic fibrosis.

LABOUR CARE

Oxygen saturation monitoring should be carried out frequently, if not continuously, and oxygen administration may be necessary. If the woman's lung function gives cause for concern, she may have central haemodynamic monitoring, and this should take place in a high-dependency environment.

An epidural is often recommended, as this may decrease the woman's oxygen requirements. Elective instrumental delivery may be carried out for the same reason. It is beneficial to avoid a general anaesthetic if a Caesarean section is needed.

POSTNATAL CARE

Breastfeeding is recommended, as always, but a check of any maternal drugs is necessary to ensure they are suitable. The nutritional demands of breastfeeding need to be considered in relation to the mother's health. There has been a suggestion that a woman with cystic fibrosis may not have normal breast milk, but although the composition may differ, it is considered adequate (Powrie, 2007).

REFERENCES

Beckmann C. The impact of pregnancy on peak flow values in women with asthma. *Br J Midwifery.* 2006; **14**(2): 62–4.

Blackburn ST. *Maternal, Fetal and Neonatal Physiology.* 3rd ed. St Louis, MO: Saunders; 2007.

Bourjeily S, Larson L, Pickard J. Asthma and other chronic pulmonary disorders. In: Rosene-Montella K, Keely E, Barbour L, *et al.*, editors. *Medical Care of the Pregnant Patient.* 2nd ed. Philadelphia, PA: ACP Press; 2008. pp. 365–82.

British Thoracic Society. *British Guideline on the Management of Asthma.* London: BTS; 2008.

Canny G. Pregnancy in patients with cystic fibrosis. *CMAJ.* 1993; **149**: 805–6.

Chung KF. *Clinicians' Guide to Asthma.* London: Arnold; 2002.

Connors PM, Ulles MM. The physical, psychological, and social implications of caring for the pregnant patient and newborn with cystic fibrosis. *J Perinat Neonatal Nurs.* 2005; **19**(4): 301–15.

Cystic Fibrosis Trust. About cystic fibrosis. 2007. Available at: www.cftrust.org.uk/ (accessed 9 December 2008).

Dack K, Cunha A, Madge S. The management of cystic fibrosis. *Pract Nurs.* 2007; **18**(9): 442–9.

de Swiet M. The respiratory system. In: Chamberlain G, Broughton Pipkin F, editors. *Clinical Physiology in Obstetrics.* 3rd ed. Oxford: Blackwell; 1998. pp. 111–28.

de Swiet M. Diseases of the respiratory system. In: de Swiet M, editor. *Medical Disorders in Obstetric Practice.* 4th ed. Oxford: Blackwell; 2002. pp. 1–28.

Dodd M, Langman H. Urinary incontinence in cystic fibrosis. *J R Soc Med.* 2005; **98**(Suppl. 45): S28–36.

Dombrowski M. Asthma and pregnancy. *Obstet Gynecol.* 2006; **108**(3 Pt. 1): 667–81.

Enriquez R, Wu P, Griffin M, *et al.* Cessation of asthma medication in early pregnancy. *Am J Obstet Gynecol.* 2006; **195**(1): 149–53.

Ezri T, Szmuk P, Evron S, *et al.* Difficult airway in obstetric anesthesia: a review. *Obstet Gynecol Surv.* 2001; **56**(10): 631–41.

Global Initiative for Asthma. *Global Strategy for Asthma Management and Prevention.* 2006. Available at: www.ginasthma.org (accessed 8 December 2008).

Hendler I, Schatz M, Momirova V, *et al.* Association of obesity with pulmonary and nonpulmonary complications of pregnancy in asthmatic women. *Obstet Gynecol.* 2006; **108**(1): 77–82.

Hilman B, Aitken M, Constantinescu M. Pregnancy in patients with cystic fibrosis. *Clin Obstet Gynecol.* 1996; **39**: 70–86.

King M, Gates A, Newman J. Maternal cystic fibrosis. *ACPWH J.* 2007; **101**: 63–9.

Mackie A, Thornton S, Edenborough F. Cystic fibrosis-related diabetes. *Diabet Med.* 2003; **20**(6): 425–36.

Minerbi-Codish I, Fraser D, Avnun L, *et al.* Influence of asthma in pregnancy on labour and the newborn. *Respiration.* 1998; **65**: 130–5.

Murphy VE, Gibson P, Talbot PI, *et al.* Severe asthma exacerbations during pregnancy. *Obstet Gynecol.* 2005; **106**(5 Pt. 1): 1046–54.

Nelson-Piercy C. Asthma in pregnancy. *Thorax.* 2001; **56**: 325–8.

Nelson-Piercy C. *Handbook of Obstetric Medicine.* 3rd ed. London: Informa Healthcare; 2006.

Powrie R. Respiratory disease. In: James D, Steer P, Weiner C, *et al.*, editors. *High Risk Pregnancy: management options.* 3rd ed. Philadelphia, PA: Elsevier; 2006. pp. 828–64.

Powrie R. Pulmonary disease in pregnancy. In: Greer IA, Nelson-Piercy C, Walters B, editors. *Maternal Medicine.* Edinburgh: Churchill Livingstone Elsevier; 2007. pp. 102–33.

Rankin J. Respiration. In: Stables D, Rankin J, editors. *Physiology in Childbearing.* 2nd ed. Edinburgh: Elsevier; 2005. pp. 239–52.

Rey E, Boulet L. Asthma in pregnancy. *BMJ.* 2007; **334**: 582–5.

Rudra C, Williams M, Frederick I, *et al.* Maternal asthma and risk of pre-eclampsia: a case-control study. *J Reprod Med.* 2006; **51**(2): 94–100.

Saker A, Benachi A, Bonnefont J, *et al.* Genetic characterization of circulating fetal cells allows non-invasive prenatal diagnosis of cystic fibrosis. *Prenat Diag.* 2006; **26**(10): 906–16.

Stenius-Aarniala BS, Hedman J, Teramo KA. Acute asthma during pregnancy. *Thorax.* 1996; **51**: 411–14.

Thibodeau GA, Patton KT. *Anatomy and Physiology.* 6th ed. St Louis, MO: Mosby Elsevier; 2007.

Turner C, Temple K, Lucassen A. Genetics. In: Peebles A, Connett G, Maddison J, *et al.*, editors. *Cystic Fibrosis Care: a practical guide.* Edinburgh: Elsevier Churchill Livingstone; 2005.

Widerman E, Millner L, Sexauer W, *et al.* Health status and sociodemographic characteristics of adults receiving cystic fibrosis diagnosis after age 18 years. *Chest.* 2000; **118**: 427–33.

Williamson C, Nelson-Piercy C. Treatment of asthma. In: Rubin P, editor. *Prescribing in Pregnancy.* 3rd ed. London: BMJ Books; 2000.

CHAPTER 7

Disorders of the digestive tract

CONTENTS

[Note: HELLP syndrome is in Chapter 5 and cystic fibrosis is in Chapter 6]

OVERVIEW OF THE DIGESTIVE SYSTEM AND CHANGES IN PREGNANCY

The digestive system's main function is to transfer nutrients, water and electrolytes from food to fuel cellular activity and provide the building blocks for renewal and development of body tissue. In pregnancy pressure from the enlarging uterus and changes mediated by oestrogen and progesterone cause anatomical and physiological adjustments that support enhanced demands for maternal and fetal nutrition. Many of the so-called minor disorders of pregnancy are attributed to changes to the digestive system, including nausea and vomiting of early pregnancy, constipation, food cravings and heartburn. Delay in the diagnosis of more serious conditions of the digestive tract may occur and, where problems exist, fetal requirements may be compromised.

The digestive system (*see* Figure 7.1) is made up of:

◗ the alimentary or gastrointestinal (GI) tract. This is a continuous fibromuscular tube lined with mucosa and surrounded by smooth muscle that extends from the mouth to the anus
◗ accessory organs, including salivary glands, the pancreas, the liver and the gall bladder.

The GI tract is regulated by the autonomic nervous system, which includes both sympathetic and parasympathetic innervations. It also has its own intrinsic network of interconnecting nerve fibres that act entirely within the walls of the digestive system. Parasympathetic stimulation increases peristaltic muscular activity and increases glandular secretion. Sympathetic stimulation, normally responsible for fight and flight responses, diverts activity away from the digestive system to more important areas and so acts in the opposite manner to the parasympathetic system. In conjunction with

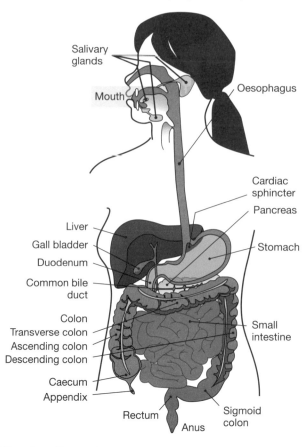

FIGURE 7.1: The digestive system

nervous responses, functions of the GI tract are regulated by various peptides, including hormones. Placental hormones including oestrogen and particularly progesterone have an impact on the digestive system (*see* Table 7.1). Gastric motility is decreased during labour in response to anxiety and pain.

TABLE 7.1: Summary of alterations to the gastrointestinal tract during pregnancy

Organ	Alteration	Significance/physiology	
General GI tract	• Increased appetite and thirst	• Changes to carbohydrate metabolism to meet demands of growing fetus	
Mouth	• Food cravings or aversions	• Dulling of sense of taste • Increased requirement of glucose and other nutrients	
	• Gingivitis (gums swollen with tendency to bleed)	• Increased blood supply to gums • Increased turnover and thinness of gum epithelial lining cells	
	• Possible increased saliva production • Increase frequency of dental caries	• 1–2 litres per day, though this is thought to be normal. Feels more because of difficulty in swallowing during periods of nausea and vomiting.	
Oesophagus	• Decreased pressure and tone of cardiac sphincter	• Heartburn caused by gastric acid reflux	
Stomach	• Decreased tone and motility with delayed gastric emptying time • Decreased gastric acidity • Pyloric sphincter incompetence	• Increased risk of gastro-oesophageal reflux and vomiting • Reflux of alkaline biliary material into stomach	
Small and large intestine	• Decreased tone and motility with prolonged intestinal transit time • Duodenal villi hypertrophy	• Facilitates absorption of essential nutrients such as iron, calcium and glucose • Increased water absorption leading to constipation • Decreased tone leads to flatulence	↑ • Relaxant effect of progesterone on smooth muscle ↓
	• Appendix and caecum displaced superiorly by growing fetus	• Complicates diagnosis of appendicitis in pregnancy	
Gall bladder	• Decreased tone and motility • Tendency to form cholesterol-based gallstones	• Volume of bile increases and emptying rate decreases	

(continued)

Organ	Alteration	Significance/physiology	
Gall bladder (*continued*)	• Tendency to retain bile salts	• Bile is more dilute, with a decreased ability to break down cholesterol • Pruritus	
Pancreas	• Increased production of insulin by islet cells	• Response to increased insulin resistance, which aids placental transfer of glucose to fetus	• Probably driven by human placental lactogen and cortisol
Liver	• Displaced by enlarging uterus • Altered production of liver enzymes, plasma proteins, bilirubin and serum lipids • Increased glycogen and triglyceride storage in hepatic cells	• Difficulties can arise in interpreting liver function tests	• Effect of oestrogen and haemodilution

Sources: Coad and Dunstall (2007); Blackburn (2007); Hytten (1991); Fagan (2002)

KEY NUTRITIONAL REQUIREMENTS FOR PREGNANCY AND LACTATION

❱ Increased intake of calories.
❱ Protein requirements increase and sources of protein should contain essential amino acids.
❱ Essential fatty acids, including omega 3, are important for fetal growth, brain and vision development.
❱ Calcium, phosphorous, magnesium required for skeletal and tissue growth.
❱ Vitamin D essential for absorption of calcium and phosphorus and mineralisation of fetal bone and teeth.
❱ Iron and folate essential for RBC production. Folic acid supplementation is recommended to reduce incidence of neural tube defects.
❱ Increased intake of vitamin E, vitamin C, thiamine, riboflavin, niacin and vitamin B6 is recommended, although routine multivitamin supplementation remains controversial.
❱ Vitamin C increases absorption of iron and is essential for tissue integrity.
❱ Low zinc levels are associated with fetal growth restriction.
❱ Iodine for increased thyroxine production.
❱ Excess vitamin A (retinol) is associated with increase in birth defects.

(Blackburn, 2007)

NAUSEA AND VOMITING

Up to 45% of women experience vomiting in early pregnancy, with the figure rising to as much as 90% for those who experience nausea alone (Blackburn, 2007). The condition is commonly called morning sickness, reflecting the fact that symptoms are generally worse before eating in the morning, but many women experience symptoms at other times or throughout the day. Nausea and vomiting of pregnancy (NVP) generally starts at around 4–5 weeks of pregnancy, with symptoms peaking at around 12 weeks, and is usually resolved by 16 weeks. Around 20% of women may experience symptoms until term (Miller, 2008). Food aversions to meat, fish, poultry and eggs often accompany NVP.

There is no established physiological cause of nausea and vomiting, but some of the factors implicated are listed in Box 7.1.

BOX 7.1: FACTORS IMPLICATED AS CAUSES OF NVP

- Human chorionic gonadotrophin (hCG). The duration of nausea roughly follows the profile of secretion of this hormone. Thyroid hormones and oestrogen may have a role, but there is no correlation between the hormone levels and symptoms (Goodwin, 2002).
- Female fetus. The maternal plasma concentration of hCG is slightly higher when the child is female, but studies have produced conflicting data on the association of a female fetus and NVP (Goodwin, 2002).
- Hormonal effects on plasma osmolarity can stimulate the vestibular (inner ear) system in susceptible individuals. Some women find relief from nausea when they lie down (Goodwin, 2002).
- Induced by effects of progesterone on the GI tract (Blackburn, 2007; Coad, et al., 2000).
- Unidentified nutritional deficiency (Coad, et al., 2000) or vitamin B6 deficiency (Neibyl and Goodwin, 2002).
- Protective reaction to prevent women eating dangerous substances. (Flaxman and Sherman, 2000).
- A psychological basis which interacts with physical and cultural factors (Blackburn, 2007), although there is more evidence that NVP causes psychological distress (Buckwalter and Simpson, 2002).

HYPEREMESIS GRAVIDARUM (HG)

HG is an uncommon disorder affecting 0.3–1.5% of pregnant women (Miller, 2008). It may represent the extreme end of the spectrum of NVP, with symptoms similarly starting at around six weeks and being resolved by 20 weeks gestation (Fagan, 2002). It is defined as prolonged and severe vomiting that results in dehydration, electrolyte imbalance, weight loss and ketosis (Blackburn, 2007; Kenyon and Nelson-Piercy, 2001). Alterations in thyroid hormones seem to have a role in HG, as does progesterone and hCG. Women with a history of eating disorders are at increased risk of HG (Kenyon and Nelson-Piercy, 2001). Kenyon and Nelson-Piercy (2001) suggest the diagnosis is based on excluding other causes of vomiting. Box 7.2 outlines other possible causes of severe protracted vomiting and indicates areas for investigation.

BOX 7.2: CAUSES OF PROTRACTED VOMITING IN PREGNANCY

- Urinary tract infection
- Pancreatitis
- Peptic ulcers
- Hyperthyroidism or Addison's disease
- Molar pregnancy
- Multiple pregnancy

Treatment of HG

Most women with HG need hospital inpatient care. It is important to rehydrate them with intravenous fluids and to consider an electrolyte imbalance. Treatment is normally done with antiemetics and occasionally steroids are needed (Fagan, 2002). Note that if steroids are taken in the antenatal period, the woman may need IV steroid cover for labour.

Nutrient supply may be compromised, with serious repercussions (Kenyon and Nelson-Piercy, 2001) and vitamin supplementation may be necessary. In particular, thiamine supplementation should be given to those with prolonged vomiting (Nelson-Piercy, 2006) to avoid Wernicke's encephalopathy. A dietician should be consulted. If the woman is feeling unwell, she is unlikely to be mobile, and thromboprophylaxis should be considered. Fetal surveillance, particularly by growth scans, is usual.

THE SMALL INTESTINE

The small intestine is divided into three sections. The *duodenum* extends beyond the pyloric sphincter in the stomach. The common bile duct empties into the duodenum. The duodenum is the primary site of iron and calcium absorption. The height of duodenal villi increases in pregnancy and, along with a longer transit time, enhances greater absorption of these and other substances. The next section of the small bowel is known as the *jejunum* and is responsible for the absorption of fats, carbohydrates and protein. The last section is the *ileum*, which is responsible for the absorption of vitamin B12 and bile salts. The surface of the small intestine forms a series of circular folds, which increases the surface area available to absorb nutrients, which is the primary function of the small intestine. The surface has a velvet appearance due to the presence of fine hair-like projections known as villi, which are where absorption takes place.

COELIAC DISEASE

Coeliac disease is intolerance to gluten, a protein found in wheat, rye, barley and oats, which affects the small intestine. Atrophy of the villi causes malabsorption due to an abnormal inflammatory response to exposure to gluten. Symptoms are variable but include recurrent attacks of diarrhoea, steatorrhoea (fat in stools), abdominal distension, flatulence and stomach cramps (Smith and Watson, 2005). Malabsorption results in lower levels of iron, vitamin B12 and folic acid. Unexplained anaemia is a common presentation for a coeliac condition.

A blood test which detects blood levels of antibodies indicative of coeliac (serum anti-endomysium antibodies: EMA) can be used, but a firm diagnosis is made by small-bowel biopsy, which shows villous atrophy and a flat mucosa. Adherence to a strict gluten-free diet will restore the normal appearance of the small bowel as the villi grow back. Most women notice relief of their symptoms when they follow the diet, providing further confirmation of the diagnosis.

Coeliac disease was once thought to be diagnosed mainly in childhood, but the UK Coeliac Society reports that the median age of diagnosis was 44 years (Hin, *et al.*, 1999), and undiagnosed coeliac disease may be frequent among pregnant women. Pregnancy has been suggested as a factor that may reveal latent coeliac disease (Corrado, *et al.*, 2002). An Italian study found that of 5055 women tested, 51 (one in 80) were found to have coeliac disease (Greco, *et al.*, 2005). It should be noted that there is geographical variation in the incidence of coeliac disease and Italy is known to be a high-incidence area, so these figures represent the higher end of the scale. Pregnancy outcome was good except for women with clinically evident disease, although anaemia was more frequent. Undiagnosed coeliac disease may present as bone pain from osteoporosis, due to malabsorption of calcium and vitamin D (Fagan, 2002).

Guidelines by the British Society of Gastroenterology (1996) recommend a routine follow-up for coeliac patients at various times, including pregnancy, although there is evidence this does not take place (McPhillips, 2000). The midwife could encourage this during the antenatal period, as stress can precipitate symptoms and pregnancy is well-known as a time of physical and psychological stress.

Management of coeliac disease

The management of coeliac disease involves permanent adherence to a strict gluten-free diet. Gluten is present in wheat, rye, barley and oats, and avoiding foods such as bread, pasta, cakes and sauces makes the diet challenging. Some people with coeliac disease can tolerate oats in their diet. However, traces of gluten can be hidden in foods such as flavoured crisps, stock cubes and beer. Food that is gluten-free must be prepared separately from food containing gluten to avoid small amounts of contamination that can set off the inflammatory process and consequent symptoms if ingested. Coeliac UK (www.coeliac.org.uk) provides comprehensive dietary information and support to coeliacs.

Coeliac disease causes distressing symptoms, and non-adherence to the diet puts the woman at risk of several long-term complications, such as small-bowel malignancy and osteoporosis (McPhillips, 2000).

If they have already been diagnosed before pregnancy (the majority), women will probably be coping very well with their diet and experience a problem only if admitted to hospital. The midwife should liaise closely with hospital catering staff to ensure she eats well in hospital. Arrangements should be made to store and prepare snacks/food she may bring with her. Prolonged breastfeeding and delay in introducing gluten to the infant's diet may reduce its incidence in offspring (Ivarsson, *et al.*, 2002).

THE LARGE INTESTINE

The large intestine extends from the ileocaecal valve to the anus. It is made up of the colon, caecum, appendix and rectum. Absorption in the large intestine mostly involves the removal of water and some electrolytes. Otherwise the large bowel is responsible for storage and the movement of the bowel contents. Micro-organisms known as gut flora inhabit the large intestine. These bacteria synthesise vitamins, including B-complex vitamins and vitamin K, which is essential for blood clotting. The bacteria are therefore beneficial in the gut, but if they escape into the peritoneal cavity, which could occur in cases of rupture (very serious), or ascend the reproductive or urinary tract, they result in infection.

INFLAMMATORY BOWEL DISEASE

Inflammatory bowel disease (IBD) is a collective term for two disorders, namely ulcerative colitis (UC) and Crohn's disease (CD). (Table 7.2 details specific features of IBD.) These are chronic conditions characterised by unpredictable periods of relapse and remission. For both conditions the cause is uncertain, although an interaction of genetic susceptibility and environmental triggers leads to an abnormal immunological reaction (Greig and Rampton, 2003). Pregnancy does not seem to impact on disease activity in IBD. About one-third of women with inactive IBD at conception can be expected to relapse during pregnancy or the puerperium. This is the same rate of relapse as in any other year. However, women are advised to plan conception when the disease is quiescent, as active disease at the time of conception is less likely to settle and is associated with miscarriage, prematurity and low birth weight (Alstead, 2002; Kornfeld, *et al.*, 1997).

Fertility in UC and inactive CD seems to be unaffected. However, fertility is reduced in women with active Crohn's disease. Women with Crohn's disease appear to delay conception, have fewer children and report higher rates of failure to conceive (Alstead, 2002). Dyspareunia, vaginal candidiasis and concerns regarding body image are reported in women with IBD (Moody, *et al.*, 1992).

Preconception care

Women who have undergone a large amount of gut resection may have malabsorption of fat, fat-soluble vitamins and B12 and have an electrolyte imbalance. They may also be avoiding certain foods because they are associated with symptoms and therefore they may lack some nutrients (Nightingale, 2007). A nutrition screen and dietician advice is valuable pre-pregnancy. Increased dosage of folic acid may be appropriate (Alstead, 2002; Nelson-Piercy, 2006).

As with all women taking regular medication, a review should be undertaken before pregnancy to ensure the drugs are safe and prescribed at the minimum dose possible, while also ensuring the best possible health of the woman. Rates of non-compliance for long-term medication may be about 50% (Hall, *et al.*, 2007), but planning for a pregnancy should be an incentive for a woman to maximise her own health.

Pregnancy care

Antenatal care for a woman with IBD should be multidisciplinary, with gastro-enterologists and perhaps dieticians working with the obstetrician and midwife. If a

TABLE 7.2: Features of ulcerative colitis (UC) and Crohn's disease (CD)

	Crohn's disease	Ulcerative colitis
Pathological features	• Affects all layers of the bowel • Rectum frequently spared • Inflammation discontinuous with presence of 'skip lesions' • Bowel wall thickened with deep ulcers and oedema • Tendency to form fistula or strictures	• Affects only the mucosa and submucosa • Rectum is always affected and spreads proximally upwards
Distribution	• Can affect any part of the GI tract and can manifest outside the GI tract as well	• Affects the large bowel only
Signs and symptoms	• Depends on the site and severity: diarrhoea, intermittent abdominal discomfort, weight loss, anorexia, anaemia, perianal disease, rectal bleeding	• Diarrhoea, multiple bowel movements, rectal passage of mucus and blood, fever, abdominal distension, anaemia, weight loss, electrolyte imbalance, hypo-albuminaemia (with oedema)
Incidence	• 5–10 per 100 000 in the UK. More common in Caucasians: the highest incidence is amongst the Jewish population (Smith and Watson, 2005)	• 10 per 100 000 • No race association

Sources: Grieg and Rampton (2003); Hall, *et al.* (2007); Loftus (2004); Nightingale (2007)

woman has an IBD nurse specialist involved in her care, this specialist may be able to provide effective continuity, support and information (Nightingale, 2007). Support groups such as the National Association for Colitis and Crohn's Disease (www.nacc.org.uk) may also be helpful at this time.

Women who have had surgery resulting in a colostomy usually do well, as do those with ileostomies, although they may, rarely, obstruct (Nelson-Piercy, 2006).

Pregnancy does not increase the chance of exacerbations, but if it does occur, it is more likely to be in the first trimester. Bowel symptoms during pregnancy are likely to be exacerbations, but a stool culture should always be checked for infection. Screening for anaemia, electrolytes, liver function and inflammatory markers should be undertaken.

Exacerbations will be treated with medication, which may include corticosteroids (which may also be taken regularly as a preventative measure). Consideration of alternative medication that is safe in pregnancy should be made. Attention must be paid to diet at this time and vitamin supplements may be given. Some women with Crohn's disease use diet as their primary intervention – if they are admitted, the midwife must ensure this can be maintained while they are in hospital (Hall, *et al.*, 2007).

Fetal surveillance is usual, especially if there is a question of nutritional deficiencies. If there are exacerbations during the pregnancy, there is a risk of intra-uterine growth restriction, or a premature delivery may result (Dominitz, *et al.*, 2002). There is some evidence of an increased risk of congenital malformations but the reason is unknown (Dominitz, *et al.*, 2002).

Some studies have demonstrated an increased number of premature deliveries (Elbaz, *et al.*, 2005; Sela, *et al.*, 2005) but others have not (Ludvigsson and Ludvigsson, 2002). The discrepancy in findings may be due to the number of women with disease activity during pregnancy included in the study, a fact that is not usually identified. It is likely that active disease is associated with prematurity and low birth weight.

Labour care

Most women are able to have a vaginal delivery; however, they have an increased risk of Caesarean section (Cornish, *et al.*, 2006). Those who have had perianal surgery in the past should have been individually assessed and a plan should have been made during the antenatal period about the mode of delivery. If steroids have been taken during pregnancy, arrangements will need to be made for IV steroids during labour.

Postnatal care

Exacerbations are common in the puerperium and may be due to the change in routine. The lifestyle adaptations that are necessary for a chronic disease, such as regular medication and attention to diet, may be challenging with a new baby, and the community midwife and health visitor should ensure that the new mother sees her own health as a priority, and perhaps help her to plan strategies to manage her time.

Breastfeeding should be encouraged, as it may protect the baby against the hereditary and immune components of inflammatory bowel disease.

IRRITABLE BOWEL SYNDROME (IBS)

IBS is the most common GI disorder. Around 10–15% of the population may have IBS and women may be affected more than men. IBS is a chronic condition causing abdominal pain and altered bowel function, which includes constipation and diarrhoea. Sufferers may also experience dyspepsia, backache, gynaecological and urinary symptoms. The syndrome lacks any biochemical markers or structural features and diagnosis is made by excluding any other pathological disorder. There is no agreement about what causes IBS, although the relationship between the autonomic nervous system and the GI tract and the intricate nature of the enteric nervous system seem to play a part. Proposed mechanisms include:

- stress-related triggers
- prolonged use of antibiotics
- altered intestinal motility
- inflammation due to infection
- abnormal perception of GI events.

(Smith and Watson, 2005)

Symptoms may increase in pregnancy (Nelson-Piercy, 2006) and diet modification (for example stool-bulking agents, increased fluid intake and an increase in dietary fibre) may help. If necessary, antispasmodic medication may be prescribed.

APPENDICITIS

The appendix is a small, finger-like projection at the bottom of the caecum. Appendicitis is the most common non-obstetric condition requiring surgery during pregnancy, with an incidence of around one in 1500 pregnancies (Anderson and Nielson, 1999). Appendicitis increases the risk of a spontaneous miscarriage and preterm labour (Blackburn, 2007; Fagan, 2002). The appendix is progressively displaced upwards in pregnancy and by around 20 weeks' gestation has reached the level of the iliac crest. By the third trimester it may be in the right upper quadrant.

Classic diagnostic signs may be absent, with guarding and rebound tenderness being milder and less well localised. Pain can be felt mainly in the right upper quadrant (Miller, 2008). Nausea and vomiting is common but is not diagnostic. Ultrasound is helpful, but visualisation is usually poor in the third trimester (Miller, 2008). An adapted MRI may also be used for diagnosis.

Although appendicitis is no more common in pregnancy, it tends to be more serious because of delays in diagnosis. There is also a suggestion that appendicitis may be a risk factor for abruption (Klatsky, *et al.*, 2008).

THE PANCREAS

The pancreas is a small gland well known for its endocrine function. Specialist cells distributed in the pancreas, known as the islets of Langerhan, produce insulin and glucagon that have an essential role in the control of blood sugar (*see* Chapter 1). The pancreas also has an exocrine function. It produces pancreatic juice, which contains enzymes that digest carbohydrates, proteins and fats. The common bile duct, coming from the liver, joins the pancreatic duct just before it enters the duodenum.

PANCREATITIS

In order to protect the pancreas from being damaged by the digestive enzymes it produces, those enzymes remain in an inactive form until they reach the duodenum. In the presence of gallstones, alcoholism and other conditions, the precursor enzymes can be activated while they are still in the pancreas, causing acute inflammation of the pancreas, known as acute pancreatitis. Chronic pancreatitis is due to repeated attacks of acute pancreatitis and is mainly associated with excessive alcohol consumption. Pancreatitis is rare, occurring in only one in 10 000, which includes men. In pregnancy it is usually associated with gallstones that block the pancreatic ampulla (Blackburn, 2007). There is some evidence that pancreatitis can be associated with pre-eclampsia (Opatrny, *et al.*, 2004) and also that it may occur suddenly in the immediate postnatal period (Fukami, *et al.*, 2003; Mechery and Burch, 2006).

Signs and symptoms include epigastric pain radiating to the back, constant abdominal pain and nausea or vomiting. Most cases resolve spontaneously if there is good supportive treatment. This includes bowel rest (perhaps parenteral nutrition), analgesics and intravenous fluids. As pancreatitis may become a life-threatening condition, care is usually undertaken in a high dependency or intensive care unit.

PANCREATIC TRANSPLANT

See Chapter 5 for a general discussion of risks and care in pregnancy for a woman with a transplant. Most transplants of the pancreas are done as part of a combined transplantation (e.g., pancreas–kidney) and successful pregnancies have been reported in these women since the late 1980s (Fuchs, *et al.*, 2007). In addition to monitoring renal function in these women, elements of diabetic care (e.g., eye examinations) should also be carried out.

THE LIVER

The liver is the most important metabolic organ in the body. The hepatic portal system brings venous blood from the intestine, and the absorbed nutrients are then processed, stored and detoxified by the liver. Box 7.3 outlines the numerous functions of the liver in addition to its role in digestion.

BOX 7.3: FUNCTIONS OF THE LIVER

- Metabolic processing of the major nutrients (carbohydrates, proteins, fats) after their absorption from the digestive tract
- Detoxification or degradation of body wastes and hormones as well as drugs. This includes the breakdown of protein, which produces the waste products urea and uric acid, which are excreted in urine
- Production of plasma proteins, including immunoglobulin A and those essential for blood clotting
- Regulation of blood sugar through storage and release of glycogen
- Removal of bacteria
- Excretion of cholesterol and bilirubin (from breakdown of red blood cells)
- Secretion of bile

ACUTE FATTY LIVER DISEASE OF PREGNANCY (AFLP)

Usually occurring in the third trimester, AFLP manifests suddenly as unexplained liver failure (Miller, 2008) and is potentially fatal. Early symptoms include nausea, acute vomiting, abdominal pain and general malaise, usually followed by hypoglycaemia, hyperuricaemia, jaundice, renal failure and coagulopathy (without thrombocytopenia). There may be signs of pre-eclampsia and/or HELLP syndrome and AFLP may be a variant of pre-eclampsia (Nelson-Piercy, 2006). Pancreatitis may also be present (Moldenhauer, *et al.*, 2004).

Diagnosis is ideally by liver biopsy, but this cannot be done if coagulopathy is present (Nelson-Piercy, 2006). MRI, CT or ultrasound scans are helpful but are not always conclusive (Nelson-Piercy, 2006). Liver function tests are abnormal, with raised transaminase and alkaline phosphatase levels and increased prothrombin time. Treatment is delivery of the baby, and supportive, with ventilation, dialysis and/or transfer to a specialist liver unit if necessary. Mortality and morbidity rates are high, but with early and prompt treatment women may recover without the need of a liver transplant (Esposti, *et al.*, 2008).

LIVER TRANSPLANT

See Chapter 5 for a general discussion of risks and care in pregnancy for a woman with a transplant. There is evidence of successful pregnancies in women with liver transplants (Nagy, *et al.*, 2003; Nelson-Piercy, 2006; Miller, *et al.*, 2000). Monitoring will largely consist of evaluation of liver function tests (*see* normal values for liver function tests during pregnancy in the appendix of Chapter 5). However, a combination of the impact of oestrogen and effect of haemodilution make interpretation of liver function tests difficult in pregnancy (Kenyon and Nelson-Piercy, 2001).

THE GALL BLADDER

Between meals, bile is diverted to the gall bladder for storage, and there it is concentrated by the absorption of water. Bile contains:

▶ water
▶ mineral salts
▶ mucus
▶ bilirubin
▶ bile salts
▶ cholesterol.

Bile does not contain digestive enzymes but rather it digests fats through the action of bile acids. Bile acids (salts) are derivatives of cholesterol. Following their participation in fat digestion and absorption, most bile salts are reabsorbed back into the blood and return to the liver via the portal vein. They are recycled many times a day via this entero-hepatic circulation. Bile acids are important for the elimination of excess cholesterol, to prevent cholesterol gallstones, to digest fat and for the intestinal absorption of fat-soluble vitamins (Esposti, *et al.*, 2008). The gall bladder is not essential for digestion, so removing it, as may occur for the treatment of gallstones, presents no problem.

CHOLELITHIASIS (GALLSTONES)

Gallstones are the second most common non-obstetric surgical problem in pregnancy. Gallstones, as the name implies, is the presence of stones or calculi in the gall bladder. Cholesterol stones, in particular, are more commonly seen in the female reproductive age group, with pregnancy being a known risk factor for the development of gallstones. The gall bladder volume is increased and emptying rate decreased in pregnancy, resulting in sluggish emptying that predisposes to stone formation (Blackburn, 2007).

Gallstones form when an excess amount of cholesterol in the bile in relation to other bile constituents, namely bile salts and lecithin, precipitates microcrystals. High cholesterol from a high-fat diet or normal increase in pregnancy, or low bile salts from poor absorption and reduced lecithin can all contribute to gallstone development. Box 7.4 lists risk factors for formation of gallstones.

ACUTE CHOLECYSTITIS

Acute cholecystitis occurs when gallstones irritate the mucous membrane of the gall bladder, resulting in inflammation that causes considerable pain. It is rare in pregnancy, with appendicitis being four to five times more likely (Blackburn, 2007). Diagnosis is usually by ultrasound (Ghumman, *et al.*, 1997). Pain is usually described as colicky, and pyrexia and shock may be present, depending on the degree of infection (Nelson-Piercy, 2006). Although surgery can be done in pregnancy, for most women conservative treatment (fasting, nasogastric drainage, intravenous hydration, antibiotics and analgesia) is effective.

BOX 7.4: RISK FACTORS FOR FORMATION OF GALLSTONES

- Increasing age
- Female sex
- Pregnancy/combined oral contraceptive pill
- Obesity
- Spinal cord injury

(Smith and Watson, 2005)

OBSTETRIC CHOLESTASIS (OC)

OC (also known as intrahepatic cholestasis of pregnancy) affects 0.5–1.5% of pregnancies in Europeans, although it is higher in certain populations from Scandinavia, Poland and Chile (Nelson-Piercy, 2006; Schutt and Minuk, 2007). Pruritus, raised serum bile acids, abnormal liver function tests and adverse fetal outcomes are the key features of OC. It tends to develop in the third trimester but resolves quickly after delivery (Esposti, *et al.*, 2008). Box 7.5 lists features of OC which aid diagnosis.

BOX 7.5: FEATURES OF OC

- Persistent pruritus
- Abnormal liver biochemistry
  — ↑ Aspartate aminotransferase (AST)
  — ↑ Alanine amniotransferase (ALT)
  — ↑ Gamma-glutamyl transferase (GGT)
  — ↑ Total bile acids
  — ↑ Alkaline phosphatase
- No other liver pathology
- Resolution postnatally

Less common symptoms of OC
- Tiredness
- Poor appetite and feeling sick
- Rarely, mild jaundice, dark urine and pale faeces

(Nelson-Piercy, 2006; RCOG, 2006; Schutt and Minuk, 2007; Williamson, 2007)

Pathophysiology

Bile salts are a constituent of bile (*see* description of gall bladder on p. 169). Cholestasis refers to reduced bile flow and excretion. In OC there is a slowing down of the transport or recycling of bile acids that results in an accumulation of bile acids in the blood. Bile acids can cross the placenta and affect the fetus (Esposti, *et al.*, 2008). The aetiology of OC is complex but an interplay of genetic factors with environmental and hormonal influences has been identified (Milkiewicz, *et al.*, 2002). (*See* Figure 7.2).

Up to 30% of women with OC have a family history of OC, but the mutations that cause this defect have mostly not been identified (Esposti, *et al.*, 2008; Milkiewicz, *et al.*, 2002). Oestrogen and progesterone slow down the rate of bile flow and some pregnant women are more sensitive to these hormonal levels. The metabolic demands of pregnancy appear to stress the liver to exceed the capacity for bile transport, uncovering the predisposition. Other factors may play a role. Hepatitis C virus infection has been found to be associated with OC (Esposti, *et al.*, 2008).

Features of OC

The pruritus of OC is usually a severe generalised itch, affecting the limbs and trunk, without an associated rash. The itch is often first noticed on the palms and soles. The itch has been described as intolerable, distressing and typically worse at night, disturbing sleep (Nelson-Piercy, 2006; Williamson, 2007). A mother who suffered from OC describes the impact of the itchiness: 'crying with frustration literally tearing at my

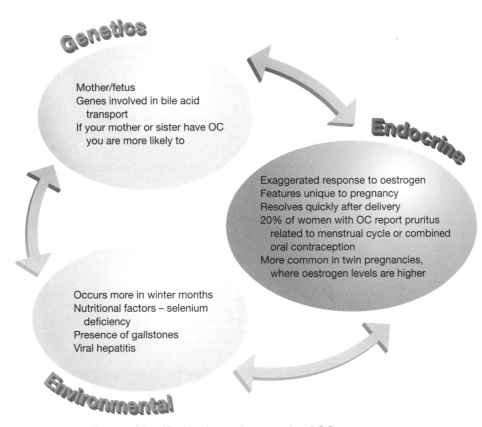

FIGURE 7.2: Factors identified in the pathogenesis of OC

Sources: Esposti, *et al.* (2008); Milkiewicz, *et al.* (2002); Nelson-Piercy (2006); Williamson (2007)

arms and legs' (Chambers, 2001, p. 18). The increase in serum bile acids is commonly thought to be the cause of the pruritus, although the mechanism is unclear. Other causes of itching in pregnancy need to be considered (Chin, 2003). Box 7.6 outlines the maternal and fetal complications of OC.

BOX 7.6: MATERNAL AND FETAL COMPLICATIONS OF OC

Maternal complications of OC
- Psychological impact of severe pruritus
- Psychological impact of stillbirth
- Sleep deprivation
- Malabsorption of vitamin K
- Post-partum haemorrhage (20%–25%)
- Increased rate of gallstones

Fetal complications of OC
- Spontaneous preterm birth
- Iatrogenic preterm birth
- Meconium-stained liquor
- Fetal distress
- Stillbirth

(Esposti, *et al.*, 2008; Williamson, 2007)

Diagnosis

Liver function tests and bile salts are measured, but if they are normal and the pruritus persists with no other reason, they should be repeated every one to two weeks as itching often precedes abnormal blood results (RCOG, 2006). Diagnosis is confirmed by exclusion of other causes of pruritus and abnormal liver function. Box 7.7 lists differential diagnosis.

BOX 7.7: DIFFERENTIAL DIAGNOSIS OF ALTERED LIVER FUNCTION TESTS IN PREGNANCY

- Hepatitis
- Cirrhosis
- Acute fatty liver disease of pregnancy
- Pre-eclampsia
- HELLP

(RCOG, 2006)

Management

See Box 7.6 for potential complications of OC. Fetal surveillance with CTGs, umbilical artery Doppler(s) and liquor volume estimation is common. However, although the risk of stillbirth is a major concern, it is difficult to predict, as intra-uterine death seems to be a sudden asphyxic event. It is not associated with suboptimal CTG or umbilical artery Doppler(s) assessments and there is no evidence of placental insufficiency, reduced liquor volume or intra-uterine growth restriction (RCOG, 2006). It is not known why fetal death occurs, although it has been proposed that bile acids may have a toxic effect on the fetal heart (Williamson, 2007). Most intra-uterine deaths occur after 37 weeks (Williamson, *et al.*, 2004). Meconium is commonly seen (Williamson, 2007).

Women are at risk of malabsorption of fat-soluble vitamins and therefore of vitamin K deficiency, and so are usually prescribed oral vitamin K daily from 32 weeks, in particular to protect against post-partum haemorrhage (Kenyon, *et al.*, 2002). Many women receive treatment with ursodeoxycholic acid for relief of the pruritus, although there is no clear evidence of its effectiveness (RCOG, 2006). Topical agents such as aqueous cream may be helpful for some women, and antihistamines may help sleep (RCOG, 2006).

Although premature labour is common, early induction of labour may also take place, usually around 37 weeks, although this will be guided by the woman's liver function test results. The woman should be given information on recognition of premature labour and how to contact help if concerns arise. The midwife should anticipate the risk of post-partum haemorrhage. In labour, close fetal monitoring is required because of the risk of fetal distress (Nelson-Piercy, 2006). The baby should receive an intramuscular dose of vitamin K soon after birth.

In the postnatal period it should be ensured that the woman's symptoms have gone and her liver function tests (LFTs) have returned to normal. She should receive information about the high recurrence rate, the increased incidence of OC in family members and the importance of avoiding oestrogen-containing contraceptives (RCOG, 2006).

Psychological concerns

The psychological and physical stress from intense itching and lack of sleep in addition to concerns for the baby make women with OC vulnerable to sustained anxiety and depression. Jenny Chambers (2001), a sufferer of OC, describes her experience of the stillbirth of two of her children and the intense frustration she experienced because of the lack of recognition and information from health professionals. She has documented the experiences of women with OC contacting a helpline. Figure 7.3 summarises the emotions women expressed and Figure 7.4 summarises what they want from health professionals and others when they are suffering. Midwives were identified by the women as an important source of support (Chambers, 2006).

Literature which may be useful for a woman with OC is available from the British Liver Trust (www.britishlivertrust.org.uk). Support and information can be accessed from Obstetric Cholestasis Support (www.ocsupport.org.uk).

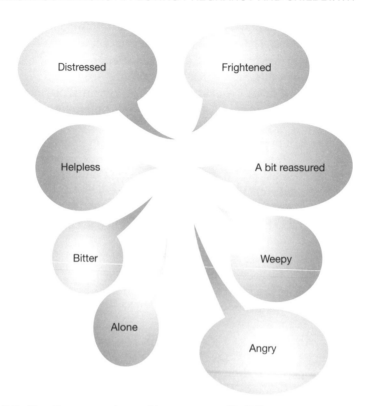

FIGURE 7.3: Emotions experienced by women with OC

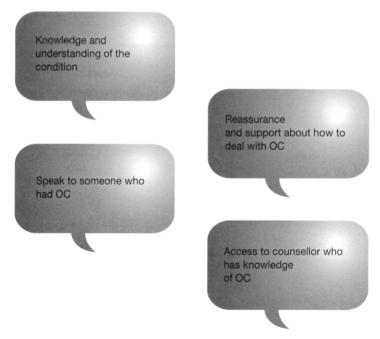

FIGURE 7.4: What women with OC want from health professionals

REFERENCES

Alstead EM. Inflammatory bowel disease in pregnancy. *Postgrad Med J.* 2002; **78**: 23–6.

Anderson B, Nielson TF. Appendicitis in pregnancy: diagnosis, management and complications. *Acta Obstet Gynecol Scand.* 1999; **78**: 758–62.

Blackburn ST. *Maternal, Fetal and Neonatal Physiology.* 3rd ed. St Louis, MO: Saunders; 2007.

British Liver Trust. *Fighting Liver Disease.* Available at: www.britishlivertrust.org.uk (accessed 9 December 2008).

British Society of Gastroenterology. *Guidelines for the Management of Patients with Coeliac Disease.* London: British Society of Gastroenterology; 1996.

Buckwalter JG, Simpson SW. Psychological factors in the etiology and treatment of severe nausea and vomiting in pregnancy. *Am J Obstet Gynecol.* 2002; **186**(5 Pt. 3): S210–14.

Chambers J. Obstetric cholestasis: a mother's experience. *Pract Midwife.* 2001; **4**(4): 18.

Chambers J. What Women Want. Abstract of lectures, Obstetric Cholestasis Conference. London: Imperial College; 19 September 2006. Unpublished.

Chin GY. Dermatoses of pregnancy. *J Paediat Obstet Gynaecol.* 2003; **29**(2): 22–7.

Coad J, Dunstall M. *Anatomy and Physiology for Midwives.* 2nd ed. Edinburgh: Elsevier; 2007.

Coad J, Al-Rasasi B, Morgan J. New insights into nausea and vomiting in pregnancy. *MIDIRS.* 2000; **10**(4): 451–4.

Coeliac UK. Home page. Available at: www.coeliac.co.uk (accessed 9 December 2008).

Cornish J, Tan E, Teare J, *et al.* A meta-analysis on the influence of inflammatory bowel disease on pregnancy. *Gut.* 2006; **56**(6): 830–7.

Corrado F, Magazzu G, Sferlazzas C. Diagnosis of celiac disease in pregnancy and puerperium: think about it. *Acta Obstet Gynecol Scand.* 2002; **81**: 180–1.

Dominitz J, Young J, Boyko E. Outcomes of infants born to mothers with inflammatory bowel disease: a population-based cohort study. *Am J Gastroenterol.* 2002; **97**(3): 641–8.

Elbaz G, Rich A, Levy A, *et al.* Inflammatory bowel disease and preterm delivery. *BJOG.* 2005; **90**(3): 193–7.

Esposti SD, Goodwin TM, Pickard J, *et al.* Liver disease. In: Rosene-Montella K, Keely E, Barbour LA, *et al.*, editors. *Medical Care of the Pregnant Patient.* 2nd ed. Philadelphia, PA: ACP Press; 2008. pp. 567–93.

Fagan EA. Disorders of the gastrointestinal tract. In: de Swiet M, editor. *Medical Disorders in Obstetric Practice.* 4th ed. Oxford: Blackwell; 2002. pp. 346–85.

Flaxman SM, Sherman PW. Morning sickness: a mechanism for protecting mother and embryo. *Q Rev Biol.* 2000; **75**(2): 113–48.

Fuchs K, Wu D, Ebcioglu Z. Pregnancy in renal transplant recipients. *Sem Perinatol.* 2007; **31**: 339–47.

Fukami T, Chaen H, Imura H, *et al.* Acute pancreatitis occurring in early postpartum period: a case report. *J Perinat Med.* 2003; **31**(4): 345–9.

Ghumman E, Barry M, Grace P. Management of gallstones in pregnancy. *Br J Surg.* 1997; **84**: 1646–50.

Goodwin T. Nausea and vomiting of pregnancy: an obstetric syndrome. *Am J Obstet Gynecol.* 2002; **186**: S184–9.

Greco L, Veneziano A, Di Donato L, *et al.* Undiagnosed coeliac disease does not appear to be associated with unfavourable outcome of pregnancy. *Gut.* 2005; **53**(1): 149–51.

Greig ER, Rampton DS. *Management of Crohn's Disease.* London: Martin Dunitz; 2003.

Hall A, Porrett T, Cox C. Diagnosis and current management of Crohn's disease. *Gastrointest Nurs.* 2007; **5**(2): 11–20.

Hin H, Bird G, Fisher P, *et al.* Coeliac disease in primary care: case-finding study. *BMJ.* 1999; **318**: 164–7.

Hytten FE. The alimentary system. In: Hytten F, Chamberlain G, editors. *Clinical Physiology in Obstetrics.* 2nd ed. Oxford: Blackwell; 1991. pp. 137–49.

Ivarsson A, Hernell O, Stenlund H, *et al.* Breast-feeding protects against celiac disease. *Am J Clin Nutr.* 2002; **75**(5): 914–21.

Kenyon AP, Nelson-Piercy C. Hyperemesis gravidarum, gastrointestinal and liver disease in pregnancy. *Curr Obstet Gynaecol.* 2001; **11**: 336–43.

Kenyon AP, Girling J, Nelson-Piercy C, *et al.* Pruritus in pregnancy and the identification of obstetric cholestasis risk: a prospective prevalence study of 6531 women. *J Obstet Gynaecol.* 2002; **22**(Suppl. 1): S15.

Klatsky P, Cronbach E, Shahine L, *et al.* Abruptio placentae in the setting of an atypical presentation of acute appendicitis. A case report. *J Reprod Med.* 2008; **53**(2): 129–31.

Kornfeld D, Cnattingius S, Ekbom A. Pregnancy outcomes in women with inflammatory bowel disease. A population-based cohort study. *Am J Obstet Gynecol.* 1997; **177**: 942–6.

Loftus EV Jr. Clinical epidemiology of inflammatory bowel disease: incidence, prevalence and environmental influences. *Gastroenterology.* 2004; **126**: 1504–7.

Ludvigsson JF, Ludvigsson J. Inflammatory bowel disease in mother or father and neonatal outcome. *Acta Paediatr.* 2002; **91**(2): 145–51.

McPhillips J. Understanding coeliac disease: symptoms and long-term risks. *Br J Nurs.* 2000; **9**(8): 479–83.

Mechery J, Burch D. Postpartum pancreatitis. *J Obstet Gynaecol.* 2006; **26**(4): 371.

Milkiewicz P, Elias E, Williamson C. Obstetric cholestasis. *BMJ.* 2002: **324**: 123–4.

Miller J, Mastrobattista J, Katz A. Obstetrical and neonatal outcome in pregnancies after liver transplantation. *Am J Perinatol.* 2000; **17**(6): 299–302.

Miller M. Gastrointestinal disorders. In: Rosene-Montella K, Keely E, Barbour LA, *et al.*, editors. *Medical Care of the Pregnant Patient.* 2nd ed. Philadelphia: ACP Press; 2008. pp. 549–66.

Moldenhauer J, O'Brien J, Barton J, *et al.* Acute fatty liver of pregnancy associated with pancreatitis: a life-threatening complication. *Am J Obstet Gynecol.* 2004; **190**(2): 502–5.

Moody GA, Probert G, Srivasta E, *et al.* Sexual dysfunction in women with Crohn's disease: a hidden problem. *Digestion.* 1992; **52**: 179–83.

Nagy S, Bush M, Berkowitz R, *et al.* Pregnancy outcome in liver transplant recipients. *Obstet Gynecol.* 2003; **102**(1): 121–8.

National Association of Colitis and Crohn's Disease. Home page. Available at: www.nacc.org.uk/content/home.asp (accessed 9 December 2008).

Nelson-Piercy C. *Handbook of Obstetric Medicine.* 3rd ed. Abingdon: Informa Healthcare; 2006.

Niebyl JR, Goodwin TM. Overview of nausea and vomiting of pregnancy with an emphasis on vitamins and ginger. *Am J Obstet Gynecol.* 2002; **186**(5 Pt. 3): S253–5.

Nightingale A. Diagnosis and management of inflammatory bowel disease. *Nurse Prescribing.* 2007; **5**(7): 289–96.

Obstetric Cholestasis Support. Home page. Available at: www.ocsupport.org.uk (accessed 9 December 2008).

Opatrny L, Michon N, Rey E. Preeclampsia as a cause of pancreatitis: a case report. *J Obstet Gynaecol Can.* 2004; **26**(6): 594–5.

Royal College of Obstetrics and Gynaecology. Obstetric Cholestasis: guideline 43. 2006. Available at: www.rcog.org.uk/resources/Public/pdf/obstetric_cholestasis43.pdf (accessed 9 December 2008).

Schutt VA, Minuk GY. Liver diseases unique to pregnancy. *Best Pract Res Clin Gastroenterol.* 2007; **21**(5): 771–92.

Sela H, Rojansky N, Hershko A. Reproduction and ulcerative colitis. A review. *J Reprod Med.* 2005; **50**(5): 361–6.

Smith G, Watson R. *Gastrointestinal Nursing.* Oxford: Blackwell; 2005.

Williamson C. Hepatic disorders. In: Greer IA, Nelson-Piercy C, Walters B, editors. *Maternal Medicine.* Edinburgh: Churchill Livingstone Elsevier; 2007. pp. 179–90.

Williamson C, Hems LM, Goulis DG, *et al.* Clinical outcome in a series of cases of obstetric cholestasis identified via a patient support group. *Br J Obstet Gynaecol.* 2004; **111**(7): 676–81.

CHAPTER 8

Disorders of the nervous system

CONTENTS
- → Epilepsy
- → Multiple sclerosis (MS)
- → Headaches

EPILEPSY

Epilepsy is a relatively common neurological condition affecting around one in 200 women attending antenatal clinics (Nelson-Piercy, 2006). The term epilepsy refers to a sudden abnormal discharge of electrical energy from cerebral neurones, which disrupts normal function. It is a group of disorders, not a single condition, and epilepsy affects each woman differently, with a range of symptoms and varying degrees of severity. There is concern for fetal well-being, particularly about congenital abnormalities associated with anti-epileptic treatment. Although in general a woman with epilepsy can expect good outcomes, her pregnancy is not without risk, as more seizures are reported in up to a third of pregnant women. The Confidential Enquiries have noted several deaths a year since 1988 in women with epilepsy (Lewis, 2007) and all authorities emphasise the need for good preconception care, as well as a high standard of care in pregnancy, labour and the puerperium from a skilled multidisciplinary team to ensure the woman's – and baby's – well-being.

PHYSIOLOGY AND PATHOPHYSIOLOGY
The neurone

Cerebral function works by the constant exchange of electrical signals along neural networks. Neurones are the cells of the nervous system, which is made up of the brain and spinal cord. These neurones gather and send information from senses such as touch and smell and send signals to effecter cells, such as muscles and glands (*see* Figure 8.1). Epileptic seizures occur when a large collection of neurones are activated simultaneously. Impulses starting in the brain cells stimulate muscle fibres to contract.

The axon is the output process of the neurone. Specialised cell junctions called

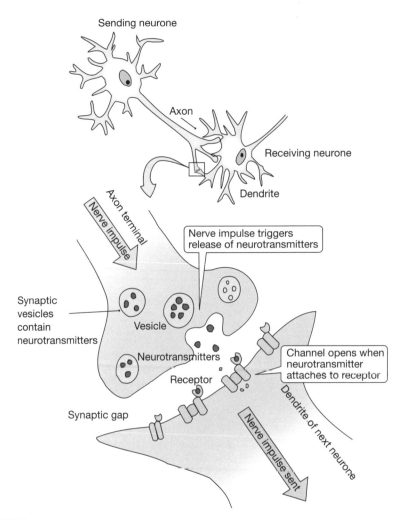

FIGURE 8.1: A neurone

synapses between the axon and other cells allow for efficient communication between cells. The input region comprises a complex arrangement of processes called dendrites. One axon (output) will synapse onto many different neurones and a dendrite will receive inputs from many neurones. Neurotransmitters are released across this synapse and once a critical point is reached an electrical (nerve) impulse (action potential) is fired down the axon. Some neurotransmitters, such as glutamate, are excitatory, triggering depolarisation of the post-synaptic membrane and thus producing an action potential. Inhibitory neurotransmitters such as gamma-aminobutyric acid (GABA) decrease the chance of post-synaptic action potential (Manford, 2003).

The excitability of individual neurones is affected by cell membrane properties, genetics, cell structure, spontaneous brain lesions or those occurring as a result of injury as well as the balance of inhibitory and excitatory neurotransmitters. In simple terms each person has a seizure threshold, which is the brain's individualised level of sensitivity to seizures, and this sensitivity is probably genetically determined. People with epilepsy have a lower-than-normal seizure threshold.

The brain

The location and extent of excessive neuronal discharge gives rise to varying symptoms and types of epilepsy. Looking at the structures of the brain gives some understanding of the different types of epilepsy. The three main areas of the brain are the cerebral cortex, the cerebellum and the brainstem, with the cerebral cortex being the area most likely to be affected by epilepsy.

The *cerebral cortex* (or cerebrum) is the main area of brain that governs behaviour and thought. It is made up of two hemispheres joined together at the base by the thick, multi-fibrous corpus callosum. Each hemisphere has four lobes – frontal, parietal, temporal and occipital. The *cerebellum* is situated just beneath the cerebral cortex and is important in controlling movement. The *brainstem* is vital to the performance of basic functions such as breathing, heartbeat and eye and tongue movements. Figure 8.2 shows key areas of the brain, denoting some aspects of function.

PREDISPOSING FACTORS IN EPILEPSY

Overall seizure threshold and hence an individual's tendency to have epilepsy, seems to be genetically determined. Everyone can have seizures given certain conditions, such as a high fever or after heavy drinking. Seizures in an infant can be outgrown as the brain develops. Epilepsy is generally classified into two types. Primary (idiopathic) epilepsy is where an inherited low convulsive threshold exists and there is no other obvious lesion. Secondary (symptomatic) epilepsy is when an identified lesion interferes with brain tissue (Lawal, 2005). Box 8.1 lists systemic causes of seizures.

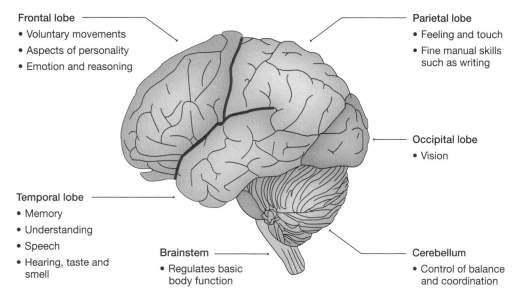

Frontal lobe
• Voluntary movements
• Aspects of personality
• Emotion and reasoning

Parietal lobe
• Feeling and touch
• Fine manual skills such as writing

Occipital lobe
• Vision

Temporal lobe
• Memory
• Understanding
• Speech
• Hearing, taste and smell

Brainstem
• Regulates basic body function

Cerebellum
• Control of balance and coordination

FIGURE 8.2: Areas of the brain

BOX 8.1: CAUSES OF SEIZURES

- Birth injury
- Brain tumours
- Head injury
- Drugs and alcohol
- Degenerative brain disease
- Metabolic imbalance
- Infection such as malaria and meningitis
- Febrile illness

(Davies, *et al.*, 2001; Lawal, 2005; WHO, 2001)

SEIZURE TRIGGERS

Seizures can be triggered by certain events and self-management of the condition seeks to minimise conditions that provoke a seizure. Pregnancy may contribute challenges to the prevention of seizures (discussed later). Some of the factors that have been identified as potential triggers to seizures are listed in Box 8.2.

BOX 8.2: TRIGGERS TO SEIZURE ACTIVITY

- Stress (including emotional stress)
- Lack of sleep
- Not taking medication. This can be a particular problem in pregnancy when women stop taking medication because they are concerned over possible harm to their babies
- Hormonal changes (catamenial epilepsy)
- Alcohol
- Lights, noises and patterns (photosensitive epilepsy)
- Intense exercise
- Hyperventilation
- Dietary factors
- Medications, including cough medicines and antidepressants
- Dehydration
- Constipation

(Lawal, 2005; Manford, 2003; Marshall and Crawford, 2006)

SEIZURES

Seizures vary from a brief lapse of attention which can go almost unnoticed to severe and prolonged convulsions which can cause injury and death. They can vary in frequency from less than one a year to several a day.

Tonic-clonic seizures, commonly known as grand mal, are probably what most people think of when epilepsy is mentioned. Women may recognise an impending seizure through some prodromal (anticipatory) symptom, such as nausea or a headache. For some the first they know about it is when they regain consciousness and see people gathered around them. During the tonic phase the woman's body initially goes rigid and she falls. Her jaw muscles contract and she may bite her tongue. Breathing stops momentarily and she may turn blue. She may be incontinent of urine and faeces. This tonic phase may last for a minute or more. The clonic phase starts immediately afterwards and involves rhythmically jerking movements lasting several seconds to minutes. Following the clonic phase is a period of recovery known as the postictal phase, where consciousness gradually returns. The woman may remain drowsy and disorientated for some time and usually has painful muscles and a bad headache. Up to 4% of women with epilepsy can experience a tonic-clonic seizure during labour or within the first 24 hours after birth (NICE, 2004a).

However, there are numerous forms of epilepsy apart from the tonic-clonic seizure described. There are also recognised phases of seizure activity. Women are advised to give information to midwives and other caregivers about the individual aspects of their epilepsy and discuss management strategies for the woman and midwife, should a seizure be predicted or observed, and the midwife should ensure this discussion takes place at the booking visit.

Classification of seizures

In *generalised seizures* discharge often occurs simultaneously throughout the cortex and consciousness is impaired. *See* Box 8.3 for description of different types of generalised seizures. *Partial or focal seizures* start in a particular part of the brain, though they may spread to the whole cortex, becoming what is known as secondary generalised seizures. *See* Box 8.4 for a description of partial seizures. Box 8.5 defines *status epilepticus*, the most serious form of seizure.

BOX 8.3: GENERALIZED SEIZURES

- *Absence* (petit mal) are blank spells that may be accompanied by little involuntary movements, such as blinking, fumbling or chewing. They usually last just a few seconds but may occur numerous times in a day and commonly begin in childhood.
- *Myoclonic.* Sudden jerky movements of whole body or of arms or legs. Usually fleeting but can occur a number of times a day.
- *Clonic.* Intermittent, rhythmical, muscular contraction and relaxation of legs, arms and sometimes the whole body, resulting in jerky movements.
- *Tonic.* A stiffening of the limbs or the whole body as a result of sustained muscular contraction. Usually causes a fall.
- *Tonic-clonic.* (*See* previous description.)
- *Atonic.* Sudden brief loss of muscle tone, causing person to fall. Sudden drop can cause injury.

(McElroy-Cox, 2007; Marshall and Crawford, 2006)

BOX 8.4: PARTIAL SEIZURES

- *Simple partial.* Affects a localised part of the brain and symptoms correspond to one of the four hemispheres (temporal, frontal, parietal, occipital) where the seizure starts. The person remains conscious and aware.
- *Complex partial.* Consciousness is impaired as a simple partial seizure spreads to areas that affect consciousness. Typically the sufferer appears to be in a trance or performing a series of movements over which they have no control (automatisms) such as chewing, scratching their head or plucking at their clothing.
- *Secondary generalised.* This results from the spread of simple or complex partial seizure throughout the brain.

(Lawal, 2005; McElroy-Cox, 2007; Marshall and Crawford, 2006)

BOX 8.5: STATUS EPILEPTICUS

Status epilepticus is a continuous prolonged seizure lasting for 30 minutes or more, or a series of seizures (> three) when there is no recovery in between. Besides having serious potential maternal effects, this can result in premature labour, rupture of membranes, abruption or fetal death (Carhuapoma, *et al.*, 2006).

ANTICONVULSANT MEDICATION

Whilst alternatives to drug management of epilepsy exist, such as lifestyle changes, surgery, mind-control therapies and use of seizure-alert dogs, drug management using anti-epileptic drugs (AEDs) remains the established treatment for most women. AEDs control seizures in up to 80% of epileptic patients, with most requiring only one drug (monotherapy). AEDs work by acting on neurones to slow down the tendency for action potential through alterations at the synaptic membrane or by the modulation of neurotransmitters, thus inhibiting the explosive bursts of electrical activity that cause seizures (Duncan, *et al.*, 2006). Box 8.6 lists common drugs used for epilepsy.

The physiological changes that occur in pregnancy influence the distribution, availability and metabolism of AEDs and adjusting medication as pregnancy progresses can be difficult (Adab and Chadwick, 2006). While it is beyond the role of the midwife to be involved in the prescription of medication, it is necessary for the midwife to be familiar with the drugs and common side effects. Midwives may get involved in discussions with women regarding the safety of drugs in pregnancy and lactation and therefore require some basic knowledge. It is essential that the woman is referred to specialist medical care for full discussion and choice. This choice will be based on balancing risks of uncontrolled convulsive seizures against possible risks to the fetus both from taking medication and from not taking it (Donaldson, 2002). Compliance with treatment is an area of concern and encouragement to explore options fully with a specialist should be given to optimise outcomes for mother and baby.

BOX 8.6: COMMON DRUGS USED FOR EPILEPSY

First-line drugs	Second-line drugs
carbamazepine **	clonazepam
phenytoin **	phenobarbitol**
ethosuximide	primidone**
lamotrigine*†	gabapentin*
sodium valproate	vigabatrin*

* New drugs. There is relatively little data upon which to base a definitive risk to the fetus (NICE, 2004b).

** Some AEDs interfere with the action of the combined oral contraceptive pill. The enzyme-inducing anti-epileptic drugs (EIAEDs) stimulate the activity of an enzyme in the liver known as P450 hepatic cytochrome. This enzyme increases the metabolism of oestrogen and progesterone, thereby lowering the blood concentrations of those drugs by 50% or more (O'Brien and Gilmour-White, 2005).

† Lamotrigine interferes with combined oral contraception, but by a different mechanism than that described above.

Teratogenicity

The area of greatest concern for the fetus is damage to it from the drugs the mother is taking to control her epileptic seizures. The incidence of fetal abnormality in the general population is around 2–3%. Most studies, including data from the UK Epilepsy and Pregnancy Register, show a twofold to threefold increased risk of major congenital malformations in babies of women with epilepsy, and this is largely attributed to medication (Breen and Davenport, 2006; Holmes, *et al.*, 2001; Morrow, *et al.*, 2006). Research into the effects of AEDs on the fetus are difficult because of small numbers, the range of different AEDs, combination therapy, questions over patient compliance with drug regimes and interaction with genetic traits which may predispose epileptic women to a higher rate of congenital malformations anyway (Breen and Davenport, 2006). Data from the UK Epilepsy and Pregnancy Register indicate that taking a single drug (monotherapy) at the lowest possible dose reduces risk. Risks rise significantly with use of valproate and combinations of more than one drug (polytherapy) (Morrow, *et al.*, 2006; NICE, 2004a; Tomson and Hiilesmaa, 2007). Box 8.7 lists some of the malformations that have been associated with AED exposure.

PRECONCEPTION CARE

Preconception care is extremely important for women with epilepsy, although there is evidence that many do not receive it (Scottish Intercollegiate Guidelines Network, 2003). Adjustments to medication should be made some time before pregnancy, where possible, to minimise risks to the fetus. However, one study found that half of women with epilepsy had not planned their pregnancy (Fairgrieve, *et al.*, 2000). This highlights the need for all those working with adolescents with epilepsy to ensure they understand the importance of good contraception and planned pregnancies.

The aim prior to conception is to achieve control of epilepsy on the lowest possible dose of a single drug, avoiding any known high-risk drugs (NICE, 2004a). New drugs may have fewer side effects but their effects on pregnancy or the fetus/baby are largely unknown (NICE, 2004b), so changing drugs needs to be done with expert help. With a sudden cessation of AEDs there is a risk of sudden unexpected death in epilepsy (SUDEP) (*see* Box 8.8) and status epilepticus (*see* Box 8.5). NICE guidelines (2004a) suggest individual counselling regarding drug regimes and their possible effect on the fetus.

BOX 8.7: NEWBORN PROBLEMS ASSOCIATED WITH AED EXPOSURE DURING PREGNANCY

- Congenital heart disease
- Neural tube defects
- Hypospadias
- Cleft lip and palate
- Fetal anticonvulsant syndrome: a range of dysmorphic features including cranio-facial features and hypoplasia of fingertips and fingernails
- Neuro-developmental delay
- Neonatal coagulopathy

(Adab and Chadwick, 2006; Fairgrieve, *et al.*, 2000; O'Brien and Gilmour-White, 2005)

BOX 8.8: SUDDEN UNEXPECTED DEATH IN EPILEPSY (SUDEP)

SUDEP is a recognised cause of death, possibly from cardiac arrhythmias, although the underlying pathophysiology is not clear. This also happens outside pregnancy and the estimation of occurrence ranges widely, the risk rising along with the severity of the epilepsy (Nilsson, *et al.*, 1999). SUDEP is not common in those whose seizure control is good (Nelson-Piercy, 2006). When a pregnant woman with epilepsy dies and no other cause of death is found, this may be the diagnosis.

Some AEDs are folate antagonists, and women taking these are recommended to take the higher dose of folic acid (5 mg) preconception and continue taking it throughout the pregnancy (NICE, 2004a). However, despite these recommendations, many studies have shown that this is not commonly done.

Some congenital abnormalities in the neonate may be related to genetics of the mother, not drugs (Donaldson, 2002), so during preconception counselling it may be valuable to take a detailed family history.

Genetic counselling concerning the specific risk of a woman passing on epilepsy to her child can be offered if the woman wishes it. The literature suggests there is about a 4–5% risk in general, but this varies according to the woman's individual condition and that of her partner.

PREGNANCY CARE
Multidisciplinary care
It is strongly recommended by the *Report on Confidential Enquiries into Maternal Deaths* (Lewis, 2007) that all women with epilepsy should be looked after in pregnancy

by specialist combined obstetric and medical/neurological teams, which seems vital, considering the complexity of many of these women's needs.

This enquiry into maternal deaths (2003–2005) (Lewis, 2007) identified 11 deaths in women with epilepsy and determined that the cause of death for six women was due to SUDEP (*see* Box 8.8). Another potentially fatal risk to women and their fetuses is status epilepticus (*see* Box 8.5), which may complicate 1–2.5% of pregnancies in women with epilepsy (Nelson-Piercy, 2006). Obesity, non-compliance with medication and learning difficulties may increase the rate of sudden death (Nelson-Piercy, 2002). However, in the 10 years from 1988–1999, 19 women with epilepsy died, but only five had poorly controlled epilepsy, and two had not fitted for two years (Nelson-Piercy, 2002), so prediction of mortality or morbidity from risk factors is difficult.

Seizure activity

For most women pregnancy does not affect the number of epileptic seizures they experience. Those women with catamenial epilepsy (related to menstrual cycle variations) can show improvement. However, about 10–30% of women will have an increase in seizure frequency (Nelson-Piercy, 2002; Swartjes and van Geijn, 1998). The likelihood of fitting during pregnancy is related to control: the longer the woman has gone without fitting pre-pregnancy, the less likely she is to fit during pregnancy, but those who normally fit about once a month are most at risk of increased seizures during pregnancy (Crawford, *et al.*, 1999; Donaldson, 2002).

When increased seizures have been noted, they can most commonly be attributed to non-compliance in medication or decreased drug levels from vomiting, reduced sleep, stress (Nelson-Piercy, 2002) or weight gain and metabolic changes (Crawford, 2002).

Drugs

Because of the risk of fits when changing drugs, the American Academy of Neurology suggests not altering drugs after 10 weeks of pregnancy, as the major fetal organs are already formed and changing drugs may precipitate seizures (Koh and DeGiorgio, 2008).

Drug dosages may need to change during pregnancy as the serum concentration levels alter due to the effect of haemodilution. During pregnancy individual women may need regular (perhaps monthly) blood tests of drug levels (the free protein-unbound anti-convulsive level may be more reliable than the total anti-convulsive level) so dosages can be altered to maintain that woman's predetermined therapeutic level (Donaldson, 2002). Testing is also useful when there is concern about toxicity or adherence (Scottish Intercollegiate Guidelines Network, 2003). However, the routine monitoring of drug levels is not helpful (Nelson-Piercy, 2006; NICE, 2004a), except for women taking phenytoin, as the levels correlate poorly with seizure control (Scottish Intercollegiate Guidelines Network, 2003).

Many women fear the potential harm the drugs they take may do to their baby. It should be ensured that women are treated as partners in their care and that they are fully informed and participate in discussions about drug changes. It has been demonstrated that counselling increases compliance with drug regimes and improves epileptic control in pregnancy (Manford, 2003).

As previously mentioned, an increased dose of folic acid should continue daily throughout the pregnancy as there is a risk of anti-convulsant-induced folate deficiency (Nelson-Piercy, 2006). It has also been suggested that supplementation with vitamin D may be useful, as some AEDs may lead to malabsorption.

Women taking AEDs have an increased risk of their baby having haemorrhagic disease of the newborn (HDN) (*see* section on *fetus/neonate* following for a full explanation). An oral dose of vitamin K (10–20 mg) from about four weeks before the expected delivery may be prescribed (Koh and DeGiorgio, 2008; Nelson-Piercy, 2006), although some believe this is necessary only for women who have an additional risk, such as those with liver disease or those who anticipate a premature delivery (Scottish Intercollegiate Guidelines Network, 2003).

Fetal assessment

The main risk identified for women with epilepsy is the increase in congenital abnormalities in the fetus. Antenatal fetal screening and diagnostic tests, where appropriate, should be offered to all women with epilepsy, together with information on their risks, and then they can – as all women should – make an informed decision that is right for them. Of particular importance is a detailed ultrasound at 18–20 weeks to rule out neural tube defects, and a repeat ultrasound (or perhaps a fetal echocardiogram) at 22 weeks to detect any cardiac anomalies. Some women need regular growth scans as IUGR is associated with some AEDs (Crawford, 2002).

Pregnancy complications

Traditionally women with epilepsy have been reported to be at increased risk of pre-eclampsia, APH and premature labour (Crawford, *et al.*, 1999; Foldvary, 2001). This, however, may no longer be true and it is now considered that women with epilepsy may not have increased pregnancy complication rates (Adab and Chadwick, 2006; Nelson-Piercy, 2006).

It has been suggested that the incidence of breech presentation is increased, perhaps because the drugs slow the fetus's movements so it does not turn to cephalic (Marshall and Crawford, 2006), but this is not well documented.

As enzyme-inducing AEDs accelerate the metabolism of steroids, if it is necessary to give steroids to a woman with threatened premature labour the dose should be increased (Scottish Intercollegiate Guidelines Network, 2003) and given over a longer time.

Midwifery advice and support

It may be appropriate for the midwife to take on the role of giving the woman advice and support in coping with specific aspects of epilepsy during pregnancy, as well as general pregnancy concerns. Initially, the nausea and vomiting of pregnancy may compromise her drug regime and this needs to be urgently addressed. Since common problems such as lack of sleep or constipation can trigger seizures (*see* Box 8.2) in some women, the midwife could advise solutions. Hyperventilation is also a trigger for a seizure and, as this is common during labour, the midwife could ensure her client knows about effective breathing techniques to counter this. It is also wise to make a plan for the problems that may arise in the postnatal period as time is often limited in the early puerperium. Appropriate reading could be suggested, not only around pregnancy and new motherhood, but also to update her, if necessary, on her condition, which she probably had first diagnosed in childhood.

Some basic advice for pregnancy
▶ Take medication regularly.
▶ Get enough sleep (naps and learn relaxation techniques).
▶ Parentcraft/yoga classes for breathing techniques.
▶ Avoid constipation.
▶ Access specific literature to learn more about condition.

LABOUR AND IMMEDIATE POSTNATAL CARE
There is a possibility of increased seizure activity during labour and triggers could include poor absorption of drugs due to the physiological changes of labour (Nelson-Piercy, 2002), sleep deprivation, hyperventilation, dehydration or stress (Scottish Intercollegiate Guidelines Network, 2003). For this reason these women should not be left alone during this time. Medication needs to be given as usual, but if the woman has a history of fitting in previous labours, perhaps this could be given rectally or intravenously during labour. NICE (2004a) consider there is only a low risk (1–4%) of seizure at this time, but this is largely unpredictable.

BOX 8.9: BASIC CARE DURING A SEIZURE

Apart from the first four of these actions, these may be carried out in any order depending on the situation and the help available.
- Call/send for help but stay with the woman.
- Maintain safety (e.g., ensure the woman does not hit her head, etc., but do not restrain her or insert anything into her mouth).
- Maintain a patent airway.
- Put her in the recovery position as soon as possible.
- Give her oxygen.
- Cannulate.
- Send bloods as appropriate (tests should include toxicology and AED levels).
- Give IV drugs, usually benzodiazepines (e.g., lorazepam, diazepam) and anticonvulsives (e.g., phenytoin) – or rectal diazepam if necessary.
- CTG if pregnant.
- Throughout, if possible, observe what is happening during the fit (e.g., cyanosis) and how long each stage lasts.

Seizures in labour
Seizures in labour can be treated with IV lorazepam or IV/rectal diazepam (Nelson-Piercy, 2006; Scottish Intercollegiate Guidelines Network, 2003). As in the care of any fit (*see* Box 8.9), attention must be paid to maintaining the woman's airway. Oxygen should be administered and attaching a saturation monitor is an easy way to monitor its effectiveness. If there is any question of eclampsia, then magnesium sulphate

is given. As soon as the woman's condition is stabilised, early delivery is considered. Status epilepticus (*see* Box 8.5) in labour is associated with maternal and fetal mortality (Scottish Intercollegiate Guidelines Network, 2003).

Analgesia

Pethidine (meperidine) is not recommended as it can trigger seizures (Koh and DeGiorgio, 2008). There are no reasons Entonox cannot be used, but hyperventilation (also known as a possible trigger for seizures) should be avoided – breathing exercises taught in the antenatal period can help. There are no contraindications to epidural analgesia and an early siting may be recommended to avoid a seizure triggered by anxiety or pain (Nelson-Piercy, 2002).

Delivery

It has been reported that there is an increased rate of instrumental and operative delivery (Fonager, *et al.*, 2000; Katz and Devinsky, 2003), possibly because of less effective contractions caused by AEDs (Pennell, 2004). However, skilful midwifery care should optimise the woman's chance of a normal birth.

POSTNATAL CARE

One to two per cent of women will have a seizure in the first 24 hours postnatal (Nelson-Piercy, 2006) and therefore close supervision should be available. In fact, the main risk for unexpected seizures may come in the puerperium in general, and it is important to prepare the woman for this, although NICE (2004a) suggests that an increase in the first few months after birth is unlikely.

AED levels need to be assessed in the postnatal period. If the dose was increased in pregnancy, it may need to be adjusted (Scottish Intercollegiate Guidelines Network, 2003). It is known that the most common complaint by all new mothers is fatigue (Bick, *et al.*, 2001). For those who are epileptic there is the danger of lack of sleep triggering seizures. A plan should be made by all women with this risk, to ensure they can schedule in naps or obtain help during the night to ensure they get enough sleep. Relaxation techniques taught in pregnancy may continue to be helpful in the puerperium.

Breastfeeding should usually be encouraged by midwives, although data on individual drugs needs to be reviewed as some are contraindicated. Generally, the level of drugs in breast milk is considered to be much less than the amount the fetus received via the placenta and therefore breastfeeding can prevent drug withdrawal by babies, by giving them minute amounts of the drug in breast milk. If the baby is not breastfed, it may show withdrawal symptoms from some maternal drugs (Donaldson, 2002).

Advice can be given to mothers, if they feel their babies seem sleepy, to try and feed before they take their medication, so the serum concentration – and therefore the drugs in the breast milk – may be less (Nelson-Piercy, 2002). Accumulation of the drugs in the neonate, especially if the baby is premature, is possible, so individual decisions on feeding must be made, in conjunction with the paediatrician, based on the condition of the baby and the drug involved.

New mothers may worry about keeping their baby safe if they have a fit. Safety leaflets are available with relevant advice (*see* Box 8.10 for some examples) and these should have been accessed from support organisations by the mother before she goes home. It is also important that the woman herself keeps as safe as possible. Recommendations have been made by the *Report on Confidential Enquiries into Maternal Deaths* (Lewis, 2001) following the deaths of women in baths, presumably following a fit, that women should shower or only bath with someone else around or in very shallow water.

BOX 8.10: EXAMPLES OF SAFETY INFORMATION FOR THE MOTHER WITH EPILEPSY

- Change or dress the baby on the floor.
- Fit a brake to the pram/pushchair which will operate if the mother lets go.
- Feed and cuddle the baby when propped up comfortably against the wall on the floor.
- Only bath the baby if someone else is there, or wipe them instead of bathing.
- Keep hot drinks, etc. away from the baby.

Extra support may be needed by those women with a learning or physical disability (Scottish Intercollegiate Guidelines Network, 2003).

Contraception

Some AEDs interfere with the action of the combined oral contraceptive pill (*see* Box 8.6) (Doggett-Jones, 2007). Effective contraception is vital for women with epilepsy as a planned pregnancy is so important, and therefore specialist advice should be sought.

FETUS/NEONATE

Perinatal mortality is higher in babies of epileptic mothers than in the general population, although improvements in the rate have been seen to occur over the years (Crawford, 2002). Babies have a higher risk of prematurity and fetal distress in labour (Crawford, 2002). Babies of epileptic women may be more vulnerable to IUGR, although this is probably associated with women taking more than one AED, indicating those with more complex epilepsy (Hvas, *et al.*, 2000). Kaaja *et al.* (2003) found no association between increased seizures in the first trimester and malformations, and other investigators have confirmed this for the duration of pregnancy (Nelson-Piercy, 2006).

It appears that the fetus is tolerant of isolated tonic-clonic (grand mal) seizures, even though during a seizure the fetus will inevitably suffer some hypoxia. Fetal bradycardia has been documented during and after maternal seizures (Donaldson, 2002; Nelson-Piercy, 2006) but there is no data on the long-term effects on the child (Nelson-Piercy, 2002). There is a possible association between seizures and fetal intracranial haemorrhage and fetal loss (Yerby, 2000). Non-convulsive seizures are believed to be of little risk to the fetus (Adab and Chadwick, 2006). Status epilepticus, where seizure is continuous, is dangerous for the mother and fetus and can result in maternal and/or fetal death.

If the mother received a sedative AED (such as lorazepam) during labour, the baby is at risk of respiratory depression initially and may need respiratory support (Manford, 2003).

It has been suggested that babies of mothers receiving EIAEDs are at risk of haemorrhagic disease of the newborn within 24 hours of birth, despite routine vitamin K for the newborn (Crawford, 2002), because of a reduction in vitamin K clotting factors caused by these drugs (Pennell, 2003). Whether the mother has received oral vitamin K in the last month of her pregnancy or not, it is very important that the baby receive 1 mg IM vitamin K following birth (NICE, 2004a). Some authorities have suggested that the baby have 1 mg vitamin K at birth, and then again at 12 hours old (Little, 2006).

If a woman has been taking AEDs during pregnancy, the neonate should receive a thorough paediatric examination to rule out congenital abnormalities, even if the woman has had full antenatal screening. Major and minor congenital abnormalities and children with cognitive impairment (Koh and DeGiorgio, 2008) are associated with anti-epileptic drugs (*see teratogenicity* earlier in this chapter).

PSYCHOSOCIAL ISSUES

Living with epilepsy may involve a constant fear of seizures, taking daily medication, perhaps not being able to drive and having uncertainties over career and relationships. Along with medical concerns of managing epilepsy, a bigger problem may be self-imposed limitations and overprotection from others (Marshall and Crawford, 2006). This aspect is important to consider as midwives seek to empower women to manage the challenges of pregnancy effectively and promote good mother/child relationships.

It must also be remembered by all midwives that new motherhood is a vulnerable and emotional time for all women, but women with epilepsy may find it particularly difficult as they may blame their disease for their 'inadequacies'. Support – in particular contact with other new mothers – may help alleviate these feelings.

MULTIPLE SCLEROSIS (MS)

Multiple sclerosis (MS) is an autoimmune neurological condition affecting young adults. Two-thirds of MS patients are women of child-bearing age (Pickard, *et al.*, 2008). Women with MS have individual symptoms with a varying degree of impairment relating to the extent and pattern of neurological damage. In addition to physical symptoms such as numbness, tingling and weakness of limbs, feelings of fatigue and an increased rate of depression add an emotional strain to the illness which may be heightened when pregnancy and parenthood are contemplated. Pregnancy is not thought to lead to an exacerbation of the illness; however, relapse in the postnatal period is more common (Vukusic, *et al.*, 2004).

MS is a particularly relevant medical condition for midwives, as women with MS will often need limited medical input from obstetricians and neurologists, but their pregnancy, birth and new-parent experience can be immeasurably improved by knowledgeable and committed midwifery care. Midwives can provide practical, sensitive and individualised care working in partnership with women and acknowledging the emotional and physical concerns of the illness.

PATHOPHYSIOLOGY

The central nervous system, which is made up of the brain and spinal cord, is composed primarily of nerve cells called neurones (*see* Figure 8.1). Each neurone is protected by a fatty white insulating substance called myelin. Myelin improves the conduction of the electrical impulses that travel along the nerves. In MS there is activation of the immune cells, CD4 and T cells, which self-attack a protein component of the myelin sheath. Scarring and oedema occurs at the site as part of the inflammatory response. Hardened areas or plaques known as sclerosis develop (Boss, 2006). Multiple lesions form in various locations seemingly randomly and hence the name multiple sclerosis. Demyelination involves the breakdown of the myelin occurring as a result of the repeated and progressive inflammatory damage described. Without this protective covering the nerves do not function as efficiently, leading to the neurological symptoms that characterise MS (*see* Figure 8.3).

The cause of the autoimmune response is unknown but it is thought to be an interaction of a genetic tendency with environmental factors (Boss, 2006; Compston, 1999; MS Trust, 2007). It is rare in tropical areas and more common in the temperate regions of Europe and North America. Proposed environmental triggers for MS include inadequate vitamin D, Epstein-Barr viral infection and smoking (Ascherio and Munger, 2008).

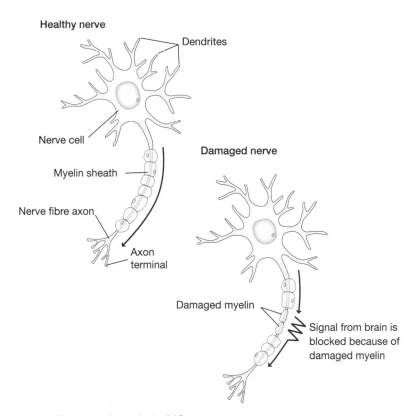

FIGURE 8.3: Damaged myelin in MS

GENETICS OF MS

MS does not exhibit a defined pattern of inheritance but 15% of people with MS will have an affected relative. There is a slightly higher incidence of MS in the children of parents with the condition. The risk of MS is about 0.1% in the whole population, compared to a risk of 3% in children born to a parent with MS (Compston, 1999).

CHARACTERISTICS OF MS

MS is characterised by periods of progression, remission and relapse (*see* Box 8.11). *Progression* describes the gradual worsening of symptoms. *Remission* is a period during which symptoms decrease and can vary from weeks to years. A *relapse* is a period of exacerbated symptoms and can occur as a result of an infection or in response to psychological or physical stress. These may be factors in postnatal relapse. Symptoms can be made worse by fever or hot environments (MS Trust, 2007; NICE, 2003).

BOX 8.11: TYPES OF MS

- *Relapsing-remitting MS (RR–MS):* The most common form of MS overall (80%), it affects the young age group and is more common in women. Symptoms come and go. Features flare up, with deterioration over a period of several days, during which new symptoms can appear and/or old ones resurface, followed by improvement (remission). Relapses occur approximately once or twice every two years.
- *Primary progressive MS:* Symptoms worsen from onset of disease, with only occasional and limited remission. This is less common (10%), and men are most likely to be affected.
- *Secondary progressive MS:* Remission gradually occurs less frequently with reduced improvement. Half those with relapsing-remitting MS develop secondary progressive MS in the first 10 years after diagnosis.
- *Benign MS:* Affects 10% of people, who do well for more than 15 years

(Boss, 2006; MS Trust, 2007; NICE, 2003)

MS is usually difficult to diagnose. Often the diagnosis is divided into possible, probable and definite, as the symptoms and investigations become gradually clearer (Robinson, *et al.*, 2000). Diagnosis is based on clinical signs, use of MRI and analysis of CSF (cerebrospinal fluid) (Pickard, *et al.*, 2008). Symptoms may first present in the puerperium (Pickard, *et al.*, 2008).

One of the first and often most persistent symptoms of MS is fatigue (other possible symptoms are listed in Box 8.12). The degree to which the woman is affected varies according to individuals, together with the type of impairment and how quickly the disease progresses, making it very difficult for a woman planning pregnancy to predict her ability to parent in the way she would perhaps wish. It has been suggested that women with MS have a high level of terminations (Taylor, 1997) and this could be seen as reflecting the uncertainty of this disease.

There is no cure for MS and treatment is aimed at alleviating symptoms and/or providing support, depending on the system(s) affected. Many consider nutrition to be an important factor and advise a diet low in saturated fat, with increased unsaturated fats (Graham, 1999). Complementary therapies are also widely used.

BOX 8.12: SYMPTOMS OF MS

- Weakness/clumsiness
- Lack of balance/gait ataxia
- Fatigue
- Loss of sexual sensation in women, impotence in men
- Inappropriate sensations of heat and cold
- Bladder dysfunction, including urgency and incontinence
- Bowel dysfunction
- Numbness, tingling and weakness of limbs
- Visual and speech disturbances
- Muscle stiffness, spasms, pain
- Cognitive difficulties (e.g., crying inappropriately)

Recent studies have confirmed that during pregnancy MS improves or at least remains stable (Vukusic, *et al.*, 2004). The risk of relapse during pregnancy decreases, although it increases transiently in the postnatal period (NICE, 2003). This improvement is thought to be related to the relative immune suppression of pregnancy that prevents fetal rejection (McKay-Moffat, 2007). However, the usual so-called minor disorders of pregnancy caused by the physiological changes of pregnancy may pose particular difficulties for a mother with MS, aggravating existing symptoms (Taylor, 1997). Fatigue and sensitivity to heat may increase. Mobility may be further impaired by weight changes affecting balance and putting increased strain on weakened limbs. Constipation and urinary symptoms of pregnancy will pose challenges to the mother with MS. Control of urine may be difficult.

PRECONCEPTION CARE

Those taking drugs (commonly muscle relaxants, immunosuppressants or anti-muscarinics) should have their medication reviewed for a potential effect on a fetus and perhaps change or modify their drugs before pregnancy (Ferrero, *et al.*, 2006).

PREGNANCY CARE

Care for the woman with MS should be multidisciplinary, including not only the midwife, obstetrician and neurologist, but also an MS nurse and perhaps occupational therapists, physiotherapists, incontinence nurses or others, according to the woman's needs.

A problem identified in the literature (McKay-Moffat and Cunningham, 2006) is the possibility of restricted communication between the midwife and woman, probably reflecting the midwife's desire to be sensitive and not cause offence. The midwife should ensure a detailed, honest dialogue takes place concerning the woman's needs and abilities, and then she will be in a position to offer appropriate help or suggest resources. This situation will be greatly improved if there is one-to-one care, so the woman and midwife can develop a trusting relationship. However, the midwife also needs to keep good records and ideally a care plan, as others will need information if involved.

Midwives can work with the woman and the relevant other agencies to help her plan for the postnatal period (Royal College of Midwives, 2000). If the woman needs help, identifying how and where she can get it can reduce anxiety and stress during pregnancy and the postnatal period, and this may perhaps reduce the severity of exacerbations (Graham, 1999). It is appropriate for the woman to meet the health visitor (and community midwife, if she is not receiving one-to-one care) to enable planning for baby care at home to begin. If the woman has a local MS nurse, the nurse may be able to introduce her to other new parents in her community, and they may be able to offer valuable advice. The resources listed at the end of this section may also be useful.

During the pregnancy it is important that the midwife and woman visit the hospital wards together to try and predict any problems (for example, with mobility aids, toilet and washing facilities, etc.) and ensure a plan is made and resources are accessed before delivery. Consideration of the possible triggers of a relapse (*see* Box 8.13), could help the midwife to provide an appropriate environment. For example, a hot environment can make symptoms worse. The woman is the expert in her needs and her suggestions will probably greatly aid her care (Seaman, 2007).

If preconception care was not carried out, a medication review should be undertaken as soon as possible. Some drugs have limited information about their safety in pregnancy and should be discontinued (Ferrero, *et al.*, 2006). However, these decisions need to be made according to individual women's needs and it is important that women should not stop prescribed medication without receiving expert advice.

There is no evidence that MS has any effect on the complications of pregnancy such as miscarriage, pre-eclampsia, gestational diabetes or premature birth, nor is there evidence that it affects the baby's birth weight or well-being (Sandberg-Wollheim, *et al.*, 2005; Dahl, *et al.*, 2005). However, many of the minor disorders of pregnancy may have an increased affect on the woman with MS. Constipation may be more likely with decreased mobility, and the usual advice and treatment may need to be started promptly. Urinary tract infections are common in pregnancy, but for a woman with MS an infection may trigger a relapse, so regular, careful screening needs to be undertaken. Fatigue is a feature of most MS sufferers, and in pregnancy this can become extreme, sometimes contributed to by increased heat sensitivity.

As many pregnancy symptoms can exacerbate or minic MS symptoms (for example, increasing size affecting balance, back pain, descent of the fetal head affecting bladder control), the midwife must reassure the woman that these can be normal pregnancy complaints. Women with MS may have altered pelvic sensation so may not feel uterine contractions (McKay-Moffat, 2007) and therefore may not recognise the onset of labour. Teaching her to palpate contractions may be useful.

LABOUR CARE

Labour care needs to be adapted to the individual woman's needs. For example, a woman with limited mobility may be vulnerable to pressure area compromise.

Distension of the bladder must be avoided. If muscle tone is poor, certain positions and pushing in the second stage may be a challenge and an instrumental delivery may be appropriate. A woman with restricted ability to abduct her hips may be limited in her delivery options and vaginal examinations may be difficult as well as possibly being painful. Having a known midwife who understands her abilities and needs with her at this time will make labour easier for both the woman and her carer.

If corticosteroids have been taken during the antenatal period, then stress dose steroids are usually given in labour.

Most authorities suggest all usual labour analgesias are acceptable (Nelson-Piercy, 2006) and, although in the past there has been some controversy over spinal analgesia, which has traditionally been avoided in women with MS, most anaesthetists now undertake regional blocks with pre-assessment and informed consent (Drake, *et al.*, 2006). There have also been reports of transcutaneous electrical nerve stimulation (TENS) causing spasms in some women (Watkiss and Ward, 2002).

The woman with MS is vulnerable to relapse induced by infection or pyrexia, so particular care needs to be taken to prevent infection.

POSTNATAL CARE

As in pregnancy, common symptoms of the puerperium (fatigue, forgetfulness, distraction) can be seen as MS symptoms, and the woman should be made aware that these feelings are normal. However, there does appear to be an increase in exacerbations in the postnatal period (Carhuapoma, *et al.*, 2006; McKay-Moffat, 2007) that occurs most often in the first three months. However, a recent study found 72% did not relapse (Vukusic, *et al.*, 2004), which was a higher figure than had previously been thought. As in many medical conditions, it was found that those who had suffered a recent relapse or had greater disability before pregnancy were more likely to have a postnatal relapse. MS can also develop for the first time following childbirth (Lorenzi and Ford, 2002).

To reduce the risk of a postnatal relapse, the midwife could note the possible contributory factors (*see* Box 8.13) and address these wherever possible. Although they are more usual in the first three months, the risk of postnatal relapse continues for almost the entire first year; therefore the woman needs to be aware that she may be vulnerable during this time and may need to access extra help.

BOX 8.13: POSSIBLE CONTRIBUTORY FACTORS TO EXACERBATIONS

- Inadequate rest
- Stress
- Infection
- Overheating
- Anaemia
- Compromised nutrition

Many women with MS have bladder problems and may fear childbirth will make these worse, although recent research has shown no difference between those with MS who had given birth and those who had not (Durufle, *et al.*, 2006).

Breastfeeding should be encouraged (as with all women), but for women with MS it may be particularly important for her to feel she is doing something positive for the baby. There is also a suggestion that those who breastfeed have a lower relapse rate in the postnatal period (Vukusic, *et al.*, 2004). If she has compromised strength in her arms, the midwife will need to be creative in helping her to find methods and positions that will make breastfeeding possible. Occupational therapy departments may be able to provide specific equipment if appropriate, and this should have been arranged during the pregnancy. However, if she is taking medication at this time, it must be reviewed for safety during breastfeeding.

Contraception choices may be limited for a woman with MS. For example, if her mobility is compromised an oral contraceptive containing oestrogen may increase her risk of thromboembolism. However, this is a vital subject for discussion and therefore care must be taken to tailor contraceptive advice to the individual woman's situation.

An increased risk of postnatal depression has been suggested (Taylor, 1997) and appropriate support should be made available by the midwife and health visitor in order to screen for and treat this condition.

PSYCHOSOCIAL ISSUES
Pregnancy can be a very anxious time for a woman with MS. The uncertainty of the progression of her disease will live with her every day, but if she has few physical signs to remind the midwife of her condition, this can be easily overlooked. The midwife needs to be particularly sensitive to seemingly irrational fears and concerns.

USEFUL RESOURCES:
▶ Disabled Parents Network (www.disabledparentsnetwork.org.uk): maternity services and support for new parents.
▶ MS Trust (www.mstrust.org.uk): fact sheets for pregnancy.
▶ MS Society (www.mssociety.org.uk).
▶ Disability, Pregnancy and Parenthood International (www.dppi.org.uk).

HEADACHES
A headache is a symptom commonly experienced by most women of child-bearing age (Von Wald and Walling, 2002). It is common in pregnancy and mostly entirely harmless, but midwives need to be alert to headache symptoms that may be indicative of a more serious complication, making appropriate referral (Carhuapoma, *et al.*, 2006). Most headaches experienced by pregnant women are tension headaches or migraines. These are termed primary headaches, where the headache is the dominant symptom. Primary headaches tend to improve in pregnancy after the 16th week, when the tiredness of pregnancy diminishes (Lowe, 2007). Pregnant women have increased vulnerability to some types of secondary headache, where the headache arises from an underlying condition (Von Wald and Walling, 2002). Box 8.14 lists possible causes of secondary headache in pregnancy, although these remain uncommon.

TENSION (OR MUSCLE CONTRACTION) HEADACHES
Tension headaches are the most common headache overall. They are bilateral, mild to moderate in intensity and are often described as squeezing or pressure-like. They are

not usually associated with nausea, but if it is present it is minimal (Lowe, 2007; Pickard and Barbour, 2008). Tension headaches are thought to be due to muscular tension and are related to periods of stress (Nelson-Piercy, 2006). They generally improve with rest and simple analgesics (Lowe, 2007). Tension headaches have not been studied much in pregnancy, so it is difficult to determine the impact of pregnancy on the incidence of tension headaches. Some writers suggest little change in their incidence (Pickard and Barbour, 2008), whilst others suggest that psychological factors and muscular skeletal changes in pregnancy increase the likelihood of such headaches (Von Wald and Walling, 2002).

BOX 8.14: POSSIBLE CAUSES OF SECONDARY HEADACHE IN PREGNANCY

- Head and neck trauma (domestic violence, road traffic accidents)
- Vascular complications (subarachnoid haemorrhage, stroke)
- Increased cerebrospinal fluid pressure
- Substance abuse/withdrawal
- Systemic infections
- Intracranial mass lesions

Conditions unique or more common in pregnancy
- Pre-eclampsia
- Idiopathic intracranial hypertension
- Cerebral venous thrombosis
- Post-dural puncture headache complicating insertion of epidural catheter

(Lowe, 2007; Nelson-Piercy, 2006; Von Wald and Walling, 2002)

MIGRAINE HEADACHES

The cause of headache pain is complex and poorly understood. Migraine is thought to be due to vasodilatation of cerebral blood vessels (Nelson-Piercy, 2006), although a combination of vascular, neurological and other influences play a role.

Migraines are described as being severe, often throbbing, usually unilateral headaches which may be accompanied by nausea and vomiting, photophobia (avoidance of light) and phonophobia (avoidance of sound). Migraines can occur rarely or several times a month and last between four and 48 hours (Pickard and Barbour, 2008; Von Wald and Walling, 2002). Migraines can be subdivided into those that are preceded by an aura and those that are not. Only 18% of migraine sufferers experience an aura, which typically lasts 20–30 minutes before the headache. This aura can be a visual disturbance, tingling and numbness of the face, speech disturbances or weakness of arms and legs (Von Wald and Walling, 2002). Migraine is more common in women, with a higher prevalence during the reproductive years. Migraines run in families, with women often reporting that their female relatives have migraines. Box 8.15 lists triggers to developing a migraine.

Migraines tend to occur less frequently overall and be less severe in pregnancy, particularly by the third trimester (Goadsby, et al., 2008). Those women whose migraines are linked to menstruation are the most likely to show improvement in pregnancy (Carhuapoma, *et al.*, 2006) and the relative hormonal stability of pregnancy is thought to bring about that improvement (Goadsby, *et al.*, 2008). However, some women experience migraine for the first time in pregnancy or puerperium (Goadsby, *et al.*, 2008). Headaches tend to worsen in the puerperium, with a third of migraine sufferers experiencing a migraine in the first week post-partum (Carhuapoma, *et al.*, 2006).

BOX 8.15: TRIGGERS TO DEVELOPING A MIGRAINE

- Dietary factors – chocolate, cheese
- Pre-menstruation
- Oral contraceptive pill
- Weather changes
- Lack of sleep

(Nelson-Piercy, 2006; Goadsby, *et al.*, 2008)

CARE ISSUES

During pregnancy many women wish to treat their headaches without medication, and strategies such as rest, ice packs and fluids could be suggested. However, many women will take a simple analgesic such as paracetamol with good results.

Although most headaches are non-threatening, if they are prolonged; of sudden, severe onset; involve a change in the level of consciousness, understanding, vision, or mobility; or are associated with trauma, high blood pressure or other signs such as pyrexia (Von Wald and Walling, 2002), then urgent attention should be sought.

When a woman has a headache, pre-eclampsia should be considered as a possible cause, although the association, according to Lowe (2007), between pre-eclampsia and headache is not as strong as many have thought. Nevertheless, a full assessment of the woman's condition should be undertaken. A history of migraine headaches may predispose a woman to pre-eclampsia, especially when this is also associated with obesity (Adeney, *et al.*, 2005).

A post-dural-puncture headache can occur following an accidental dural puncture during the insertion of an epidural. The pain is related to posture, occurring or worsening when becoming upright. The woman will be cared for lying flat, and if the headache persists, it is usually treated with a blood patch (Thew and Paech, 2008).

One study which considered persistent postnatal headaches found 47% were tension/migraine headaches, 24% were associated with pre-eclampsia, 16% were post-dural-tap headaches and the remainder (13%) needed further investigation with cerebral imaging (Stella, *et al.*, 2007). Although headaches are common and usually benign, midwives need to take women's complaints seriously. Headaches which are persistent should be referred for medical opinion.

REFERENCES

Adab N, Chadwick D. Management of women with epilepsy during pregnancy. *Obstet Gynaecol.* 2006; **8**(1): 20–5.

Adeney K, Williams M, Miller R, *et al.* Risk of preeclampsia in relation to maternal history of migraine headaches. *J Matern Fetal Med.* 2005; **18**(3): 167–72.

Ascherio A, Munger K. Epidemiology of multiple sclerosis: from risk factors to prevention. *Semin Neurol.* 2008; **28**(1): 17–28.

Bick D, MacArthur C, Knowles H, *et al. Postnatal Care.* Edinburgh: Elsevier Health Sciences; 2001.

Boss BJ. Alterations of neurological function. In: McCance KL, Huether SE, editors. *Pathophysiology: the biological basis for diseases in adults and children.* 5th ed. St Louis, MO: Elsevier Mosby; 2006. pp. 547–604.

Breen DP, Davenport RJ. Teratogenicity of anti-epileptic drugs. *BMJ.* 2006; **333**: 615–16.

Carhuapoma J, Tomlinson M, Levine S. Neurological disorders. In: James DK, Weiner CP, Steer PJ, *et al.*, editors. *High Risk Pregnancy: management options.* 3rd ed. Philadelphia, PA: Elsevier Saunders; 2006. pp. 1061–97.

Compston A. The genetic epidemiology of multiple sclerosis. *Philos Trans R Soc Lond B Biol Sci.* 1999; **354**(1390): 1623–34.

Crawford P. Epilepsy and pregnancy. *MIDIRS.* 2002; **12**(3): 327–1.

Crawford P, Appleton R, Betts T, *et al.* Best practice guidelines in the management of women with epilepsy. *Seizure.* 1999; **8**: 201–17.

Dahl J, Myhr K, Daltveit A, *et al.* Pregnancy, delivery and birth outcome in women with multiple sclerosis. *Neurology.* 2005; **65**: 1961–3.

Davies A, Blakeley AGH, Kidd C. *Human Physiology.* Edinburgh: Churchill Livingstone; 2001.

Doggett-Jones S. Contraception for women with epilepsy. *Pract Nurs.* 2007; **33**(4): 32–7.

Donaldson JO. Neurological disorders. In: de Swiet M, editor. *Medical Disorders in Obstetric Practice.* 4th ed. Oxford: Blackwell; 2002. pp. 486–500.

Drake E, Drake M, Bird J, *et al.* Obstetric regional blocks for women with multiple sclerosis: a survey of UK experience. *Int J Obstet Anesth.* 2006; **15**(2): 115–23.

Duncan JS, Sander JW, Sisodiya SM, *et al.* Adult epilepsy. *Lancet.* 2006; **367**: 1087–100.

Durufle A, Nicholas B, Petrilli S, *et al.* Effects of pregnancy and childbirth on the incidence of urinary disorders in multiple sclerosis. *Clin Exp Obstet Gynaecol.* 2006; **33**(4): 215–18.

Fairgrieve S, Jackson M, Jonas P, *et al.* Population based, prospective study of the care of women with epilepsy in pregnancy. *BMJ.* 2000; **321**: 674–5.

Ferrero S, Esposito F, Pretta S, *et al.* Fetal risks related to the treatment of multiple sclerosis during pregnancy and breastfeeding. *Expert Rev Neurother.* 2006; **6**(12): 1823–31.

Foldvary N. Treatment issues for women with epilepsy. *Neurol Clin.* 2001; **19**: 409–25.

Fonager K, Larsen H, Pedersen L, *et al.* Birth outcomes in women exposed to anticonvulsant drugs. *Acta Neurol Scand.* 2000; **101**: 289–94.

Goadsby PJ, Goldberg J, Silberstein SD. Migraine in pregnancy. *BMJ.* 2008; **336**: 1502–4.

Graham J. *Multiple Sclerosis and Having a Baby: everything you need to know about conception, pregnancy and parenthood.* Rochester, VT: Healing Arts Press; 1999.

Holmes, LB, Harvey EA, Coull BA, *et al.* The teratogenicity of anticonvulsant drugs. *N Eng J Med.* 2001; **344**(15): 1132–8.

Hvas C, Henriksen T, Ostergaard JR. Birth weight in offspring of women with epilepsy. *Epidemiol Rev.* 2000; **22**: 275–82.

Kaaja E, Kaaja R, Hiilesmaa V. Major malformations in offspring of women with epilepsy. *Neurology.* 2003; **60**(4): 575–9.

Katz J, Devinsky O. Primary generalized epilepsy: a risk factory for seizures in labor and delivery? *Seizure.* 2003; **12**: 217–19.

Koh S, DeGiorgio C. Epilepsy. In: Rosene-Montella K, Keely E, Barbour LA, *et al.*, editors. *Medical Care of the Pregnant Patient.* 2nd ed. Philadelphia, PA: ACP Press; 2008. pp. 622–40.

Lawal M. Management and treatment options for epilepsy. *Br J Nurs.* 2005; **14**(16): 854–8.

Lewis G, editor. *Why Mothers Die 1997–1999. The Fifth Report of the Confidential Enquiries into Maternal Deaths in the UK.* London, RCOG; 2001.

Lewis G, editor. The Confidential Enquiry into Maternal and Child Health (CEMACH). *Saving Mothers' Lives: reviewing maternal deaths to make motherhood safer 2003–2005. The Seventh Report on Confidential Enquiries into Maternal Deaths in the UK.* London, CEMACH; 2007.

Little B. *Drugs and Pregnancy: a handbook.* New York: Hodder Arnold; 2006.

Lorenzi A, Ford H. Multiple sclerosis and pregnancy. *Postgrad Med J.* 2002; **78**(922): 460–4.

Lowe SA. Neurological disease in pregnancy. In: Greer IA, Nelson-Piercy C, Walters B. *Maternal Medicine.* Edinburgh: Churchill Livingstone Elsevier; 2007. pp. 250–63.

McElroy-Cox C. Caring for patients with epilepsy. *Nurse Pract.* 2007; **32**(10): 34–40.

McKay-Moffat S. The interaction between specific conditions and the childbirth continuum. In: McKay-Moffat S, editor. *Disability in Pregnancy and Childbirth.* Edinburgh, Churchill Livingstone Elsevier, 2007. pp. 159–88.

McKay-Moffat S, Cunningham C. Services for women with disabilities: mothers' and midwives' experiences. *Br J Midwifery.* 2006; **14**(8): 472–7.

Manford M. *Practical Guide to Epilepsy.* Burlington, MA: Butterworth Heinemann; 2003.

Marshall F, Crawford P. *Coping with Epilepsy.* 2nd ed. London: Sheldon Press; 2006.

Morrow J, Russell A, Guthrie E, *et al.* Malformation risks of anti-epileptic drugs in pregnancy: a prospective study from the UK Epilepsy and Pregnancy Register. *J Neurol Neurosurg Psychiatry.* 2006; **77**: 193–8.

Multiple Sclerosis Trust. *Multiple Sclerosis Information for Health and Social Care Professionals.* Letchworth Garden City: Multiple Sclerosis Trust; 2007.

National Institute for Clinical Excellence (NICE). *Multiple Sclerosis: management of multiple sclerosis in primary and secondary care: NICE guideline 8.* London: NICE; 2003.

National Institute for Clinical Excellence (NICE). *The Epilepsies: the diagnosis and management of the epilepsies in adults and children in primary and secondary care: NICE guideline 20.* London: NICE; 2004a.

National Institute for Clinical Excellence (NICE). *Epilepsy (Adults) – Newer Drugs: NICE technology appraisal 76.* London: NICE; 2004b.

Nelson-Piercy C. Epilepsy in pregnancy. In: MacLean A, Neilson J, editors. *Maternal Morbidity and Mortality.* London: RCOG Press; 2002. pp. 289–99.

Nelson-Piercy C. *Handbook of Obstetric Medicine.* 3rd ed. Abingdon: Informa Healthcare; 2006.

Nilsson L, Farahmand B, Persson P, *et al.* Risk factors for sudden unexpected death in epilepsy: a case-controlled study. *Lancet.* 1999; **353**: 888–93.

O'Brien MD, Gilmour-White SK. Management of epilepsy in women. *Postgrad Med J.* 2005; **81**: 278–85.

Pennell P. Antiepileptic drug pharmacokinetics during pregnancy and lactation. *Neurology.* 2003; **61**: 35–42.

Pennell P. Pregnancy in women who have epilepsy. *Neurol Clin.* 2004; **22**: 799–820.

Pickard J, Barbour LA. Headaches. In: Rosene-Montella K, Keely E, Barbour LA, *et al.*, editors. *Medical Care of the Pregnant Patient.* 2nd ed. Philadelphia, PA: ACP Press; 2008. pp. 609–12.

Pickard J, Larson L, Lee R. Nerve compression syndromes, multiple sclerosis and myasthenia gravis. In: Rosene-Montella K, Keely E, Barbour LA, *et al.*, editors. *Medical Care of the Pregnant Patient*. 2nd ed. Philadelphia, PA: ACP Press; 2008. pp. 641–9.

Robinson I, Neilson S, Rose F. *Multiple Sclerosis at Your Fingertips*. London: Class Publishing; 2000.

Royal College of Midwives. Position Paper 11a: *Maternity Care for Women with Disabilities*. London: RCM; 2000.

Sandberg-Wollheim M, Frank D, Goodwin T, *et al*. Pregnancy outcomes during treatment with interferon beta-1a in patients with multiple sclerosis. *Neurology*. 2005; **65**: 802–6.

Scottish Intercollegiate Guidelines Network (SIGN). *Guideline 70: Diagnosis and Management of Epilepsy in Adults*. Edinburgh: SIGN; 2003.

Seaman S. Multiple sclerosis and childbirth. *Pract Midwife*. 2007; **10**(9): 16–21.

Stella C, Jodicke C, How H, *et al*. Postpartum headache: is your workup complete? *Am J Obstet Gynecol*. 2007; **196**(4): 318.e1–318.e7.

Swartjes J, van Geijn H. Pregnancy and epilepsy. *Eur J Obstet Gynecol Reprod Biol*. 1998; **79**: 3–11.

Taylor M. Multiple sclerosis and midwifery care. In: Karger I, Hunt SC, editors. *Challenges in Midwifery Care*. London: Macmillan; 1997. pp. 146–64.

Thew M, Paech M. Management of postdural puncture headache in the obstetric patient. *Curr Opin Anaesthesiol*. 2008; **21**(3): 288–92.

Tomson T, Hiilesmaa V. Epilepsy in pregnancy. *BMJ*. 2007; **335**: 769–3.

Von Wald T, Walling AD. Headache during pregnancy. *Obstet Gynecol Surv*. 2002; **57**(3): 179–85.

Vukusic S, Hutchinson M, Hours M, *et al*. Pregnancy and multiple sclerosis (the PRIMS study): clinical predictors of post-partum relapse. *Brain*. 2004; **127**(6): 1353–60.

Watkiss K, Ward N. Pregnancy and parenthood. *Nurs Stand*. 2002; **17**(3): 45–53.

World Health Organization. *Epilepsy: aetiology, epidemiology and prognosis*. Fact Sheet 165. 2001. Available at: www.who.int/mediacentre/factsheets/fs165/en/ (accessed 11 December 2008).

Yerby M. Quality of life, epilepsy advances and the evolving role of anticonvulsants in women with epilepsy. *Neurology*. 2000; **55**(5 Suppl. 1): 21–31.

CHAPTER 9

Autoimmune disorders

CONTENTS

IMMUNITY, CHANGES IN PREGNANCY AND AUTOIMMUNITY

The immune system is a complex network of specialised cells, tissue, organs and chemical signals interacting together to provide a defence against pathogens. There are two aspects to the system: innate immunity (or in-built immunity), which is present all the time and acts as a first line of defence (*see* Box 9.1) and adaptive immunity.

BOX 9.1: COMPONENTS OF THE INNATE SYSTEM

- Barriers – skin, normal bacterial flora, lysozymes, pH, mucous membranes
- Phagocytes (neutrophils and macrophages)
- Natural killer cells (NK)
- Complement system

Adaptive immunity (specific or acquired immunity) responds specifically to particular antigens (an antigen is any substance perceived by the body as foreign). Adaptive immunity is the type of immunity that, rather than being present at birth, develops throughout life. The foreign pathogens are attacked by T lymphocytes. B lymphocytes and other specialised immune system cells act in concert with T lymphocytes to produce antibodies that attach to the antigen directly. Antibodies also stimulate the release of special chemical mediators in blood (e.g., complement or interferon) that further aid antigen destruction.

CHANGES TO THE IMMUNE SYSTEM DURING PREGNANCY

Changes to the immune system during pregnancy represent a balancing act between tolerating the 'foreignness' of the fetus and the need to protect mother and fetus from pathogenic invasion. There is enhancement of certain immune mechanisms and suppression of others.

AUTOIMMUNITY

The immune system that protects the body from invasion of foreign pathogens works on the ability to distinguish biological 'self' from 'non-self'. When this well-regulated process goes wrong it results in autoimmunity. In SLE and other autoimmune diseases the antibodies produced to ward off foreign invaders like bacteria and viruses start attacking the body's own tissues. Autoimmune diseases are characterised by typical (although widely varying) signs and symptoms that are confirmed by blood tests that show the presence of auto-antibodies. These auto-antibodies can be responsible for tissue damage, although in some cases they are simply present and confirm the existence of an autoimmune process (Porter and Branch, 2006).

The pathophysiological mechanisms that lead to autoimmune diseases are unknown but a combination of environmental, genetic and host factors need to be present to trigger the full expression of the disease. The incidence varies between populations, with one recent review indicating the highest prevalence among Afro-Caribbean women in the UK (Danchenko, *et al.*, 2006).

Autoimmune diseases are more common in women of child-bearing age and it seems that oestrogens promote disease, whilst androgens are protective. However, some autoimmune diseases deteriorate in pregnancy and some improve. It seems the effect of pregnancy depends on whether the autoimmune disease is cell-mediated (innate) or due to auto-antibodies (adaptive). Diseases such as rheumatoid arthritis and multiple sclerosis have strong cellular pathophysiology and generally show improvement in pregnancy. In contrast, diseases featuring auto-antibody production, such as SLE and Graves disease, tend to increase in severity in pregnancy (Porter and Branch, 2006).

SYSTEMIC LUPUS ERYTHEMATOSUS (SLE)

SLE is an autoimmune, connective tissue disorder that can affect any body system and thus presents with a broad range of symptoms. It predominantly affects women of child-bearing age. The outcome of pregnancy is optimistic for many women with SLE, particularly for those in remission at conception. However, in some forms of SLE (particularly those with antiphospholipid antibodies) and when major organ damage (especially the kidney) is involved, complications of pregnancy and further organ damage with enhanced morbidity and even mortality may occur.

FEATURES OF SLE

SLE is characterised by the presence of auto-antibodies:
▶ anti-nuclear antibody (ANA)
▶ antibody to double-stranded DNA (dsDNA).

Other auto-antibodies that may be found are included in Box 9.2.

BOX 9.2: ANTIBODIES FOUND IN SLE

- Anti-nuclear antibody (ANA)
- Antibody to double-stranded DNA (dsDNA)
- Anti-smooth-muscle antibody (SM)
- Anti-Ro/SSA
- Anti-La/SSB
- Anti-ribonucleoprotein (RNP)
- Anticardiolipin (ACA)*
- Lupus anticoagulant (LAC)*

(Nelson-Piercy and Rosene-Montella, 2008; Molad, 2006)

* Up to 40% of women with SLE have antiphospholipid antibodies (Mackillop, *et al.*, 2007). *See* section on APS later in this chapter.

Autoimmune tissue damage leads to a wide array of individual symptoms, with profound fatigue being experienced by most sufferers. Pyrexia, weight loss and muscle and joint pain are also common symptoms (*see* Table 9.1 for list of symptoms). Like other autoimmune diseases, SLE is characterised by periods of remission and relapse. Periods of relapse are known as flares.

TABLE 9.1: Range of signs and symptoms in SLE

Area	Signs and symptoms
Generalised symptoms	Fatigue, aching, fever, weakness, weight gain
Skin	Rashes: photosensitive rash, characteristic butterfly rash on both cheeks and nasal bridge; nose, mouth ulcers; hair loss
Joints	Pain, redness, swelling, arthritis, arthralgia, tendonitis, myositis
Kidneys	Proteinuria, hypertension, oedema. Lupus nephritis is a serious complication of SLE
Blood	Haemolytic anaemia, leukopenia, thrombocytopenia
Reproductive	Menorrhagia, amenorrhoea, preterm delivery, pre-eclampsia, fetal loss, thrombosis
Heart and lungs	Shortness of breath, cough, pleurisy, pericarditis, peritonitis, endocarditis
Nervous system	Convulsions, psychosis, neuropathies, headaches or migraine, lupus cerebritis

SLE is controlled by drugs – the type and dosage depending on the individual symptoms and degree of illness (*see* Box 9.3 for some examples).

BOX 9.3: COMMON DRUGS USED WITH SLE

- *Glucocorticoids*: maternal side effects – immunosuppression, weight gain, acne, striae, hirsutism, osteonecrosis, gastrointestinal ulceration, increased risk of pre-eclampsia, increased risk of glucose intolerance in pregnancy. Fetal side effects – placental insufficiency, IUGR.
- *Anti-malarials*, such as hydroxychloroquine, are commonly used to treat SLE. Although they have previously been considered unsafe in pregnancy because of concern about teratogenicity, more recent research has demonstrated they may not only be relatively safe (Motta, *et al.*, 2002) but also may be superior to glucocorticoids (Levy, *et al.*, 2001) during pregnancy.
- *Cytotoxic agents* have only limited data concerning their effects on the fetus or pregnancy, but it is generally considered that these drugs should be avoided in pregnancy. If a woman needs a cytotoxic agent to control her disease, careful counselling regarding the potential risks, balanced against her needs, should be carried out on an individual basis.
- *Nonsteroid anti-inflammatory drugs (NSAIDs)* are used commonly to treat to symptoms of SLE outside pregnancy, but their chronic use should be avoided at all stages of pregnancy. These drugs cross the placenta and block progesterone synthesis and fetal anomalies have been associated with their use (Porter and Branch, 2006).

DIAGNOSIS

Diagnosis is suspected by clinical signs (*see* Table 9.1), the most common of which are fatigue, pyrexia and arthralgia/arthritis, and these symptoms affect most SLE sufferers (90% have joint pain with swelling) (Nelson Piercy, 2006). Diagnosis is confirmed by detection of circulating auto-antibodies. The American Rheumatism Association has strict guidelines for diagnosis, including four clinical signs, together with laboratory criteria (Silver, *et al.*, 2008), but if a woman does not meet these criteria, although she may not have the diagnosis of SLE, she may have a 'lupus-like disease' and benefit from specialist care (Porter and Branch, 2006).

Lupus sometimes appears for the first time in pregnancy or in the first three months post-partum. Unfortunately diagnosis may be particularly difficult at this time due to the overlap of pregnancy signs and symptoms.

COMPLICATIONS OF SLE IN PREGNANCY

Box 9.4 is a summary of possible complications of SLE that are associated with pregnancy.

Fetal loss

Pregnancy loss is greater in those with SLE (Porter and Branch, 2006), probably between 11–34%, with a larger number being second- and third-trimester losses (Cortes-Hernandez, *et al.*, 2003; Georgiou, *et al.*, 2000). The degree of control of the disease, plus the presence of renal complications, influence the rate of pregnancy loss (de Swiet, 2002). Fetal death is also associated with the presence of antiphospholipid antibodies (*see* later in this chapter).

BOX 9.4: SUMMARY OF COMPLICATIONS OF SLE ASSOCIATED WITH PREGNANCY

- Fetal loss
- Intra-uterine growth restriction (IUGR)
- Premature delivery
- Neonatal lupus
- Pre-eclampsia
- Identification and management of flares in pregnancy, including difficulty in distinguishing pre-eclampsia from renal nephritis flare
- Deterioration of any existing renal impairment
- Thrombosis (with APS)
- Pulmonary hypertension

Premature delivery and IUGR

Studies have shown an increase in the rate of premature birth (up to 30%) and IUGR (up to 50%) for woman with SLE (Molad, *et al.*, 2005.).

Premature birth is associated with antiphospholipid antibodies, chronic hypertension and disease activity (Georgiou, *et al.*, 2000). However, in a recent study some women with active disease did continue their pregnancy to term (Kiss, *et al.*, 2002). It should be noted that much of the preterm birth is iatrogenic following complications, for example, pre-eclampsia (Porter and Branch, 2006).

IUGR may occur as a result of complicating factors such as renal compromise, hypertension and pre-eclampsia (Porter and Branch, 2006).

Neonatal lupus

Neonatal lupus is a rare condition and can involve dermatological, haematological or cardiac anomalies. The most common presentation of neonatal lupus is cutaneous neonatal lupus, where the newborn develops a characteristic rash at around two weeks old (Mackillop, *et al.*, 2007). Cardiac neonatal lupus, a more serious condition, may involve congenital complete heart block, and diagnosis is usually made antenatally when a fetal bradycardia (60–80 bpm) is identified. In severe cases the fetus will die, but less severely affected fetuses may respond to medication given to the mother, although they may need a pacemaker following birth (Buyon, *et al.*, 1998). Assessment of the presence of anti-Ro antibodies and anti-La antibodies may help to determine whether neonatal lupus is likely in the fetus, although anti-Ro antibodies seem to be associated only with fetal congenital heart block, not other adverse outcomes (Brucato, *et al.*, 2002). The risk to all mothers with SLE of having a baby with neonatal lupus is thought to be < 5% (Porter and Branch, 2006), but those with a positive antibody screen have a potentially raised risk (Porter and Branch, 2006). Delivery in a hospital with neonatal cardiac facilities is recommended. Mothers of babies with neonatal lupus may have no symptoms, but most will eventually develop SLE (Silver, *et al.*, 2008).

Flares in pregnancy

There is controversy concerning whether pregnancy is associated with increases of disease activity known as flares. The rate of flares during pregnancy differs between studies, because most studies include women not in remission before pregnancy, and many use different criteria for defining flares (Buyon, *et al.*, 1999; Ruiz-Irastorza, *et al.*, 2004). The general consensus is that the rate of flares probably increases and that the post-partum period seems to be a time of increased susceptibility (Mackillop, *et al.*, 2007; Mok and Wong, 2001). The rate of flares during pregnancy has been estimated in the range of 15–60% (Molad, *et al.*, 2005; Porter and Branch, 2006). Women who discontinue maintenance drugs or who have had a history of more than three severe flares before pregnancy are more likely to flare in pregnancy (Porter and Branch, 2006). Stress of the delivery and fatigue from looking after the newborn, combined with loss of the natural immunosuppressive effects of pregnancy, may be responsible for the increased risk of a disease flare after delivery (Lupus UK, 2005).

Flare symptoms can be confused with common symptoms of pregnancy and vice versa. Serious flares involving the kidney, heart and central nervous system do occur.

Renal complications and pre-eclampsia

There is an increased risk of pre-eclampsia for women with SLE, especially in those with pre-existing hypertension, nephritis and the presence of antiphospholipid antibodies (Yee, *et al.*, 2007).

Lupus nephritis is a common and more serious complication of SLE (about 50%), and it is diagnosed by renal biopsy when the urine shows blood and protein. Where lupus is quiescent prior to pregnancy and renal status is optimal, women can expect good fetal and maternal outcomes (Mackillop, *et al.*, 2007). However, a severe flare in pregnancy is life-threatening and the drugs used to treat it may have toxic effects on the fetus.

There is some evidence that pregnancy worsens renal function in those with pre-existing lupus nephritis (Mackillop, *et al.*, 2007), but if the disease is well controlled prior to pregnancy and renal function is normal, pregnancy can be successful (Julkunen, 2001; Oviasu, *et al.*, 1999). Proteinuria, elevated serum creatinine, hypertension and thrombocytopenia in the second half of pregnancy are found both in a relapse of SLE and pre-eclampsia.

See Chapter 5 for further discussion of renal disease in pregnancy.

Pulmonary hypertension

Pulmonary hypertension has been found in up to 10% of women with SLE, and this may predate or develop after their SLE diagnosis. This is a particularly dangerous complication in pregnancy and there is an increased risk of mortality (McMillan, *et al.*, 2002) (*see* Chapter 3, *Eisenmenger's syndrome and pulmonary hypertension*).

PRECONCEPTION CARE

For most women with SLE, fertility is unaffected (Mok and Wong, 2001); however, irregular menstrual cycles and anovulatory cycles are more common during flares. The drug cyclosposphamide, which is used for the treatment of lupus nephritis, is associated with female infertility when used for long periods (Mok and Wong, 2001).

In the past women were thought to be putting themselves at risk if they became pregnant and with pregnancy losses being more common for women with SLE, they were advised to avoid pregnancy. Care for women with SLE certainly presents challenges, but careful individual assessment and care by an experienced team will improve the possibility of a successful pregnancy. For women with uncomplicated SLE the risk in pregnancy is comparable to that in the general population (Mackillop, *et al.*, 2007). In a recent study of 267 pregnancies in 203 women with SLE the live birth rate was 86% (31% were premature). Women with lupus are advised to delay pregnancy until the lupus is well controlled on drugs that can be continued in pregnancy. Pregnancy is generally more successful if the woman is in remission (Georgiou, *et al.*, 2000; Nelson-Piercy, 2006). Women with SLE should receive counselling from an obstetrician with experience of SLE concerning potential obstetric problems (pre-eclampsia, IUGR, premature birth, pregnancy loss) plus the risk of flares and neonatal lupus. Deterioration of renal function is a concern for those with renal disease. *See* Box 9.5 for a list of factors associated with adverse outcomes. This will be a time of anxious decision-making for the woman and her family. Clear information based on individual assessment given in a supportive manner with the opportunity to ask further questions for clarification is essential.

BOX 9.5: FACTORS ASSOCIATED WITH ADVERSE OUTCOMES IN PREGNANCY

- Increased disease activity
- Hypertension
- Renal impairment
- Antiphospholipid, anti-Ro or anti-La antibodies
- Central nervous system involvement

(El-Sayed, *et al.*, 2002; Mackillop, *et al.*, 2007)

A general health assessment for anaemia, thrombocytopenia and renal function plus assessment of antiphospholipid antibodies, lupus anticoagulant and anticardiolipin should be made (Nelson-Piercy, 2006). A drug review is necessary. Glucocorticoids are the most common treatment for women with SLE and can be given as maintenance treatment or used only to treat a flare. If the disease is stable, the dosage may be reduced to see if it can be safely withdrawn. Otherwise the maintenance dose can be continued during pregnancy, although there are potential side effects for the fetus, in particular the likelihood of IUGR.

PREGNANCY CARE

Multidisciplinary care in a combined clinic, including physician specialists in connective tissue disease, is the recommended model. Frequent visits are often necessary, dependent on the woman's condition: more if flares, hypertension, proteinuria, clinical IUGR or APS are present. At booking the midwife should make detailed notes of how the SLE manifests itself. Flares tend to follow similar patterns (Mackillop, *et al.*, 2007) and this will be helpful in distinguishing changes in pregnancy from flares. Taking time to understand how the woman is affected will be the basis for individualised care. A supportive midwife who listens, takes the woman's concerns seriously and refers appropriately is vital.

Monitoring for hypertension and proteinuria are essential. Although the risk of women with SLE developing pre-eclampsia is uncertain, it is increased and those with lupus nephritis are at particular risk (Porter and Branch, 2006), along with those women with a history of chronic hypertension, secondary APS and chronic steroid use (Porter and Branch, 2006). The challenge when caring for women with SLE in pregnancy is distinguishing the flares from complications of pregnancy such as pre-eclampsia. To assess conditions, various serological markers to evaluate SLE may be used, but many do not give an accurate result (Porter and Branch, 2006). Anti-dsDNA titers elevation may be the most specific, preceding flares in more than 80% of cases (Ho, et al., 2001). Elevations have been shown to correlate with the necessity for preterm delivery (Tomer, et al., 1996). This test is particularly useful if the woman has hypertension, proteinuria and multi-organ dysfunction – symptoms which are common to both a SLE flare and pre-eclampsia (Porter and Branch, 2006).

The midwife may suggest the woman performs her own urinalysis for protein at home in addition to regular monitoring by the multidisciplinary team. Knowledge of symptoms of pre-eclampsia such as headaches, visual disturbance and epigastric pain and recognition of premature labour will assist the woman to seek timely access to health professionals. Information about whom to contact and how to do so also needs to be given.

Fetal surveillance, including growth scans, regular liquor volume measurement and dopplers to assess well-being, is usual (Porter and Branch, 2006).

Flares occurring during pregnancy can be mild or severe. They can commonly be treated with the introduction or increase in glucocorticoids orally, although severe exacerbations will be treated more aggressively with IV regimes.

There is no good evidence to commence treatment prophylactically in pregnancy (Porter and Branch, 2006), but if a woman has active disease or raised anti-dsDNA, the use of glucocorticoids have been shown to improve the outcome (Georgiou, et al., 2000).

Repeated screening for gestational diabetes for those taking glucocorticoids is recommended (suggested at 22–24 weeks, 28–30 weeks and 32–34 weeks)(Porter and Branch, 2006). Requirements for thromboprophylaxis should be assessed. The midwife can give information on preventing thrombosis, such as leg exercises and elevation, avoiding periods of immobility and keeping well hydrated. See the section on Thromboembolic disease in Chapter 4 for further discussion.

LABOUR CARE

Depending on the woman's condition, labour care may be routine. If there was any concern about fetal growth or condition, continuous electronic fetal monitoring would be recommended. TED stockings may be used, especially if the woman is relatively immobile.

Women taking steroids may have adrenal insufficiency and need doses of glucocorticoids IM /IV prescribed for labour and/or at Caesarean section (Porter and Branch, 2006).

A flare may occur in labour, and acute administration of steroids (probably IV) will be necessary.

POSTNATAL CARE

Women with lupus often suffer from severe tiredness and fatigue. The midwife should discuss strategies with the woman to cope with the demands of the postnatal period. The mother will need help to look after her newborn baby and any other children. Furthermore, as there may be an increased risk of flares in the postnatal period it is recommended women with SLE, as with any other debilitating chronic disease, have a plan for who will care for the baby if she does become seriously ill.

If the woman was receiving maintenance medication in pregnancy, then the dose may need adjusting. If she is receiving steroids, the effect this may have on the immune system at this vulnerable time of healing (Boyle, 2006) should be remembered. Many drugs commonly taken by women with SLE are safe when breastfeeding, but all drugs should be checked for the most up-to-date information prior to advising the woman. Contraception containing oestrogen may not be suitable for women with SLE and midwives should ensure these women have access to experts for advice.

ANTIPHOSPHOLIPID SYNDROME (APS)

APS (also known as Hughes syndrome) is an autoimmune disease that primarily affects women. The concern for midwives and women with APS is that it is associated with a considerable risk of thrombosis in pregnancy and a higher rate of fetal loss (ACOG, 2005; Shehata and Nelson-Piercy, 2001). Women with APS produce antibodies to their own phospholipids and proteins. Phospholipids (which the antibodies target) are an integral component of cell membranes. The membrane coating of platelets, the endothelial lining of blood vessels, or clotting proteins in the blood are implicated (Porter and Branch, 2006; Hughes, 2001).The two antibodies involved are:

▶ anticardiolipin
▶ lupus anticoagulant.

These antibodies cause endothelial activation and thrombus formation. Lupus anti-coagulant is confusingly named, as it is associated with the tendency to form a clot, not to prolong bleeding time, as the name implies (de Swiet, 2002). Diagnosis of the syndrome is made based on laboratory findings of these antibodies along with clinical features of vascular thrombosis and/or pregnancy complications (Greer and Walker, 2007). It is worth noting that cardiolipin cross-reacts with the Wasserman reaction test for syphilis and therefore women with APS may get a false positive result for syphilis on booking bloods where this test is still used (Robson and Hodgett, 2008).

APS may exist as an isolated condition (primary APS) or in combination with other autoimmune diseases (secondary APS), most commonly SLE (*see* Figure 9.1).

The mechanism by which APS causes thrombosis is not fully understood (Shehata and Nelson-Piercy, 2001). However, the association between antiphospholipid antibodies, thrombosis and pregnancy loss is well-established, with higher titres of anticardiolipin antibodies correlating with a greater risk to the fetus (de Swiet, 2002).

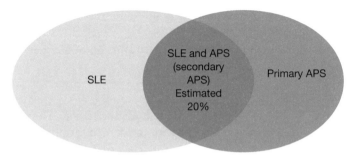

FIGURE 9.1: The association between SLE and APS
Sources: ACOG (2007); Hughes (2001)

The usual triggers for thrombosis are the same in APS, with pregnancy being one of them (Box 9.6 lists common triggers for thrombosis: *see* section on *Thromboembolic disease* in Chapter 4 for further discussion). However, the presence of antiphospholipid antibodies can cause thrombosis at any time without obvious triggers. In addition, infection has been suggested as a possible trigger in APS.

BOX 9.6: TRIGGERS FOR THROMBOSIS

- Smoking
- Immobility (e.g., long flights)
- Dehydration
- Contraceptive pill
- Pregnancy

Correct identification of women with APS is important as effective treatment with heparin can reduce the risk of thrombosis and improve pregnancy outcome (Petri and Qazi, 2006). APS complications in pregnancy are primarily related to abnormalities of the decidual spiral arteries resulting in abnormal placental function as a result of thrombus formation (Porter and Branch, 2006). In addition, thrombus formation can occur in any part of the body, giving rise to a broad spectrum of possible presentations of APS. Box 9.7 lists the possible complications of APS seen in pregnancy.

PRECONCEPTION CARE

As with all medical conditions, women with APS should be informed of the general pregnancy risk (*see* Box 9.7). Those with APS pulmonary hypertension, which is very dangerous in pregnancy, should be counselled as to the risk (de Swiet, 2002). If it has not recently been undertaken, a full medical assessment should be made, with particular attention to potential anaemia and renal function. If the woman is taking warfarin this should be discontinued because of potential teratogenicity, and LMWH should be commenced.

BOX 9.7: COMPLICATIONS OF APS IN PREGNANCY

Those related directly to pregnancy are:
- recurrent early pregnancy loss
- second- and third-trimester fetal loss
- severe, early-onset (less than 34 weeks) pre-eclampsia
- intra-uterine growth restriction
- deep vein thrombosis.

General complications that may occur in pregnancy:
- thrombosis in internal organs – kidneys, brain, eye, liver
- blotchiness of skin from skin vein thrombosis, leg ulcers
- ischaemic stroke, transient cerebral ischaemia
- headaches, seizures, memory loss, multiple sclerosis-type symptoms
- thrombosis to heart valves and coronary arteries
- low platelet count and bruising.

(ACOG, 2005; Nelson-Piercy, 2006; Greer and Walker, 2007; Hughes, 2001; Woodward, 2007)

PREGNANCY CARE

In those with a history of recurrent miscarriage, prophylactic heparin and low-dose aspirin can reduce fetal loss by 50% (Empson, *et al.*, 2002). The evidence is less clear for the reduction of other adverse effects such as pre-eclampsia and placental insufficiency; however, these women are also often treated with the same regime (ACOG, 2005). Heparin is usually administered from early in the first trimester, usually when the fetal heart is identified (at about six weeks), together with low-dose aspirin (usually when pregnancy is confirmed, although some suggest the aspirin could be commenced preconception) (de Swiet, 2002; Empson, *et al.*, 2002).

Women who receive heparin will usually use LMWH, where it is thought the risk of osteoporosis is less than with standard heparin (Silver, *et al.*, 2008). However, it may still be appropriate to consider calcium and vitamin D supplements and increased weight-bearing exercise such as walking. The midwife will assist in instructing and supporting the woman in self-administering LMWH injections. Assistance in obtaining the right equipment (e.g., a sharps bin for needle disposal) and regular prescription may be needed in addition to information about side effects such as bruising and bleeding gums.

Antenatal care involves frequent appointments to monitor fetal well-being and screen for pre-eclampsia and thrombosis. Serial ultrasound for growth is usually carried out from 18 weeks, and later amniotic fluid estimation and doppler assessment may be done as necessary. There is also some evidence that frequent contact with supportive health professionals may improve the outcome for a woman who has had recurrent miscarriages (Regan, 2001).

LABOUR CARE

Due to the increased risk of pre-eclampsia, thrombosis and fetal distress (uteroplacental insufficiency), labour should be monitored closely.

There is no evidence on the best regime for anticoagulation but the principle is to discontinue anticoagulants in time to prevent excess bleeding at delivery and allow for an epidural or spinal if necessary, but not stop it too soon and risk thrombosis. If the woman is at very high risk, she may have IV heparin in labour until 4–6 hours before delivery, then recommence 4–6 hours postnatal (12 hours post-Caesarean section) (Porter and Branch, 2006).

Thromboembolic stockings should be fitted and the midwife should encourage regular change of position and leg and deep-breathing exercises.

POSTNATAL CARE

If there is a history of thrombosis, it is recommended that anticoagulation begin in the postnatal period as soon as possible (Ginsberg, *et al.*, 2001). Anticoagulation therapy is usually continued for 6–8 weeks in the puerperium as the risk of thrombosis remains (Branch and Khamashta, 2003). Contraceptives containing oestrogen are contraindicated (Porter and Branch, 2006).

REFERENCES

American College of Obstetricians and Gynecologists (ACOG). Antiphospholipid syndrome. ACOG Practice Bulletin. *Obstet Gynecol.* 2005; **106**(5): 1113 21.

Boyle M. *Wound Healing in Midwifery.* Oxford: Radcliffe Publishing; 2006.

Branch D, Khamashta M. Antiphospholipid syndrome: obstetric diagnosis, management and controversies. *Obstet Gynecol.* 2003; **101**: 1333–44.

Brucato A, Doria A, Frassi M, *et al.* Pregnancy outcome in 100 women with autoimmune diseases and anti-Ro/SSA antibodies: a prospective controlled study. *Lupus.* 2002; **11**(11): 716–21.

Buyon J, Hiebert R, Copel J, *et al.* Autoimmune-associated congenital heart block: demographics, mortality, morbidity and recurrence rates obtained from a national neonatal lupus registry. *J Am Coll Cardiol.* 1998; **31**: 1658–66.

Buyon J, Kalunian K, Ramsey-Goldman R, *et al.* Assessing disease activity in SLE patients during pregnancy. *Lupus.* 1999; **8**: 677–84.

Cortes-Hernandez J, Ordi-Ros J, Labrador M, *et al.* Predictors of poor renal outcome in patients with lupus nephritis treated with combined pulses of cyclophosphamide and methylprednisolone. *Lupus.* 2003; **12**(4): 287–96.

Danchenko N, Satia JA, Anthony MS. Epidemiology of systemic lupus erythematosus: a comparison of worldwide disease burden. *Lupus.* 2006; **15**: 308–18.

de Swiet M. APS, SLE and other connective tissue diseases. In: de Swiet M, editor. *Medical Disorders in Obstetric Practice.* 4th ed. Oxford: Blackwell; 2002. pp. 267–81.

El-Sayed Y, Lu E, Genovese M, *et al.* Central nervous system lupus and pregnancy: 11-year experience at a single center. *J Matern Fetal Med.* 2002; **12**(2): 99–103.

Empson M, Lassere M, Craig J, *et al.* Recurrent pregnancy loss with antiphospholipid antibody: a systematic review of therapeutic trials. *Obstet Gynecol.* 2002; **99**: 135–44.

Georgiou P, Politi E, Katsimbri P, *et al.* Outcome of lupus pregnancy: a controlled study. *Rheumatol.* 2000; **39**: 1014–19.

Ginsberg JL, Creer I, Hirsh J. Use of antithrombotic agents during pregnancy. *Chest.* 2001; **119**(Suppl. 1): S122–31.

Greer I, Walker I. Thrombosis and hemostasis. In: Greer I, Nelson-Piercy C, Walters B, editors. *Maternal Medicine: medical problems in pregnancy.* Edinburgh: Churchill Livingstone Elsevier; 2007. pp. 146–70.

Ho A, Magder L, Barr S, *et al.* Decreases in anti-double-stranded DNA levels are associated with concurrent flares in patients with systemic lupus erythematosus. *Arthritis Rheum.* 2001; **44**: 2342–9.

Hughes G. *Hughes Syndrome: a patient's guide.* London: Springer Verlag; 2001.

Julkunen H. Pregnancy and lupus nephritis. *Scand J Urol Nephrol.* 2001; **35**: 319–27.

Kiss E, Bhattoa H, Bettembuk P, *et al.* Pregnancy in women with systemic lupus erythematosus. *Eur J Obstet Gynecol Reprod Biol.* 2002; **101**(2): 129–34.

Levy R, Vilela V, Cataldo M, *et al.* Hydroxychloroquine (HCQ) in lupus pregnancy: double-blind and placebo-controlled study. *Lupus.* 2001; **10**: 401–4.

Lupus UK. The importance of planning pregnancy in SLE. Reproduced from *National Magazine.* 2005. Available at: www.lupusuk.org.uk/planningpregnancyinsle.asp (accessed 12 December 2008).

Mackillop LH, Germain SJ, Nelson-Piercy C. Pregnancy plus: systemic lupus erythematosus. *BMJ.* 2007; **335**: 933–6.

McMillan E, Martin W, Waugh J, *et al.* Management of pregnancy in women with pulmonary hypertension secondary to SLE and anti-phospholipid syndrome. *Lupus.* 2002; **11**(6): 392–8.

Mok CC, Wong RWS. Pregnancy in systemic lupus erythematosus. *Postgrad Med J.* 2001; **77**: 257–65.

Molad Y. Systemic lupus erythematosus and pregnancy. *Curr Opin Obstet Gynecol.* 2006; **18**(6): 613–17.

Molad Y, Borkowski T, Monselise A, *et al.* Maternal and fetal outcome of lupus pregnancy: a prospective study of 29 pregnancies. *Lupus.* 2005; **14**(2): 145–51.

Motta M, Tincani A, Faden D, *et al.* Antimalarial agents in pregnancy. *Lancet.* 2002; **359**: 524–5.

Nelson-Piercy C. *Handbook of Obstetric Medicine.* 3rd ed. Abingdon: Informa Healthcare; 2006.

Nelson-Piercy C, Rosene-Montella K. Systemic lupus erythematosus. In: Rosene-Montella K, Keely E, Barbour L, *et al.*, editors. *Medical Care of the Pregnant Patient.* 2nd ed. Philadelphia, PA: ACP Press; 2008. pp. 513–20.

Oviasu E, Hicks J, Cameron J. The outcome of pregnancy in women with lupus nephritis. *Lupus.* 1999; **1**: 19–15.

Petri M, Qazi U. Management of antiphospholipid syndrome in pregnancy. *Rheum Dis Clin North Am.* 2006; **32**: 591–607.

Porter TF, Branch DW. Autoimmune diseases. In: James D, Steer P, Weiner C, *et al.*, editors. *High Risk Pregnancy: management options.* Philadelphia, PA: Elsevier; 2006. pp. 949–85.

Regan L. *Miscarriage: what every woman needs to know.* 2nd ed. London: Orion; 2001.

Robson SE, Hodgett S. Autoimmune disorders. In: Robson SE, Waugh J, editors. *Medical Disorders in Pregnancy.* Oxford: Blackwell; 2008. pp. 137–46.

Ruiz-Irastorza G, Khamashta M, Gordon C, *et al.* Measuring systemic lupus erythematosus activity during pregnancy: validation of the lupus activity index in pregnancy scale. *Arthritis Rheum.* 2004; **51**: 78–82.

Shehata HA, Nelson-Piercy C. Connective tissue and skin disorders in pregnancy. *Curr Obstet Gynaecol.* 2001; **11**: 329–5.

Silver RM, Cowchock SZ, Rosene-Montella K. Antiphospholipid antibody syndrome. In: Rosene-Montella K, Keely E, Barbour L, *et al.*, editors. *Medical Care of the Pregnant Patient.* 2nd ed. Philadelphia, PA: ACP Press; 2008. pp. 521–33.

Tomer Y, Viegas O, Swissa M, *et al.* Levels of lupus autoantibodies in pregnant SLE patients: correlations with disease activity and pregnancy outcome. *Clin Exp Rheumatol.* 1996; **1**(4): 275–80.

Woodward S. Antiphospholipid (Hughes) syndrome. *BJNN.* 2007; **3**(1): 16–18.

Yee CS, Gordon C, Khamashta M. Immunological diseases. In: Greer A, Nelson-Piercy C, Walters B, editors, *Maternal Medicine: medical problems in pregnancy.* Edinburgh: Churchill Livingstone Elsevier; 2007. pp. 191–7.

CHAPTER 10

Thyroid disease

CONTENTS
→ The thyroid gland
→ Thyroid function in pregnancy
→ Hyperthyroidism (thyrotoxicosis)
→ Hypothyroidism
→ Post-partum thyroiditis (PPT)

Thyroid disease is the second most common endocrine disorder found in pregnant women. The incidence of thyroid disorders increases with increasing maternal age (Lao, 2007).

There are many identified pregnancy complications (*see* Box 10.1) associated with thyroid dysfunction, which may occur in both hyperthyroidism and hypothyroidism (Lao, 2007). However, if women have their condition well controlled, there should be a satisfactory outcome.

THE THYROID GLAND

The thyroid is a butterfly-shaped gland located in the neck just below the larynx (*see* Figure 10.1). It produces two hormones, tri-iodothyronine (T3) and thyroxine (T4), which regulate metabolism throughout the body.

Levels of thyroid hormones are regulated by feedback via the pituitary and hypothalamus. Together they release thyroid-stimulating hormone (TSH) to instruct the thyroid to make more T3 and T4. Figure 10.2 shows the negative feedback regulation of the secretion of thyroid hormones.

In theory, if thyroid hormones are low, then TSH should be high. Conversely if levels of T3 and T4 are adequate, then TSH will be low.

Normal production of thyroid hormones (T3 and T4) is dependent on:
▶ an adequate supply of dietary iodine
▶ a normally functioning thyroid gland
▶ a functioning pituitary gland producing adequate TSH
▶ a functioning hypothalamus producing adequate TRH.

Thyroid tissue is composed of secretory cells (known as follicular cells) which are arranged into hollow spheres that form a functional unit called a follicle. These spheres contain colloid, a thick sticky protein material which is mostly made up of thyroglobulin, a precursor of the thyroid hormones. These follicles serve as both a factory and warehouse for thyroid hormones. The basic ingredients for thyroid hormone production are tyrosine, derived from thyroglobulin, and iodine taken from the diet. Iodine is found in seafood, vegetables grown in iodine-rich soil and iodised table salt. Iodine in the diet is reduced to iodide and is absorbed through the small intestine. TSH influences the thyroid gland to promote the uptake of iodide.

BOX 10.1: ADVERSE OUTCOMES ASSOCIATED WITH THYROID DISORDERS

- Miscarriage
- Premature labour
- Pre-eclampsia
- Intra-uterine growth restriction (IUGR)
- Fetal distress
- Lactation difficulty
- Postnatal depression

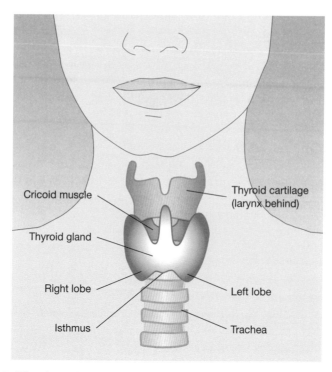

FIGURE 10.1: The thyroid gland

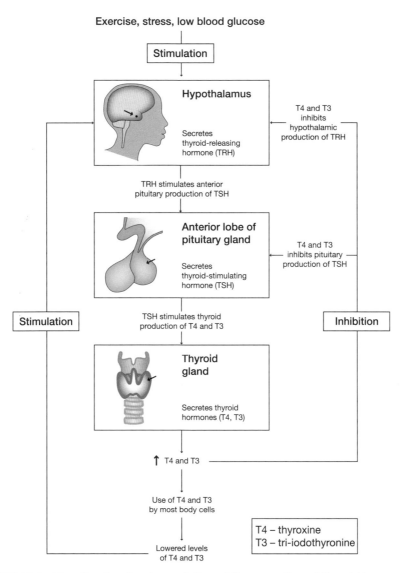

FIGURE 10.2: Negative feedback regulation of the secretion of thyroid hormones
Sources: Higgins (2007); Waugh and Grant (2006)

More than 99% of the T4 and T3 that circulate in the blood are bound to specific proteins, mostly thyroxine-binding globulin (TBG). In this bound form the hormones are inactive. Free (unbound) T3 and T4 are the physiologically active forms. Carrier proteins (TBG) allow maintenance of a stable pool of thyroid hormones from which the active, free hormones can be released for uptake by target cells when required. Thyroid hormones are required by all cells in the body and enter cells through membrane transporter proteins. About 90% of the thyroid hormone released from the thyroid gland is in the form of T4, yet T3 is about four times more potent in its biological activity. T4 is converted to T3 by being stripped of one of its iodides in the liver, kidney or muscle. T3 is therefore the major biological active form of thyroid hormones, even though the thyroid gland secretes mostly T4.

Active thyroid hormones are delivered to the cells, where they act to speed cellular metabolic reactions leading to an increase in basal metabolic rate. Some of these metabolic effects include lipid metabolism, carbohydrate metabolism and heat production. Thyroid hormones increase the response of target cells to catecholamines (epinephrine and norepinephrine) and hence promote sympathetic nervous system effects. For example, thyroid hormone increases heart rate and the force of cardiac muscle contraction to increase cardiac output. Normal growth and development are dependent on the thyroid function. Brain development is strongly dependent on an adequate supply of thyroid hormone and this is particularly important for the developing fetus (Pop and Vulsma, 2005). Variations in thyroid hormones lead to alterations in the mental state. Too little thyroid hormone (hypothyroid) can cause mental sluggishness, while too much (hyperthyroid) induces anxiety and nervousness. *See* Table 10.1 for a comparison of features of hyperthyroidism and hypothyroidism, and *see* Box 10.2 for explanation of terms.

TABLE 10.1: Features of abnormal secretion of thyroid hormones

Hyperthyroidism (↑T3 and T4)	Hypothyroidism (↓T3 and T4)
Increased basal metabolic rate	Decreased metabolic rate
Weight loss with good appetite	Weight gain and poor appetite
Anxiety, physical restlessness, nervousness, excessively emotional	Easily fatigued, mental sluggishness, depression, lethargy, psychosis
Hair loss	Dry skin, brittle hair
Fast pulse, heart palpitations	Slow, weak pulse
Intolerance to heat, warm sweaty skin	Dry cold skin, poor tolerance to cold Puffy appearance on face, hands and feet (myxoedema)
Diarrhoea	Constipation
Exophthalmos (protrusion of the eyes) in Graves' disease	
Oligomenorrhea or amenorrhoea	Anovulation

Sources: Jones and Huether (2006); Sherwood (1994); Waugh and Grant (2006)

GOITRE

A goitre (enlarged thyroid tissue) may appear in either hypothyroidism or hyperthyroidism. Differentiated thyroid carcinoma is one of the most common cancers in women of child-bearing age, and since it can grow rapidly in pregnancy, it must be ruled out when a goitre is discovered (Lao, 2007). In labour a large goitre may compromise airway management in an emergency situation and an anaesthetic consultation should be carried out in the antenatal period. Surgery (sub-total thyroidectomy) may be undertaken in the second trimester (Becks and Burrow, 2000) if necessary.

BOX 10.2: EXPLANATION OF TERMS

- Euthyroid(ism): normal thyroid activity
- Hyperthyroid(ism): overactive thyroid
- Hypothyroid(ism): underactive thyroid
- Goitre: enlargement of the thyroid gland – *see* above
- Thyrotoxicosis: the clinical syndrome that results from hyperthyroidism and often used as a synonym for hyperthyroidism
- Myxoedema: the syndrome that results from severe hypothyroidism
- Cretinism: a devastating and preventable condition characterised by deaf–mutism, intellectual deficiency and spastic motor disorder

---

THYROID FUNCTION IN PREGNANCY

A number of physiological changes occur to the thyroid function in pregnancy, with an important relationship existing between maternal and fetal thyroid function. Iodine crosses the placenta and thyroxine (T4) is transferred, but only in the first trimester. T3 and TSH do not cross at all. The fetal thyroid begins functioning at the end of the first trimester and prior to that the fetal brain development is dependent on maternal T4, which is converted intracellularly to T3 (Girling, 2006).

Changes to maternal thyroid function in pregnancy include:

- a marked increase in TBG
- increased TBG leads to an increase in TSH and enhanced production and secretion of total thyroid hormone
- fetal requirements for thyroid hormones
- increased demand for iodine
- hCG has a thyroid-stimulating effect
- de-iodination of thyroid hormones in the placenta to facilitate passage of iodine to the fetus.

Thyroxine-binding globulin (TBG)

As described above, TBG binds the thyroid hormones T4 and T3, keeping them in an inactive form. The concentration of TBG increases almost three times in the first half of pregnancy due to the effects of oestrogen, which boosts the synthesis and decreases the clearance of TBG (Girling, 2006; Kenyon and Nelson-Piercy, 2005).

With the increased number of binding sites available for the thyroid hormones, TSH acts to increase total thyroid, mostly T4, in the blood (Ramsey, 1998) but the levels of free T4 and T3 remain the same (Girling, 2006). Consequently, assessing levels of free T3 and T4 are more reliable than measuring total T3 and total T4 in serum thyroid function tests in pregnancy (Girling, 2006).

Fetal requirements for thyroid hormone

Fetal mental development is dependent on adequate amounts of thyroid hormone. Deficiencies can lead to impaired growth and irreversible mental retardation. The fetal gland begins synthesising thyroid hormone after 12 weeks' gestation. Prior to this the fetus is dependent on maternal supply of T4. It is during this early time that thyroid hormones are most important to fetal brain development, although it continues and thyroid hormone is important in later gestation.

Demand for iodine

Pregnancy is characterised by a significant demand for iodine with thyroid iodine uptake increasing. However, more iodine is excreted through renal clearance subsequent to the increased glomerular filtration rate of pregnancy and there is transfer of iodine to the developing fetus (Blackburn, 2007; Girling, 2006; Ramsey, 1998). The thyroid gland compensates for the increased loss of iodine by enlarging. Kenyon and Nelson-Piercy (2005) suggest a physiological goitre (enlarged thyroid) may be seen on ultrasound, but it would not be apparent when looking at the woman. A goitre that is clinically apparent suggests an iodine deficiency or some other kind of pathology. In women with severe iodine deficiency, trapping mechanisms override fetal demand, conserving iodine for maternal use but resulting in fetal cretinism (poor growth and mental retardation).

Human chorionic gonadatrophin (hCG)

HCG and TSH share a similar structure and have similar receptors, giving hCG thyroid-stimulating features. HCG is thought to stimulate the thyroid gland during early pregnancy. In situations where there is increased hCG, such as multiple pregnancy, trophoblastic disease (molar pregnancy) and hyperemesis gravidarum, hCG may overstimulate the TSH receptors, resulting in a transient biochemical hyperthyroidism. Two-thirds of women with hyperemesis have abnormal thyroid function tests but do not have thyroid disease (Kenyon and Nelson-Piercy, 2005).

De-iodination of thyroid hormones in the placenta

A group of enzymes controls the metabolism of T4 to the more active T3 and can deactivate both back to inactive compounds. They are important for the local regulation of thyroid hormone concentrations. One of these enzymes, known as de-iodinase III, occurs in the placenta and its concentration increases with gestation. It works to inactivate T4 and T3, removing molecules of iodine that are then easily transported to the fetus (Girling, 2006). The fetal requirement for iodide increases in the second and third trimester as fetal thyroid levels rise.

THYROID ACTIVITY IN LABOUR AND THE PUERPERIUM

In response to the increased energy requirement of the contracting uterine muscle, levels of total and free T3 increase during labour.

With delivery of the placenta and consequent reduction in oestrogen, the production of TBG decreases, as does the renal excretion of iodine. Gradually over 4–6 weeks the changes to thyroid function of pregnancy are reversed (Ramsey, 1998). Thyroid hormones are secreted in breast milk (Blackburn, 2007) and may delay the development of hypothyroidism in some infants with this disorder. Early detection and treatment of congenital hypothyroidism is essential to prevent profound morbidity and is included on the newborn blood spot screening programme for the neonate.

THYROID FUNCTION TESTS DURING PREGNANCY

Assessment of clinical features of thyroid status is more difficult during pregnancy and post-partum as many of the diverse signs and symptoms of pregnancy overlap with features of an alteration of thyroid function. However, for midwives identification and referral of women at risk is important because of the potential damaging effects of poor thyroid control during pregnancy, as well as long-term health issues.

The parameters for many laboratory tests to assess thyroid function are altered in pregnancy, predominantly due to the increased TBG and changes as the pregnancy progresses. Girling (2006) highlights the need for further research to establish accurate reference ranges for thyroid function tests.

Diagnosis of thyroid disorders should ideally take place before conception, as some diagnostic tools and treatments are unadvisable in pregnancy. Radioactive iodine studies for diagnosis, monitoring levels of drugs to establish the minimal effective dosage and surgery should be undertaken before pregnancy. It is suggested that after radioactive iodine treatment, pregnancy is delayed for one year (Lao, 2007).

HYPERTHYROIDISM (THYROTOXICOSIS)

Hyperthyroidism is thought to affect about 1% of pregnant women (Keely and Barbour, 2008) and Graves' disease probably accounts for 85% of these cases.

Graves' disease (or Basedow's disease) is the main cause of hyperthyroidism (Kenyon and Nelson-Piercy, 2005) in pregnant women. This is an autoimmune disorder (*see* Chapter 9) in which thyroid-stimulating immunoglobulins attach themselves and activate TSH receptors on thyroid follicles. This causes overproduction of thyroid hormones and results in symptoms of hyperthyroidism. It is characterised by goitre, exophthalmos (one or both eyes protruding), non-pitting oedema and fatigue. Most diagnoses of Graves' disease have been made pre-pregnancy, but if the first diagnosis is during pregnancy, these women often present with hyperemesis (Lao, 2007). During pregnancy those with Graves' disease may need adjustments to their medication in the first one to two months and in the postnatal period, as symptoms often increase at these times (Casey and Leveno, 2006). If a woman has a family history of Graves' disease, then it may be advisable for her to have her thyroid function tested (Lao, 2007).

Diagnosis will be suspected by the signs and symptoms (*see* Table 10.1) and diagnosed on laboratory tests: the presence of thyroid-stimulating antibodies, increased free T4 and/or T3 and decreased TSH. An ultrasound will also be undertaken.

Treatment is medical, using thionamides (*see* Box 10.3). Beta blockers may also be prescribed for some women, usually only for a limited time, to control tremors and tachycardia (Lao, 2007).

If control of the thyrotoxicosis is good, then the outcome for both mother and baby should be uncomplicated. However, untreated or poorly controlled thyrotoxicosis is associated with miscarriage, stillbirth, IUGR, abruption, pre-eclampsia, infection, preterm labour and increased perinatal mortality (Kenyon and Nelson-Piercy, 2005) and can even result in heart failure or thyroid storm (*see* Box 10.4).

BOX 10.3: THIONAMIDES

Thionamides cross the placenta but are not thought to cause congenital abnormalities, although propylthiouracil is preferred for use in pregnancy (Marx, *et al.*, 2008) The medication may protect the fetus, as thyrotoxicosis itself may cause congenital abnormality (Girling, 2006). Medication intake or absorption during pregnancy may be compromised by nausea and vomiting or iron/calcium supplement intake (Girling, 2006). Babies whose mothers were taking thionamides during pregnancy may have transient hypothyroidism, which usually resolves within the first week. Breastfeeding during thionamide medication is thought to be safe, but if increased levels of drugs are needed, then divided doses and infant monitoring should be carried out (Girling, 2006).

BOX 10.4 THYROID STORM

Thyroid storm (or thyrotoxic crisis) may present with a variety of serious symptoms and, although it is rare, it is an acute and life-threatening event. Labour and delivery may predispose to it as well as infection and trauma, usually in those in whom the thyroid disease is less well controlled. Symptoms include tachycardia, tremor, pyrexia, diarrhoea and vomiting, dehydration, delirium, fits and coma. Heart failure can occur if there is cardiomegaly from excessive thyroxine. Treatment is medication and system support in an ICU or emergency setting.

PREGNANCY CARE

If manifesting for the first time in pregnancy, thyrotoxicosis usually occurs in the late first or early second trimester and can be hard to diagnose, as many of the signs and symptoms (*see* Table 10.1) are common in pregnant women. Weight loss despite increased appetite, persistent tachycardia or tremor may be among the more reliable signs and symptoms.

Regular blood tests to assess thyroid function in pregnancy (and probably an increased number for those newly diagnosed) are usual and about 30% of women can discontinue their medication towards the end of pregnancy as the immune suppressive effect of pregnancy leads to reduced antibody levels (Harborne, *et al.*, 2005; Kenyon and Nelson-Piercy, 2005).

Radioactive iodine is contraindicated during pregnancy and lactation. Surgery is best avoided but may be carried out if medical treatment fails, if a goitre causes pressure symptoms or if there is a suspicion of cancer of the thyroid (Girling, 2006).

There is a risk of fetal or neonatal thyrotoxicosis (Peleg, *et al.*, 2002) and this may be suspected in the antenatal period by fetal heart auscultation (> 160 bpm persistently) and confirmed on ultrasound (fetal goitre with or without IUGR) (Wallace, *et al.*, 1995). If suspected, this will need careful monitoring as an increased fetal mortality rate (Smith, *et al.*, 2001) has been identified, as well as other complications (Kenyon and Nelson-Piercy, 2005). Fetal thyrotoxicosis can be treated by maternal medication titrated against the fetal heart rate (Lao, 2007). Testing maternal TSH receptor auto-antibodies may predict fetal or neonatal thyrotoxicosis (Glinoer, 1998).

POSTNATAL CARE

In the puerperium symptoms often reappear, and for those who have discontinued their drugs due to the immunosuppressive benefit of pregnancy, assessment may show a need for the medication to be recommenced.

Breastfeeding is usually recommended, but if drugs are prescribed, these need to be reviewed for safety.

HYPOTHYROIDISM

The main cause of hypothyroidism is iodine deficiency, and treatment is simple with a single oral dose of iodine annually or the iodination of drinking water, salt or flour (Girling, 2006). This is no longer a factor in the UK, due to salt iodization, but world-wide is the cause of preventable mental retardation in a condition called cretinism.

Most cases of hypothyroidism in the UK are the result of autoimmune destruction of thyroid tissue. There are two main types, atrophic autoimmune thyroiditis and Hashimoto's thyroiditis (chronic autoimmune thyroiditis). In the atrophic form there is destruction of the gland, with atrophy and fibrosis. In Hashimoto's, damage leads to goitre formation where the thyroid is enlarged but function is poor. Those who have had thyroid surgery or radioactive iodine treatment for hyperthyroidism may also become hypothyroid, needing lifelong thyroxine replacement therapy (Perry, 2003).

Hypothyroidism may affect up to 1% of pregnant women (Kenyon and Nelson-Piercy, 2005). It is characterised by an increased TSH and decreased free T4 (Casey and Leveno, 2006).

Hypothyroidism can become evident for the first time in pregnancy, as those with subclinical undiagnosed disease may not be able to meet the extra demand on the thyroid for the increased metabolic rate of pregnancy (Table 10.1).

PRECONCEPTION CARE

There is much controversy about the effect of maternal hypothyroidism on fetal brain development (Casey and Leveno, 2006; Kenyon and Nelson-Piercy, 2005). However, since maternal T4 crosses to the fetus in the first trimester, where it is thought to be necessary for fetal brain development, it is recommended that T4 therapy is optimised before conception or as early in pregnancy as is possible.

PREGNANCY CARE

Drug dose changes may not be necessary during pregnancy if doses were adequate pre-pregnancy (Chopra and Baber, 2003), although one study found 45% of women needed increased medication (Harborne, *et al.*, 2005). If the woman is taking thyroxine it should be noted that taking iron or calcium supplements at the same time will reduce absorption, and advice should be to take them at least two hours apart (Keely and Barbour, 2008).

Risks associated with hypothyroidism include miscarriage, pre-eclampsia, abruption, low birth weight, stillbirth, premature birth (Casey and Leveno, 2006), increased rates of gestational hypertension (Kenyon and Nelson-Piercy, 2005) and, rarely, myxoedema coma (*see* Box 10.5). However, those who are well controlled should have a reduced level of complications. Hypothyroidism may affect the neonate as the transfer of maternal antibodies may occur, but this is very rare (Kenyon and Nelson-Piercy, 2005).

BOX 10.5: MYXOEDEMA COMA

This is a very rare consequence of undiagnosed or untreated hypothyroidism. It is characterised by hypothermia, bradycardia, depressed deep tendon reflexes and altered consciousness; hyponatremia, hypoglycaemia, hypoxia and hypercapnia.

(Kenyon and Nelson-Piercy, 2005)

Biochemical changes suggesting hypothyroidism can occur with severe pre-eclampsia; however, medication is not usually necessary and spontaneous recovery occurs after delivery, although the thyroid function should be monitored in the postnatal period (Lao, 2007).

POSTNATAL CARE
In the puerperium, hypothyroidism may predispose to postnatal depression. Medication should return to the pre-pregnancy dose, although this may need assessment if a substantial amount of weight was gained during pregnancy (Keely and Barbour, 2008). Postnatal testing with a TSH test is usual at 6–8 weeks.

POST-PARTUM THYROIDITIS (PPT)
It is suggested that PPT occurs in 5–10% of pregnancies (Stagnaro-Green, 2000), although other authorities have found a much lower incidence (Girling, 2006). It is an autoimmune disorder and there is an increased risk for those with thyroid antibodies in the first trimester, insulin-dependent diabetes (up to 25% may develop PPT [Casey and Leveno, 2006]) and a past history of this disorder. Onset is usually within the first few months postnatal. Most women progress through hyperthyroidism and hypothyroidism, then symptoms spontaneous resolve, usually within 12 months (Casey and Leveno, 2006). Presenting symptoms may include depression and memory impairment (Casey and Leveno, 2006). Treatment for the hyperthyroidism and hypothyroidism may be necessary (Gallas, *et al.*, 2002; Stuckey, *et al.*, 2001). It is suggested that up to 30% of these women will go on to develop permanent hypothyroidism (Casey and Leveno, 2006), therefore a yearly follow-up should be carried out (Stagnaro-Green, 2000) and increased monitoring performed after future pregnancies as reoccurrence is likely (Keely and Barbour, 2008).

REFERENCES
Becks G, Burrow G. *Thyroid Disorders and Pregnancy*. London, ON: Thyroid Foundation of Canada; 2000.

Blackburn ST. *Maternal, Fetal and Neonatal Physiology*. 3rd ed. St Louis, MO: Saunders; 2007.

Casey B, Leveno K. Thyroid disease in pregnancy. *Obstet Gynecol*. 2006; **108**(5): 1283–92.

Chopra I, Baber K. Treatment of primary hypothyroidism during pregnancy: is there an increase in thyroxine dose requirement in pregnancy? *Metabolism*. 2003; **52**: 122–8.

Gallas P, Stolk R, Bakker K, *et al*. Thyroid dysfunction during pregnancy and in the first post-partum year in women with diabetes mellitus type 1. *Eur J Endocrinol*. 2002; **1**(47): 443–51.

Girling J. Thyroid disorders in pregnancy. *Curr Obstet Gynaecol*. 2006; **16**: 47–53.

Glinoer D. The systematic screening and management of hypothyroidism and hyperthyroidism during pregnancy. *Trends Endocrinol Metab*. 1998; **9**: 403–11.

Harborne L, Alexander C, Thomson A, *et al*. Outcomes of pregnancy complicated by thyroid disease. *Aust N Z J Obstet Gynaecol*. 2005; **45**(3): 239–42.

Higgins C. *Understanding Laboratory Investigations for Nurses and Health Professionals*. 2nd ed. Oxford: Blackwell; 2007.

Jones RE, Huether SE. Alterations of hormonal regulation. In: McCance KL, Huether SE, editors. *Pathophysiology: the biological basis for diseases in adults and children*. 5th ed. St Louis, MO: Elsevier Mosby; 2006. pp. 683–734.

Keely E, Barbour L. Thyroid disorders. In: Rosene-Montella K, Keely E, Barbour L, *et al.*, editors. *Medical Care of the Pregnant Patient*. 2nd ed. Philadelphia, PA: ACP Press; 2008. pp. 253–70.

Kenyon A, Nelson-Piercy C. Thyroid disease. In: James D, Steer P, Weiner C, *et al.*, editors. *High Risk Pregnancy*. 3rd ed. Philadelphia, PA: Elsevier; 2005. pp. 1005–17.

Lao T. Thyroid disorders in pregnancy. In: Greer I, Nelson-Piercy C, Walters B, editors. *Maternal Medicine: medical problems in pregnancy*. Edinburgh: Churchill Livingstone Elsevier; 2007. pp. 73–7

Marx H, Amin P, Lazarus J. Hyperthyroidism and pregnancy. *BMJ*. 2008; **336**: 663–7.

Peleg D, Cada S, Peleg A, *et al*. The relationship between maternal scrum thyroid-stimulating immunoglobulin and fetal and neonatal thyrotoxicosis. *Obstet Gynecol*. 2002; **99**: 1040–3.

Perry M. Hypothyroidism: more common in women. *Pract Nurs*. 2003; **14**(7): 316–19.

Pop VJ, Vulsma T. Maternal hypothyroxinaemia during (early) gestation. *Lancet*. 2005; **365**: 1604–6.

Ramsey ID. The thyroid gland. In: Chamberlain G, Broughton Pipkin F, editors. *Clinical Physiology in Obstetrics*. 3rd ed. Oxford, Malden, MA: Blackwell; 1998. pp. 374–84.

Sherwood L. *Fundamentals of Physiology*. 2nd ed. Minneapolis, MI: West; 1994.

Smith C, Thomsett M, Choong C, *et al*. Congenital thyrotoxicosis in premature infants. *Clin Endocrinol*. 2001; **54**: 371–6.

Stagnaro-Green A. Recognizing, understanding and treating post-partum thyroiditis. *Endocrinol Metab Clin North Am*. 2000; **29**(2): 417–30.

Stuckey B, Kent G, Allen J. The biochemical and clinical course of post-partum thyroid dysfunction: the treatment decision. *Clin Endocrinol*. 2001; **54**: 377–83.

Wallace C, Couch R, Ginsberg J. Fetal thyrotoxicosis: a case-report and recommendations for prediction, diagnosis and treatment. *Thyroid*. 1995; **5**: 125–8.

Waugh A, Grant A. *Ross and Wilson: anatomy and physiology in health and illness*. 10th ed. Edinburgh: Elsevier Churchill Livingstone; 2006.

CHAPTER 11

Eating disorders

CONTENTS
→ Obesity
→ Underweight – restricted eating disorders

OBESITY

Obesity rates in the UK are reaching epidemic proportions. The 2007 CEMACH report *Saving Mothers Lives* emphasised the serious impact of obesity in pregnancy:

> Obesity appears to carry a greater risk of death . . . the magnitude of this risk means that obesity represents one of the greatest and growing overall threats to the childbearing population of the UK. (Lewis, 2007)

Younger women from socially deprived areas and some groups of immigrant women are most at risk of obesity. Obesity may have a genetic component to its cause, but ultimately weight gain results from low levels of physical exercise coupled with intake of energy-dense, high-fat food that is readily available.

Obesity is associated with significant health risks that are compounded by pregnancy. Weight gain above recommended levels in pregnancy with lack of weight loss post-partum contributes to a greater body mass index (BMI) in subsequent pregnancies. Preconception weight loss is ideal; however, the introduction of healthy eating and lifestyle issues can be started during pregnancy, and the postnatal period may be an optimum time for intervention.

DEFINITION

Obesity is an accumulation of excess body fat whereby energy intake (food) exceeds energy expenditure (metabolism and exercise) (Serci, 2007; 2008). Obesity is a disease that results in multiple organ pathology predisposing to chronic diseases (*see* Box 11.1) (Lean, 2003; Reece, 2008). The BMI is the standard classification for defining weight (*see* Box 11.2) as a risk factor and it is recommended that all women have their BMI calculated at booking (NICE, 2008). Excess fat on the abdomen (central fat distribution) is associated with greater risk of cardiovascular disease and diabetes and therefore waist measurement is commonly used to assess these health risks in the general population. Even with a normal BMI, a waist measurement of > 88 cm is a risk factor for disease (NICE, 2006). This is obviously of limited use in pregnancy, although it can perhaps be useful in pre-pregnancy assessment. Symptoms associated with obesity are listed in Box 11.3.

BOX 11.1: GENERAL COMPLICATIONS OF OBESITY

- Sleep apnoea
- Oedema
- Cellulitis
- Osteoarthritis
- Gall bladder disease
- Anaesthetic and surgical hazards
- Venous thrombosis
- Cardiovascular disease
- Diabetes
- Breast, ovarian, endometrial and colon cancer
- Infertility
- Psychological problems – lack of self esteem, discrimination

(Lean, 2003; Reece, 2008; Wilding, 2007)

BOX 11.2: BODY MASS INDEX (BMI)

Weight (kg) divided by height squared (m2)
- Under 18.5:   underweight
- 18.5–24.9:   healthy/normal
- 25.0–29.9:   overweight
- 30.0–34.9:   obese (1)
- 35.0–39.9:   obese (2)
- > 40.0:   obese (3)/morbidly obese/grossly obese

EPIDEMIOLOGY

A growing problem in obesity has been clearly identified by many sources. It has been shown that 3.2% of 20 year olds were obese in 1995, but in 2005 the number was 16% (Abayomi, *et al.*, 2007). Predictions are made that by 2010 one-third of UK adults will be obese (Sattar, 2007). Figures vary in different areas, but some have recently identified that 28% of pregnant women are overweight and 20.9% are obese (Yu, *et al.*, 2006).

PHYSIOLOGY OF WEIGHT GAIN
Energy balance

Weight gain occurs when energy intake consumed as food and drink exceeds the energy that is utilised by exercise and other metabolic body processes. Energy in food is measured as kilocalories (kcals) (usually shortened to calories) or kilojoules. The recommended calorie intake changes with age and lifestyle but it is generally considered to be around 2000 kcals for women of child-bearing age (British Nutrition Foundation, 2004).

BOX 11.3: SYMPTOMS ASSOCIATED WITH OBESITY

- Shortness of breath on minor exertion
- Difficulty in sleeping
- Low back, hip and knee pain
- Tiredness
- Chronic unhappiness
- Stress incontinence
- Menstrual disturbances and infertility
- Hirsutism
- Increased sweating contributing to skin problems

(Lean, 2003; Ogden, 2003)

The amount of energy used is also measured as calories. The body uses large amounts of energy just to maintain body functions such as breathing and cardiac function. This is known as the basal (or resting) metabolic rate (BMR) and varies according to gender (men have a higher BMR), age and weight. Contrary to common belief, people with higher weight have a higher BMR, although the energy needs of obese-prone individuals may be lower before or during the process of weight gain and may be a contributing factor in their weight gain (Lean, 2003; Yu, *et al.*, 2006). BMR accounts for 50–75% of energy expenditure, so even if an individual stays in bed all day, large amounts of energy to maintain body function are still needed. A further 10% of energy expenditure is in thermogenesis, the energy required to maintain warmth, for digestion of food and for response to stress (Yu, *et al.*, 2006). The remainder of energy expenditure is on physical activity, which includes the energy expended for daily activities as well as more vigorous activity that is required for manual work and sport.

Weight gain can result from relatively small cumulative balance over a period of time. Wilding (2007) gives the example that a 100 kcal excess daily (equivalent to a very small chocolate bar) will lead to an accumulation of 36 500 kcal of energy over a year. This excess energy is mostly stored as fat and will result in a 5.1 kg gain in weight. Looking at it more positively, 30 minutes of walking per day will use up 100 kcal. However, weight gain is a complex process that needs to be considered beyond just energy intake and expenditure. It incorporates excess or unregulated appetite, consideration of gene-nutrient interaction, the impact of exercise and complex social, cultural and medical factors (Lean, 2003).

Adipose tissue
Obesity is characterised by an increase in the number and/or size of fat cells (adipocytes). Extra calories from carbohydrates, protein and fat are converted into fat stores in

adipose (fat) tissue. Thus energy storage is the primary function of adipose tissue but it also has a role in regulating blood sugar, thermal insulation, and the protection of organs as well as metabolic and immune functions. There are two types of adipose tissue: brown adipose tissue (mostly in newborns) and white adipose tissue (WAT), the main type of human fat. Women typically store more fat than men, which is partly influenced by oestrogen. The different deposits of WAT fat, that is, whether it is central or subcutaneous, have different functions and while an increase in total body fat is associated with an increase in morbidity and mortality generally, it is excess fat located around the abdomen that makes the obese individual more at risk of heart disease and diabetes (Ogston, 2006). Fats in these different locations differ in the substances they secrete, which may explain the different morbidity (Powell, 2007).

Adipokines is the term used to describe the factors produced and secreted by adipose tissue. Over 100 have been identified, although the function of many is not understood. Leptin is an adipokine that was discovered in 1994, and it has a role in control of appetite, regulation of glucose, bone formation, regulation of puberty, immunity and inflammatory process. Adiponectin is another substance produced by fat cells. It has anti-athergenic properties and plays a role in regulating insulin sensitivity; levels of adiponectin decrease in obesity and this is associated with increased risk for diabetes and cardiac disease (Kiess, *et al.*, 2008; Powell, 2007).

The number of fat cells determines levels of obesity. Childhood obesity predisposes to continuing obesity throughout life. This is partly explained by attitudes and behaviour regarding diet and exercise, which are conditioned in childhood, as well as any genetic predisposition. However, when obesity occurs during this developmental stage it seems there is an increase in the number of fat cells, which sets the pattern for future obesity (Shaw, *et al.*, 2005).

Appetite

Appetite is a strong survival force set for evolutionary reasons to prevent weight loss and promote weight gain. Appetite should match physical activity to keep weight stable. However, in people with sedentary lifestyles the regulation between appetite and food requirements is lost (Lean, 2003). Eating is a conditioned response that is rewarded with pleasurable feelings. Eating should be in response to appetite, but a variety of external, contextual and social cues result in eating in the pre-appetite phase (Ogden, 2003). Eating results in a feeling of fullness known as satiety and is controlled by the hypothalamus through a complex interaction of hormones. Hunger is triggered when energy levels fall and is suppressed after eating. Leptin is produced by adipose tissue in the well-fed state. It sends messages to the hypothalamus to indicate suppression of food intake and stimulation of energy expenditure (Ockenden, 2007). Leptin should control appetite regulation; however, it is found in excess levels in obese people, where it seems there is a resistance to its effects (Kiess, *et al.*, 2008). The stomach has a feedback mechanism via the sympathetic nervous system to indicate when it is full, while the hormone ghrelin indicates when the stomach is empty (Wilding, 2007).

Appetite can be stimulated by medication, including corticosteroids, antipsychotics, antidepressants, valproate (for epilepsy) and progesterone (Lean, 2003; Wilding, 2007).

OBESITY AND THE ENVIRONMENT

Obesity is strongly influenced by environmental factors. Changing patterns of work and activity, changes to food supply and social and cultural influences have contributed to increases in levels of obesity.

Physical activity

The decrease in physical activity is seen as a major factor contributing to increasing levels of obesity (Department of Health, 2004a). Studies have repeatedly shown that women are less physically active than men at any age (Wilding, 2007). Physical activity is important because it is the main way to increase energy expenditure. The recommended guide for exercise is 30 minutes of brisk walking or equivalent five times per week (Department of Health, 2004a), but the Health Survey for England in 2003 found that only 30% of women of reproductive age were achieving this (Department of Health, 2004b). Physical activity assists in weight loss and also in maintaining weight loss, although the energy expended seems to only partly explain why it works. Physical activity also seems to be associated with improved ability to control appetite (Fox, 2005). Lean (2003) proposes that activity produces some unknown chemical that allows leptin to enter the brain and diminish appetite. Additionally, self-confidence may be improved with exercise, which may impact on control of food intake (Fox, 2005).

Diet

Despite numerous government publications about balanced diet and healthy eating, obesity levels are getting worse. Access to fast food, an expanded food range, preference for foods high in fat and effective advertising of unhealthy foods are just some of the areas blamed for unhealthy eating habits (Shaw, *et al.*, 2005). A balanced diet contains the nutrients required for healthy body function in appropriate proportion. The UK government recommendations are explained simply using the 'eat well' plate and the recommendations contained in the eight tips for eating well (Food Standards Agency, 2007). The principles of a healthy diet involve balance, moderation and variety.

National surveys show that the typical diet in the UK contains 11% protein, 37% fat and 48% carbohydrates (Hoare and Henderson, 2004). However, it is recognised that collecting accurate data about food intake is difficult, with under-reporting of intake by up to 1000 kcal per day (Lean, 2003; Macdiarmid and Blundell, 1998). The dramatic increase in the fat content of the UK diet since the Second World War has been seen as one of the contributing factors to increased rates of obesity (Obesity Resource Information Centre, 2000). Fat has the highest-density energy of all nutrients, although a certain amount (up to 30%) of fat in the diet is essential. There are different types of dietary fat. Saturated fat (found in animal products) is associated, when consumed to excess, with heart disease, whereas polyunsaturated fats and in particular omega 3 polyunsaturated fat appear to have a role in improved health.

The consumption of carbonated drinks and alcohol has also been implicated as an area of concern in the UK diet, as these drinks can add significantly to energy intake. Intake of carbonated soft drinks and fast food is linked with weight gain and the development of Type 2 diabetes (Pereira, *et al.*, 2005).

Social

Weight gain in the developing world may be seen as a sign of wealth, whereas in modern western society obesity seems to be more aligned with social deprivation. This trend is most marked in women (Department of Health, 2004b). Vulnerable obese women living in poor social circumstances have other associated problems that contribute to health risk, including poor housing, smoking and lack of leisure activity. Poor knowledge of diet, lack of access to quality food and preference for cheap accessible food that tends to have a high fat content further predispose this group to obesity. Low levels of physical activity and a sudden increase in the amount of fat consumed (meat and butter) alongside elements of social deprivation contribute to weight gain in immigrant women in the UK (Lean, 2003). Teenagers are identified as another group vulnerable to developing obesity because of their irregular meal times, access to fast food and physical inactivity (Serci, 2007).

BIOLOGICAL DETERMINANTS OF OBESITY

Obesity tends to run in families. Children with two obese parents have an 80% risk of becoming obese compared to less than 10% in children with two lean parents (Ogden, 2003). This association is partly explained by environmental factors, as families share the same influences on diet and lifestyle. However, studies of identical twins reared apart and adopted children have provided evidence of a role for genetics in determining obesity (Ogden, 2003). Genetic predisposition is complex and may influence metabolic rate, appetite regulation, the distribution and number of fat cells or a preference for a sedentary lifestyle. Conversely, a genetic tendency to obesity does not explain the increase in obesity over the last 50 years, where environmental influences are evident and yet the gene pool is essentially unchanged. There are some medical conditions with genetic components that are associated with weight gain. These are listed in Box 11.4.

BOX 11.4: GENETIC-BASED CONDITIONS ASSOCIATED WITH WEIGHT GAIN

- Metabolic X syndrome
- Rare defect of the 'ob gene' which regulates leptin
- Prader-Willi syndrome
- Bardet-Biedel syndrome
- FTO, PMO and POMC gene mutation
- Hypothyroidism, diabetes, polycystic ovarian syndrome

(Lean, 2003; Ockenden, 2007; Ogden, 2003; Wilding, 2007)

Polycystic ovarian syndrome (PCOS)

PCOS is a collection of signs and symptoms involving disturbance of the reproductive, endocrine and metabolic function that occurs in up to 25% of women to a variable degree. It affects approximately 50% of South Asian women, compared to 15–25% of white UK women (Balen, 2007). Key features are listed in Box 11.5.

BOX 11.5: KEY FEATURE OF PCOS

- Menstrual cycle disturbances
- Polycystic ovaries
- Hyperandrogenism
- Obesity
- Impaired glucose tolerance
- Hyperinsulinaemia
- Increased risk of cardiac disease and Type 2 diabetes

(Balen, 2007)

Polycystic ovaries can exist without the clinical signs, although these can surface with weight gain and commonly improve with weight loss. Even modest weight loss (5–10% of body weight) can achieve improvements in insulin sensitivity and regulation of the menstrual cycle and can increase the likelihood of a healthy pregnancy (Norman, *et al.*, 2004).

WEIGHT MANAGEMENT OPTIONS

As part of their health promotion role, midwives need to be involved in advising weight management before, during and after pregnancy. While there are particular considerations during pregnancy and lactation (discussed below), goals of weight management outside pregnancy include avoiding weight gain, having a healthy, balanced diet and keeping physically active. Successful weight loss involves behavioural and cognitive changes and a weight loss programme that sets realistic targets for gradual weight loss, includes exercise and provides support. The National Institute for Health and Clinical Excellence provides evidence-based guidance for health professionals for the management of obesity (NICE, 2006). Midwives need to be conversant with these principles and provide support and information for women where relevant. Referral to a dietician, private-sector slimming group or physician specialising in weight management may be appropriate. An interesting initiative in Wales, in which midwives are referring to, and working with, a slimming club for the benefit of pregnant members may prove to have valuable outcomes (Anon, 2007). Pharmacological agents for management of obese adults are contraindicated in pregnancy and breastfeeding.

Increasingly women are having bariatric surgery, either for general improvement of their health or specifically to combat infertility issues, which aims to reduce and maintain weight loss through restricting food intake and preventing its absorption. The three most common surgical procedures for obesity are laparoscopic gastric bypass, laparoscopic adjustable gastric bands and open gastric bypass (Colquitt, *et al.*, 2005). These procedures may cause nutritional problems, in particular where large parts of the small intestine are bypassed, which may lead to malabsorption of essential proteins, vitamins and minerals. Ideally a nutritional evaluation pre-pregnancy should be carried out. If necessary, a band may be adjusted during pregnancy (Dixon, *et al.*, 2005; Stotland, 2009). Those who have had bariatric surgery are generally recommended to avoid pregnancy for at least the first year during the time of rapid weight loss, although it has recently been shown that those who became pregnant within the first 12 months had no increased rates of malnutrition, adverse fetal outcomes or pregnancy complications (Dao, *et al.*, 2006).

WEIGHT GAIN IN PREGNANCY

Weight gain in pregnancy is normal and is made up of weight from the fetus and the placenta as well as amniotic fluid and accumulation of maternal fat deposits. An average weight gain of 12.5 kg is expected in pregnancy (Serci, 2008), although recommended weight gain is dependent on a woman's baseline BMI. Weight loss is not recommended during pregnancy, even for women who are obese, because of concern over nutrient requirements for fetal development (Bodnar, 2007).

Many women report that their weight problems stem from around the time of childbirth. A large Swedish study examined weight change from the beginning of a woman's first pregnancy to the beginning of the second pregnancy. Weight gain between pregnancies was strongly associated with poorer outcomes for mother and baby even in women of normal weight (Villamor and Cnattingius, 2006). A number of successive pregnancies may mean weight is gained progressively. Post-partum weight retention is related to excessive weight gain in pregnancy, low socioeconomic status, parity and high pre-pregnancy BMI. It is argued that the extra calorie requirements for lactation (often given as 200 calories) are not required, as women may be less active at this time and have lower BMR (Amorim, *et al.*, 2007). Poor weight gain in pregnancy is also harmful and is associated with preterm birth and low infant birth weight (Walsh and Murphy, 2007).

Government advice on healthy eating in pregnancy and breastfeeding does not provide a specific recommended calorie intake, taking a broader view of diet and advising a reduction in food containing high levels of fat and sugar. A balance of nutrients, reducing salt, including oily fish and appropriate vitamin and fluid intake is advised. Emphasis is on meeting the extra energy requirements of pregnancy through eating nutritious foods (Food Standards Agency (FSA), 2002; 2007). Pregnant women are encouraged to remain physically active in pregnancy. Most women want to achieve the best for their babies, so pregnancy may prove a powerful motivator to achieve lifestyle changes (Walsh and Murphy, 2007).

COMPLICATIONS OF OBESITY IN PREGNANCY

The combination of the physiological changes of pregnancy with the pathological impact of obesity, particularly on the cardiac and respiratory system, makes it unsurprising that so many complications occur, including the increased risk of death. There are many specific risks in pregnancy, birth and the puerperium (*see* Box 11.6) for those who are overweight, both when conceiving with an increased BMI or gaining excessive amounts of weight in pregnancy. The degree of risk is directly related to the degree of overweight (Serci, 2007): for example, it has been suggested that the risk of pre-eclampsia doubles with each 5–7 BMI unit increase in pre-pregnancy BMI (O'Brien, *et al.*, 2003).

BOX 11.6: COMPLICATIONS ASSOCIATED WITH OBESITY AROUND THE TIME OF CHILDBIRTH

- *Maternal:* infertility, increased miscarriage rate, gestational or Type 2 diabetes mellitus, hypertension and pre-eclampsia, thromboembolic disease, worsening sleep apnoea, increased interventions in labour including higher Caesarean section rate, post-partum haemorrhage, increased infection risk, reduced breastfeeding.
- *Fetal:* congenital abnormalities (especially NTD), macrosomia, IUGR, intra-uterine death, stillbirth, neonatal death, future health considerations.

Infertility

Infertility has been reported to be increased in those who are overweight and obese, despite having a normal menstrual cycle (Gesink Law, *et al.*, 2007; Nelson and Fleming, 2007) and it has been suggested that about half of overweight women have polycystic ovarian syndrome (*see* earlier in this chapter) or signs of polycystic ovaries, compared to 30% of lean women (Hart, *et al.*, 2004), which could be one explanation.

Pregnancy loss

Increased rates of early and/or recurrent miscarriage have been associated with obesity (Lashen, *et al.*, 2004). This could be at least partly related to the increased number of congenital abnormalities (discussed later in this section). There has also been an increased pregnancy loss identified with obese women undergoing infertility treatment (Fedorsak, *et al.*, 2000), and a weight loss prior to starting this treatment can improve outcomes (Clark, *et al.*, 1998).

Late fetal death/stillbirth is increased in the morbidly obese and is perhaps more than three times more likely (Cedergren, 2004; Chu, *et al.*, 2007; Galtier-Dereure, *et al.*, 2000; Salihu, *et al.*, 2007). Other studies agree (Stephansson, *et al.*, 2001) and also show an increased neonatal death rate (Kristensen, *et al.*, 2005), although some have not demonstrated this (Galtier-Dereure, *et al.*, 2000). It is suggested that a combination of rapid growth induced by excess insulin in the fetuses of obese women along with limitations of the placenta to make available enough oxygen to meet fetal requirements may lead to hypoxia and fetal death (Yu, *et al.*, 2006).

Thromboembolic disease

The risk of thromboembolic disease is increased (Robinson and Yu, 2007) in obese women. The incidence of thromboembolic disease is reported to increase from 0.04% with a BMI < 25 to 0.07% with a BMI of 25–30 and 0.08% with a BMI > 30 (Sebire, *et al.*, 2001). Reduced mobility associated with obesity increases venous stasis, which results in sluggish venous return and enhances propensity for clot formation (Bothamley, 2002). Inadequate anticoagulation, taking account of body weight, has also been highlighted as contributing to thrombosis in this group (Lewis, 2007).

Cardiac and other medical complications

Obesity has substantial effect on cardiac, respiratory, endothelial and vascular function. An increase in weight will require increased cardiac output and increased blood volume. Enlargement of the left ventricle and increased heart rate increases function and cardiac output, but with less time for myocardial perfusion. Conduction and contraction of the ventricles can be further compromised when fat deposits in the tissue of the heart exist (Yu, *et al.*, 2006).

As well as increased rates of chronic cardiac dysfunction, rates of proteinuria and non-alcoholic fatty liver disease also rise (Catalano, 2007). In addition oxygenation and ventilation are impaired in obesity, resulting in chronic hypoxia and hypercapnia and possibly pulmonary hypertension. Related to this is an increased incidence of obstructive sleep apnoea (Catalano, 2007; Saravanakumar, *et al.*, 2006) and this can worsen as the upper airways become narrower in pregnancy, especially during the third trimester, and lead to hypertension and/or IUGR (Izci, *et al.*, 2006; Roush and Bell, 2004).

Obese pregnant women have been shown to have a marked rise in serum insulin, deranged lipids, a low-grade inflammatory response and microvascular endothelial impairment (Ramsay, *et al.*, 2002). Women who are obese have an increased risk of developing gestational diabetes and, in fact, may already have undiagnosed Type 2 diabetes mellitus (*see* Chapter 1).

There is an increased risk of hypertension and pre-eclampsia (Robinson and Yu, 2007) in obese women. The risk of pre-eclampsia has been shown to increase from 3.9% with a BMI of 20–5 to 13.5% with a BMI of > 30 (Bodnar, *et al.*, 2005). It has also been proposed that a waist measurement at less than 16/40 of > 80 cm can predict hypertension and pre-eclampsia (Sattar, *et al.*, 2001).

Fetal congenital abnormalities

There are many studies demonstrating an increased number of various congenital abnormalities associated with maternal obesity (Waller, *et al.*, 2007; Watkins, *et al.*, 2003). The fetal congenital malformations found in association with maternal obesity are probably of similar aetiology to the glucose-mediated malformations associated with diabetes and studies may include women with undiagnosed Type 2 diabetes. In obesity there is extra insulin, increased insulin resistance, fetal hyperinsulinaemia and chronic hypoxia, even in the absence of diabetes. This combination of factors may possibly cause malformation (Yu, *et al.*, 2006).

It has also been suggested that the increased neural tube defect (NTD) rate may be due to decreased levels of folic acid reaching the fetus as the obese mother has increased metabolic demands and possibly a diet poor in folate (Werler, *et al.*, 1996). However, the studies regarding congenital abnormalities are contradictory (Gate and Ramsay, 2007). There is also a difficulty in ultrasound assessment of obese women (Yu, *et al.*, 2006), and if abnormalities are not identified, the women will not have had the choice to terminate these pregnancies.

Complications in the fetus, infant and beyond

The risk of fetal macrosomia rises after a 17 kg pregnancy weight gain (Cedergren, 2004; Cogswell, *et al.*, 1995), even without the presence of maternal diabetes (Yu, *et al.*,

2006). There has also been an increased rate of meconium aspiration and fetal distress demonstrated in the pregnancies of morbidly obese women (Cedergren, 2004).

A long-term effect on growth, body shape, energy regulation and weight in infants (Oken and Gillman, 2003) from maternal overnutrition has been suggested, as well as an association with obesity and insulin resistance in later life (Ravelli, *et al.*, 1998).

ROLE OF THE MIDWIFE

Despite the growing numbers of obese women and an increasing awareness as to their risk status, there are few guidelines for midwives. However, one midwife has recently published the care pathways she has set up in her practice, and these could be considered a valuable resource for other midwives (Richens, 2008a; Richens, 2008b).

There may also be a role for midwives to become involved in support programmes involving education in healthy eating and exercise. A study by Claesson *et al.* (2008a) found women valued this intervention. There is also clearly a role for the midwife in general counselling and support. Although it is a sensitive subject, and midwives may feel awkward initiating a discussion on weight with an obese woman, there is evidence that most women appreciate the support of a midwife (Claesson, *et al.*, 2008a; Richens, 2008a).

The midwife plays a vital part in all aspects of the woman's care, as detailed in the sections following. However, in general midwives may not have specialist skills in the physical management of obese women, for example, moving and handling with special lifting equipment or pressure-area care.

As the numbers of these women increase, perhaps consideration should be made of having a named or specialist midwife who could ensure a bariatric programme is set up and kept relevant, and could educate other midwives on the specific needs of obese women (Richens, 2008a). As many hospitals now have a hospital programme, this specialist midwife could also liaise with these experts, ensuring that the maternity unit had access to the necessary additional skills and equipment.

PRECONCEPTION CARE

An increased dose of folic acid is recommended for women with a BMI > 40 (Yu, *et al.*, 2006), to be continued into pregnancy as usual. As the rate of Type 2 diabetes is increased in obese women (Dunne, 2005) and it is estimated that 30–50% of adults with Type 2 diabetes are undiagnosed (Gate and Ramsay, 2007), testing and diagnosis before pregnancy would allow blood sugars to be stabilised before conception.

Ideally a weight-reduction programme would be undertaken before pregnancy to reduce the risk of complications. This could be arranged through community weight-loss programmes, referral to dieticians or doctors for individual help or bariatric surgery.

PREGNANCY CARE

NICE (2008) recommends all women are weighed and measured as soon as possible in pregnancy, usually at the booking appointment, and the BMI calculated. If a woman falls into the high-risk category, it is recommended that antenatal care is offered by a multidisciplinary team, including an obstetrician, dietician, any other relevant specialist (e.g., cardiac or diabetic) and the midwife, who is vital for both co-ordinating services and offering important support and professional care.

As in all care of women around childbirth, advice should be adapted to the woman's individual needs and risks at the different times of the pregnancy. However, increased visits will be necessary to screen for pregnancy-induced hypertension, pre-eclampsia, gestational diabetes mellitus and thromboembolic disease.

The increased dose of folic acid commenced preconception should be continued for women with a BMI > 40 (Yu, *et al.*, 2006) or commenced as soon as possible in pregnancy. As increased weight is a risk factor for gestational diabetes mellitus, glucose tolerance testing is recommended and perhaps repeated more than once in the pregnancy. Low-dose aspirin may be given if there are other clinical risk factors for pre-eclampsia (Gate and Ramsay, 2007). Thromboprophylaxis may also be considered during pregnancy if additional risk factors are present (Gate and Ramsay, 2007).

Recommended weight-gain advice during pregnancy for obese women varies. Most authorities advise against losing weight during pregnancy and emphasise that adequate nutrition levels in obese women may be compromised (Galtier, *et al.*, 2008). There is some research demonstrating satisfactory outcomes when obese women have a very small weight gain (≤ 7 kg) in pregnancy (Claesson, *et al.*, 2008b; Kiel, *et al.*, 2007) but careful supervision is necessary so the woman does not become nutritionally deficient and the risk of a small-for-dates fetus remains a concern. Others have noted that a weight gain of 10 kg seems to be statistically associated with the best obstetric outcomes (Yu, *et al.*, 2006). It is recommended that diet is planned, with the assistance of a dietician if possible, to ensure necessary nutrients are received (Yu, *et al.*, 2006), and working with the woman in partnership is necessary to obtain the best result (Cogswell, *et al.*, 1999).

Exercise can help to reduce the risk of pre-eclampsia and gestational diabetes, and it can also prevent too much weight gain. There is evidence that exercise in pregnancy is not harmful (Carpenter, 2000), and a target for activity could be > 30 minutes moderate exercise five times a week (Zaninotto, *et al.*, 2006); however, the health of each woman needs to be individually and carefully assessed before this is suggested.

Detailed anomaly scans, together with serum screening, are offered in view of the increased incidence of congenital abnormalities in women who are obese. However, adipose tissue can absorb ultrasound energy and in obesity the image quality may be compromised (Hendler, *et al.*, 2004). CVS and amniocentesis may also be appropriate, but these are more difficult procedures in an obese woman (Irvine and Shaw, 2006), so the risks of failure or complications may be raised. Pre-labour assessment of women with a BMI > 40 should be made to check their ability to abduct their hips for possible instrumental delivery or McRoberts manoeuvre (Yu, *et al.*, 2006).

Anaesthetic review is recommended. It has been suggested that antenatal education regarding anaesthetic implications of obesity is not part of pregnancy care (Dresner, 2007), and a survey of obstetricians suggests that discussion of obstetric and neonatal complications of obesity in pregnancy and labour may not routinely occur (Mhyre, *et al.*, 2007). It is understood that this may be a difficult subject to broach (Heslehurst, *et al.*, 2007) and sensitivity is necessary, but every woman requires the information to be able to make informed choices, and all midwives should ensure women in their care receive this.

LABOUR CARE

During the antenatal period, as with any other high-risk woman, there should have been a multidisciplinary plan made for labour, and this should have included anaesthetic services. The advantage of continuity of midwifery care is to allow one person to ensure that all appropriate assessments were made during pregnancy, any follow-up necessary (e.g., cardiac testing) was made, and the results were disseminated to other members of the multidisciplinary team. The midwife could also ensure anaesthetic services were involved in planning any elective procedure or were made aware when the woman was admitted in labour. Given the potential for high-risk situations, this labour may inevitably be highly medicalised, but the skilful midwife can do much not only to ensure a high standard of safe physical care, but also to create the atmosphere that will result in a psychologically satisfying experience for the woman and her partner.

There is an increased risk of labour interventions for obese women (Robinson and Yu, 2007). An increased rate of preterm birth at less than 33 weeks' gestation has also been reported (Bhattacharya, *et al.*, 2007), and this may be related to the higher rate of maternal medical complications or concern if there is difficulty in monitoring fetal well-being.

Pre-pregnancy obesity is associated with the increased risk of preterm prolonged rupture of membranes (Nohr, *et al.*, 2007). Increased risk of abruption related to increased BMI (Bhattacharya, *et al.*, 2007) has also been reported. The rate of induction of labour is increased with increased weight (Bhattacharya, *et al.*, 2007; Sebire, *et al.*, 2001). There is also evidence that obese women attempting a vaginal birth after Caesarean section are about 50% less successful than those of a normal weight (Juhasz, *et al.*, 2005).

It has been shown (after correcting for associations such as macrosomia, nulliparity, induction of labour and diabetes) that overweight and obese women have an increased Caesarean section rate (Ehrenberg, *et al.*, 2004). There may be a sixfold increase in Caesarean section rate with a BMI over 30 (Kaiser and Kirby, 2001) and each unit rise in BMI may increase the risk of Caesarean section by 7% (Brost, *et al.*, 1997). Labour dystocia (failure to progress) has been identified in studies as a common cause for the increased risk of Caesarean section (Reece, 2008; Sheiner, *et al.*, 2004) and it has been suggested that there could be a physiological cause, such as suboptimal contractions and increased fatty tissue in the pelvis (Barau, *et al.*, 2006). CTG monitoring may be difficult, as increased adipose tissue between the external transducer and the fetus may lead to a poor-quality trace (Yu, *et al.*, 2006). This difficulty in assessing the fetal well-being in labour could also result in extra instrumental or Caesarean section deliveries.

A Caesarean section is a more difficult procedure in an obese woman, and this inevitably makes its duration longer (Irvine and Shaw, 2006). A longer operating time usually leads to an increased blood loss and contributes to a longer hospital stay (Hall and Neubert, 2005) as well as possible health compromise. Instrumental deliveries have also been reported to be more challenging for the operator, and it may be harder to identify and suture vaginal or cervical lacerations (Irvine and Shaw, 2006).

An early epidural may be recommended for a woman who is morbidly obese, as insertion may be difficult, and it would be an advantage to have a working epidural should a Caesarean section be required, as a general anaesthetic in obese women has an increased risk of failed or difficult intubations (Soens, *et al.*, 2008). Spinal and epidural insertion, as well as intubation, are more difficult in obese women and may therefore need more time (Saravanakumar, *et al.*, 2006). However, the advantages of an early epidural need to be weighed against the potential restriction of mobility and possible slowing of labour progress. There also may be poor peripheral access, so early cannulation may be necessary.

Obesity increases the risk of gastro-oesophageal reflux, so policies on fasting and appropriate drugs to reduce gastric secretions should be followed (Dresner, 2007).

Obese women are often prescribed prophylactic anticoagulation drugs, which need to be given in an appropriate weight-related dose, timed with labour and the potential of regional analgesia, and also with the removal of an epidural catheter post-delivery. It is also important that the right size of TED stockings is available, and forward planning done antenatally should ensure this is not a problem.

Should the use of the operating theatre be required, it is important to note that operating theatre tables have a maximum weight tolerance and this may be different when lithotomy is used. Plans made in the antenatal period should ensure the right equipment is available when an obese woman is in labour.

Maternity beds may need an appropriate high-weight tolerance, and this should be checked both on the labour and antenatal and postnatal wards during pregnancy. If labour is anticipated to be prolonged, for instance, if the woman is being induced, with an epidural and intravenous infusions which will compromise mobility, and following Caesarean section in particular, a pressure-reducing mattress should be used.

POSTNATAL CARE

An obese woman, depending on her previous health and labour events, may well need high-dependency care following delivery. She may have ongoing medical problems from the pregnancy, such as pre-eclampsia, and she has an increased risk of post-partum haemorrhage (Bhattacharya, *et al.*, 2007).

An increased risk of infection from all sites – chest, genital, wound, urinary tract and pyrexia of unknown origin – is present in obese women (Sebire, *et al.*, 2001; Yu, *et al.*, 2006). Causes are varied; for example, respiratory complications may be caused by reduced mobility (Sararanakumar, *et al.*, 2006) or prolonged surgery. The increased risk of wound infections may be because of compromised wound healing due to obesity (Boyle, 2006). Following Caesarean section, obese women are more likely to have a drain as subcutaneous drains can reduce wound complications (Allaire, *et al.*, 2000). All women who are nutritionally compromised are susceptible to infection, so particular attention needs to be paid to diet both antenatally and in the postnatal period.

Thromboembolic risk continues into the postnatal period and is increased with increased weight (Sebire, *et al.*, 2001). Thromboprophylaxis may be commenced, or continued, and early ambulation encouraged, together with graduated compression stockings, passive exercises, deep breathing and referral to a physiotherapist as necessary.

Involution may be hard to evaluate if the woman is obese (Richens, 2008a). A careful observation of lochia may be necessary in order to assess well-being.

A systematic review of the literature (Amir and Donath, 2007) found that breast-feeding rates are reduced in obese women, for intention, initiation and duration. The reasons are varied and can be biological, psychological, behavioural, cultural or a combination of these factors. There may be mechanical difficulties in breastfeeding, as finding a comfortable position may be problematic. There is also evidence of a reduced prolactin response in obese women (Rasmussen and Kjolhede, 2004), so additional care and support may be necessary, especially if the baby is macrosomic and needs extra feeding. Maternal weight loss postnatally can be compromised if she is not breastfeeding or if there is early discontinuation of breastfeeding.

Following a sensible weight-loss diet can be difficult in the puerperium, as an organised lifestyle and new baby are usually incompatible. However, advice, referral and support should be offered wherever possible, and these can be seen not only as a contribution to long-term health, but also as preconception care for the next pregnancy. Glazer *et al.* (2004) showed that women who lost 10 lb (4.5 kg) between pregnancies had a reduced risk of gestational diabetes, but those who gained 10 lb had an increased risk. The risk of pre-eclampsia in a subsequent pregnancy also fell in women who had lost > 1 BMI unit between pregnancies (Villamor and Cnattingius, 2006), and it has been suggested that if overweight, even a modest reduction in weight (e.g., 4.5 kg) could reduce the risk of pre-eclampsia by half (Bodnar, *et al.*, 2005; Gate and Ramsay, 2007).

Achieving pre-pregnancy weight by about six months after birth appears to reduce the risk of obesity later in life and improves outcomes in subsequent pregnancies (Villamor and Cnattingius, 2006). While further research is required, a small preliminary systematic review of six trials involving 245 women suggests that diet and exercise during this time helps women lose weight without being detrimental to mother or baby (Amorim, *et al.*, 2007). However, government advice for breastfeeding mothers is not to try to lose weight but to establish healthy eating habits and physical activity that will help them lose weight gradually (FSA, 2002).

PSYCHOSOCIAL ISSUES

There is no firm evidence to suggest that obese people differ psychologically from non-obese people (Shaw, *et al.*, 2005). However, they generally do not like their obese state and while depression is attributed to obesity, studies are conflicting about rates of clinical depression (Ogden, 2003; Shaw, *et al.*, 2005). Obese people may have low self-esteem and a poor self-image. This is likely to arise from the negative stereotyping they are subjected to. Job prospects may also be affected by obesity (Shaw, *et al.*, 2005). Alternatively, weight loss is associated with an improved self-esteem and sense of well-being (Kushner and Foster, 2000). There is also a clear association between obesity and social deprivation (Heslehurst, *et al.*, 2007). Excess weight gain is three times more likely in low income groups (Yu, *et al.*, 2006) and less money is associated with increased use of cheaper foods (high in sugar and fat) and less activity (NICE, 2006).

Behavioural and cognitive therapies are the most commonly used psychological therapies for weight loss. Behavioural treatments provide adaptive strategies to control overeating and manage lapses in diet as well as to increase motivation to exercise. Techniques include stimulus control, the setting of goals and self-monitoring. Cognitive techniques can be added to behavioural therapy and seek to help the individual identify adverse thinking patterns and mood states that contribute to weight gain. Commercial weight-loss programmes integrate therapy techniques with education, social support and problem-solving to facilitate weight loss (Shaw, *et al.*, 2005). Behavioural and cognitive-behavioural strategies, when combined with diet control and exercise, have been shown to enhance weight reduction (Shaw, *et al.*, 2005).

A primary influence on nutritional intake is education and in her public health role the midwife could perhaps address this.

UNDERWEIGHT – RESTRICTED EATING DISORDERS
EPIDEMIOLOGY
Underweight is considered to be a BMI < 18.5 (*see* Box 11.2) and involves 3–10% of the UK population (Abayomi, *et al.*, 2007). Restricted eating disorders (*see* Box 11.7 for definitions) are estimated to involve about 5% of women (Ratnaike, 2007). Worldwide, anorexia is widespread but bulimia is more usual in western countries (Micali, 2007). Anorexia is estimated to occur primarily in teenagers and younger women, while bulimia sufferers are usually slightly older (NICE, 2004), but overall the vast majority of restricted eating disorders occur in women during their reproductive years, making it a very relevant subject for midwives. Underweight is associated with younger age and the estimate of possible malnutrition is up to 20% of teenagers (Abayomi, *et al.*, 2007), which adds to the other risks for teenage pregnancy.

BOX 11.7: DEFINITIONS OF RESTRICTED EATING DISORDERS

- *Anorexia nervosa* is a refusal to maintain body weight over the minimal level considered normal for age and height, an intense fear of gaining weight or becoming fat while being underweight, a distorted body image, and in post-menarcheal women, amenorrhea. It is usually divided into two types:
  — restrictive (types and amounts of food severely limited)
  — binge-eating and purging (using self-induced vomiting, diuretics, enemas or laxatives) (American Psychiatric Association, 2000).
- *Bulimia nervosa* is an eating disorder characterised by binge eating and purging, occurring at least twice a week. Sufferers are usually of normal weight or slightly underweight or overweight (Lavender, 2007).
- *Atypical eating disorders not otherwise specified:* these conditions do not meet the criteria of anorexia or bulimia, but involve abnormal eating behaviour. There are several suggested subgroups. The numbers suffering from these conditions are not known.

FEATURES OF WOMEN WITH A RESTRICTED EATING DISORDER
The causes of eating disorders are complex and appear to be a combination of genetic, neurochemical, psychological and sociocultural factors (Perry, 2002; James, 2001; Zerbe, 2007). Table 11.1 lists the risk factors associated with eating disorders.

Up to 40% of women with restricted eating disorders have an underlying affective disorder (Ward, 2008), and restricted eating disorders are one of the mental health issues that may be influenced by culture-related risk factors (Douki, *et al.*, 2007). Women with anorexia may demonstrate symptoms such as depression, anxiety or obsessive behaviour, as well as serious manifestations such as self-harming or suicidal tendencies (American Psychiatric Association, 2000; Mazzeo, *et al.*, 2006). Women with anorexia tend to isolate themselves, whereas women with bulimia may be quite sociable and outwardly appear to self-assured, hiding their lack of self-confidence and low self-esteem (Orbanic, 2001).

TABLE 11.1: Risk factors associated with eating disorders

Family factors	Positive family history of eating disorders, family dysfunction and childhood maltreatment
Psychological factors	Perfectionism, low self-esteem, depression
Social factors	Female gender, younger age, middle/upper-class socioeconomic status
Occupations	Models, athletes, actresses and dancers
Stressful life events	Domestic violence and rape, childhood sexual abuse, unresolved mourning

Sources: Kondo and Sokol (2006); Morgan, *et al.* (1999); Zerbe (2007)

Physical complications of anorexia nervosa and bulimia are summarised in Table 11.2 and Table 11.3, respectively. Impaired cardiac function has been reported to be as high as 10–21% for woman with eating disorders (James, 2001). Severe anorexia may result in reduced cardiac muscle mass, leading to impaired contractility with reduced cardiac output. In addition, the reduced mass can cause the cardiac valves to sag, with subsequent mitral valve prolapse (Perry, 2002). Electrolyte imbalance, particularly low potassium, can result in cardiac irregularities. Women who use syrup of ipecac (a medication that induces vomiting) can experience symptoms of chest pain, muscle weakness, shortness of breath and tachycardia and are at risk of cardiomyopathy, which can be fatal (James, 2001). Prolonged use of laxatives with a purging type of eating disorder may cause malabsorption, further complicating electrolyte and nutrient balance (Steffan, *et al.*, 2007). Despite the many potential complications of eating disorders, physical findings may be normal, particularly in women with normal weight who have bulimia nervosa.

COMPLICATIONS OF RESTRICTED EATING DISORDERS IN PREGNANCY

There is much research on the effects of restricted eating disorders on both the pregnant woman and the fetus/infant; however, many of the findings do not agree. Some research has shown that those with a history of anorexia may still be at increased risk of pregnancy and birth complications such as miscarriage, premature birth and low-birth-weight babies (Mitchell and Bulik, 2006), although other research has not (Franko, *et al.*, 2001). When research shows conflicting findings, it is likely that different populations were studied; for example, some studies only considered those who were hospitalised, which would be at the extreme end of the disease.

The effects of the maternal eating disorder also depend on the type of disorder. For example, a low birth weight is associated with anorexia and increased miscarriage with

TABLE 11.2: Physical complications of anorexia nervosa

Organ system	Signs and symptoms	Findings
Whole body	Lethargy, drowsiness, malnutrition	Low BMI
Central nervous system	Poor concentration, depressed, irritable	
Cardiovascular	Palpitations, chest pain, dizziness, coldness of extremities	ECG changes, low blood pressure, bradycardia
Skeletal	Bone pain, swollen joints	Arrested skeletal growth, pathological fractures, osteoporosis
Muscular	Weakness and muscle ache	Muscle-wasting, muscle enzyme abnormalities
Reproductive	Absence of menstrual periods, loss of libido	Arrested sexual development, reduced oestrogen
Endocrine	Fatigue, cold intolerance	Low body temperature, low thyroid hormones
Haematological	Fatigue, bruising	Anaemia, decreased folate and B12 levels, thrombocytopenia
Gastrointestinal	Vomiting, abdominal pain, bloating, constipation	Abdominal distention
Urinary	Pitting oedema	Renal dysfunction
Skin	Change in hair	Lanugo

Sources: American Psychiatric Association (2000); James (2001)

bulimia (Micali, 2007). However, overall reduced pre-pregnancy weight and reduced weight gain in pregnancy has been associated with many fetal and infant complications (*see* Box 11.8).

It should also be noted that not just the calorie but also the maternal nutritional intake (in particular protein, vitamins and minerals) during the first trimester is correlated with birth weight (Abayomi, *et al.*, 2007) and will also influence other outcomes. Nutrient stores may be severely reduced in bulimia, although the woman may appear to have a healthy weight. Foods commonly used to binge on are usually sweet and high in fat and carbohydrate, which tend to be easy to swallow and vomit (Thompson, 2000). Women with bulimia may demonstrate symptoms such as irritability, depression or obsession, which can be signs of reduced nutrient levels (American Psychiatric Association, 2000).

Women with eating disorders appear to be prone to a number of obstetric complications in addition to those already mentioned relating to the fetus. Box 11.9 lists these. Again the evidence is limited and sometimes conflicting.

TABLE 11.3: Physical complications of bulimia

Organ system	Signs and symptoms	Findings
Cardiovascular	Weakness, palpitations	Cardiac abnormalities
Gastrointestinal	Abdominal pain, vomiting, constipation and bowel irregularities.	Gastro-oesophageal erosions, oesophagitis, gastro-oesophageal reflux
Reproductive	Fertility problems, scant menstrual periods	May have low oestrogen levels
Metabolic	Weakness, irritability, poor skin tone	Dehydration, electrolyte disturbances
Mouth and pharynx	Dental decay, swollen cheeks, inflammation of pharynx	Enlarged salivary glands
Skin	Callus formation on knuckles	

Sources: American Psychiatric Association (2000); James (2001); Orbanic (2001); Kondo and Sokol (2006)

BOX 11.8: FETAL/INFANT COMPLICATIONS ASSOCIATED WITH RESTRICTED EATING DISORDERS

- Intra-uterine infection
- Increased breech presentation
- Premature birth
- Low birth weight/IUGR
- Low Apgar scores
- Admission to neonatal unit
- Cleft lip/palate
- Microcephaly

(Abayomi, *et al.*, 2007; Hjern, *et al.*, 2006; Kouba, *et al.*, 2005; Lavender, 2007; Micali, *et al.*, 2007)

PRECONCEPTION CARE
Fertility

Older studies suggested that fertility is reduced in those who have a history of anorexia, but more recent work has not shown this association (Hjern, *et al.*, 2006). Of particular relevance to midwives is the high number of unplanned pregnancies in anorexic women (Morgan, *et al.*, 2006). It is important that these women understand that amenorrhea does not mean anovulation, and they may well ovulate unexpectedly, especially when receiving treatment. Women with bulimia rarely have a fertility problem as they are usually around a normal weight and are more likely to be in a sexual relationship than is a woman with anorexia (Micali, 2007). However, they are prone to unplanned pregnancies as menstrual irregularities are common (Morgan, *et al.*, 1999).

BOX 11.9: MATERNAL COMPLICATIONS ASSOCIATED WITH RESTRICTED EATING DISORDERS

- Miscarriage
- Hyperemesis gravidarum
- Anaemia
- Hypertension and/or pre-eclampsia
- Preterm labour
- Instrumental delivery and Caesarean section
- Delayed wound healing
- Psychological upset
- Postnatal depression

(Franko, *et al.*, 2001; Kouba, *et al.*, 2005; Little and Lowkes, 2000; Ward, 2008)

PREGNANCY CARE
Enquiring about restricted eating disorders

Booking is an opportunity to screen for eating disorders and could be the start of curing a woman, who may now be motivated to change because of the pregnancy, provided the midwife can identify there is a need and provides the appropriate support and referrals. Use of the eating disorder examination questionnaire (EDE-Q) may be helpful (Mond, *et al.*, 2004) but it should probably be used only by those with experience and knowledge. Symptoms in women who it is suggested should be screened for eating disorders are listed in Box 11.10.

BOX 11.10: CONSIDER SCREENING FOR EATING DISORDERS IF THE WOMAN HAS

- a low BMI
- an inappropriate concern about weight or weight gain
- previously used extreme weight control tactics
- erratic food consumption patterns
- gastrointestinal symptoms
- signs of repeated vomiting or starvation
- psychological problems.

(Morrill and Nichols-Richardson, 2001; NICE, 2004)

Although shame and secrecy result in a reluctance to reveal her situation (Ratnaike, 2007) and this probably increases in pregnancy when most women want to be seen as caring for themselves and their baby, a non-judgemental attitude from midwives can encourage a woman to disclose. Continuity of midwifery care may also be effective, as although the woman may not disclose at booking, if the subject is brought up she may then think about it and talk to a known midwife later. However, if an eating disorder is confirmed, care needs to be undertaken by the multidisciplinary team (Franko and

Spurrell, 2000). No matter how supportive or caring a midwife is, a woman with an eating disorder needs someone who is an expert and who will be a resource for her for longer than the pregnancy and puerperium, although during this time the midwife, especially if continuity can be maintained, is a vital member of the team.

It has been suggested that about two-thirds of women with anorexia improve during pregnancy, but one-third worsen (Birmingham and Beumont, 2004). In women with bulimia, symptoms often reduce in pregnancy but then return in the postnatal period (Blais, *et al.*, 2000).

It is possible that women are taking drugs that are not safe in pregnancy (Ward, 2008); for example, amphetamines are often abused for appetite suppression, and this subject must be addressed. Laxatives are also often misused, and this may result in serious nutrient deficiencies (Becker, *et al.*, 1999). There is also an increased incidence of hyperemesis associated with bulimia (Franko and Spurrell, 2000), so nutritional screening and support may be advisable. Ideally every woman with an eating disorder should have access to a dietician throughout her pregnancy and at least the puerperium, although long-term support may be necessary.

Cardiac screening may also be considered, as cardiac changes often occur in severe eating disorders, especially when there has been a weight loss of 30% or more (Becker, *et al.*, 1999), and these may be long-lasting and may impact on the pregnancy. Women with eating disorders may well have anaemia and hypertension or pre-eclampsia, which have been suggested to be more common (Little and Lowkes, 2000). Increased routine screening may therefore be necessary.

If the woman is depressed or expressing suicidal thoughts, which is not uncommon in some eating disorders (American Psychiatric Association, 2000), the midwife needs to make an urgent referral, and the woman may need admission for specialist help (James, 2001).

Weight should be monitored throughout the pregnancy, but some women find this distressing, and an open and honest discussion with the woman could help the midwife to develop strategies, for instance weighing the woman with her back to the scales. As with most women, working in partnership can be supportive and validating (Little and Lowkes, 2000), resulting in good outcomes. Positive reassurance by the midwife, with the emphasis on the health of the baby, rather than the increasing weight of the baby, may be effective.

LABOUR CARE

Increased complications in labour have been reported, such as premature rupture of membranes, more infection and increased rates of instrumental and operative deliveries. As it is possible that this woman has reduced nutrient levels and an IUGR fetus, these complications are understandable. Labour care needs to reflect her condition and specific needs, such as continuous fetal heart monitoring if the baby is known to be small, or cannulation in anticipation if the woman has anaemia.

POSTNATAL CARE

When undertaking routine postnatal care for women with eating disorders, the midwife should be aware of the increased potential for infection when levels of nutrients are low during the time of postnatal healing (Boyle, 2006).

Women with eating disorders have been known to report more difficulties in breastfeeding and cease earlier (Larrson and Andersson-Ellstron, 2003). Since these women will often experience an exaggerated sense of self-consciousness and awareness of their bodies, it is understandable that breastfeeding may be difficult for them. The midwife should also be aware of the potential danger of laxatives or other drugs in the breast milk.

The new mother may demonstrate an unrealistic assessment of her baby's needs, such as concerns over an 'overweight' baby or inadequate feeding (Russell, *et al.*, 1998; Stein, *et al.*, 1994). Research on children of women with eating disorders demonstrated that they tend to weigh less than those in the control group, and the child's weight is associated with the mother's concern about her own body shape (Stein, *et al.*, 1994).

Although many women decrease binging, vomiting and abuse of laxatives during pregnancy, most return postnatally (Blais, *et al.*, 2000; Kouba, *et al.*, 2005; Rocco, *et al.*, 2005). Morgan *et al.* (1999) studied bulimic women and found that despite symptoms improving during pregnancy most of them relapsed in the first 12 months after the birth, and over half experienced more severe symptoms than they did pre-pregnancy. Increased involvement with an eating disorders expert may be appropriate in the postnatal period. This underlines the importance of referral antenatally, as midwives may no longer be involved and need to prevent the woman having to make new relationships with a support person at this vulnerable time.

Many studies have demonstrated an increased rate of postnatal depression associated with eating disorders (Franko, *et al.*, 2001; Mitchell and Bulik, 2006). This may be associated with previous affective disorders (Franko and Spurrell, 2000) and the stresses of new motherhood together with dealing with the urge to regain a sense of control (after the 'loss of control' of pregnancy). Extra postnatal support by the midwife, health visitor or community mental health team may be necessary.

Caring for women with restrictive eating disorders can be challenging for the midwife, and accessing one of the following websites may provide extra information.

▶ National Centre for Eating Disorders: www.eating-disorders.org.uk
▶ Eating Disorders Association: www.edauk.com
▶ Anorexia and Bulimia Care (ABC): www.anorexiabulimiacare.co.uk

REFERENCES

Abayomi J, Watkinson H, Topping J, *et al.* Obesity and underweight among first trimester pregnant women. *Br J Midwifery.* 2007; **15**(3): 143–7.

Allaire A, Fisch J, McMahon M. Subcutaneous drain vs suture in obese women undergoing Caesarean delivery. A prospective, randomized trial. *J Reprod Med.* 2000; **45**: 327–31.

American Psychiatric Association. Practice guideline for the treatment of patients with eating disorders. *Am J Psychiatry.* 2000; **157**(1): 1–39.

Amir L, Donath S. A systematic review of maternal obesity and breastfeeding intention, initiation and duration. *BMC Pregnancy Childbirth.* 2007; **7**: 9.

Amorim AR, Linne YM, Lourenco PMC. Diet or exercise, or both, for weight reduction in women after childbirth. *Cochrane Database Syst Rev.* 2007; **1**: CD005627.

Anon. Obese mums given healthy lifestyle advice. *Pract Midwife.* 2007; **10**(9): 13.

Balen AH. Polycystic ovary syndrome, obesity and reproductive function. In: Baker P, Balen

A, Poston L, *et al.*, editors. *Obesity and Reproductive Health.* London: RCOG Press; 2007. pp. 69–80.

Barau G, Robillard P, Hulsey T, *et al.* Linear association between maternal pre-pregnancy body mass index and risk of Caesarean section in term deliveries. *BJOG.* 2006; **113**: 1173–7.

Becker A, Grinspoon S, Herzog D. Current concepts: eating disorders. *N Engl J Med.* 1999; **340**(14): 1092–1097.

Bhattacharya S, Campbell D, Liston W, *et al.* Effect of body mass index on pregnancy outcomes in nulliparous women delivering singleton babies. *BMC Public Health.* 2007; **7**: 168.

Birmingham C, Beumont P. *Medical Management of Eating Disorders.* Cambridge: Cambridge University Press; 2004.

Blais M, Becker A, Burwell R, *et al.* Pregnancy: outcome and impact on symptomatology in a cohort of eating-disordered women. *Int J Eat Disord.* 2000; **27**: 140–9.

Bodnar L. Maternal obesity and adverse pregnancy outcomes: the role of nutrition and physical activity. In: Baker P, Balen A, Poston L, *et al.*, editors. *Obesity and Reproductive Health.* London: RCOG Press; 2007.

Bodnar L, Ness R, Markovic N, *et al.* The risk of preeclampsia rises with increasing prepregnancy body mass index. *Ann Epidemiol.* 2005; **15**: 475–82.

Bothamley J. Thromboembolism in pregnancy. In Boyle M, editor. *Emergencies Around Childbirth.* Oxford: Radcliffe Publishing; 2002.

Boyle M. *Wound Healing in Midwifery.* Oxford: Radcliffe Publishing; 2006.

British Nutrition Foundation. *Nutrient Requirements and Recommendations 2004.* Available at: www. nutrition.org.uk/upload/Nutritient%20Requirements%20and%20recommendations%20 pdf(1).pdf (accessed 12 December 2008).

Brost B, Godenberg R, Mercer B, *et al.* The preterm prediction study: association of Caesarean delivery with increases in maternal weight and body mass index. *Am J Obstet Gynecol.* 1997; **177**: 333–7.

Carpenter M. The role of exercise in pregnant women with diabetes mellitus. *Clin Obstet Gynecol.* 2000; **43**: 56–64.

Catalano P. Management of obesity in pregnancy. *Obstet Gynecol.* 2007; **109**(2 Pt. 1): 419–33.

Cedergren M. Maternal morbid obesity and the risk of adverse pregnancy outcome. *Obstet Gynecol.* 2004; **103**(2): 219–24.

Chu S, Kim S, Lau J, *et al.* Maternal obesity and risk of stillbirth: a meta-analysis. *Am J Obstet Gynecol.* 2007; **197**(3): 223–8.

Claesson I, Josefsson A, Cedergren M, *et al.* Consumer satisfaction with a weight-gain intervention programme for obese pregnant women. *Midwifery.* 2008a; **24**: 163–7.

Claesson I, Sydsjo G, Brynhidsen J, *et al.* Weight gain restriction for obese pregnant women: a case-controlled intervention study. *BJOG.* 2008b; **115**(1): 44–50.

Clark A, Thornley B, Tomlinson L, *et al.* Weight loss in obese infertile women results in improvement in reproductive outcome for all forms of fertility treatment. *Hum Reprod.* 1998; **13**: 1502–5.

Cogswell M, Serdula M, Hunderford D, *et al.* Gestational weight gain among average-weight and overweight women – what is excessive? *Am J Obstet Gynecol.* 1995; **172**: 705–12.

Cogswell M, Scanlon K, Fein S, *et al.* Medically advised, mother's personal target, and actual weight gain during pregnancy. *Obstet Gynecol.* 1999; **94**: 616–22.

Colquitt J, Clegg A, Loveman E, *et al.* Surgery for morbid obesity. *Cochrane Database Syst Rev.* 2005; **4**: CD003641.

Dao T, Kuhn J, Ehmer D, *et al.* Pregnancy outcomes after gastric-bypass surgery. *Am J Surg.* 2006; **192**: 762–6.

Department of Health. *At Least Five a Week: evidence on the impact of physical activity and its relationship to health. A report from the chief medical officer.* London: Department of Health Publications; 2004a.

Department of Health. *Health Survey for England 2003.* London: Department of Health; 2004b.

Dixon J, Dixon M, O'Brien P. Birth outcomes in obese women after laparoscopic adjustable gastric banding. *Obstet Gynecol.* 2005; **106**: 965–72.

Douki S, Ben Zineb S, Nacef F, *et al.* Women's mental health in the Muslim world: cultural, religious, and social issues. *J Affect Disord.* 2007; **102**(1–3): 177–89.

Dresner M. Obesity and anaesthesia. In: Baker P, Balen A, Poston L, Sattar N, editors. *Obesity and Reproductive Health.* London: RCOG Press; 2007. pp. 175–80

Dunne F. Type 2 diabetes and pregnancy. *Semin Fetal Neonatal Med.* 2005; **10**(4): 333–9.

Ehrenberg H, Durwald C, Catalano P, *et al.* The influence of obesity and diabetes on the risk of Caesarean delivery. *Am J Obstet Gynecol.* 2004; **191**: 969–74.

Fedorsak P, Storeng R, Dale P, *et al.* Obesity is a risk factor for early pregnancy loss after IVF or ICSI. *Acta Obstet Gynecol Scand.* 2000; **79**: 43–8.

Food Standards Agency (FSA) Eating for breastfeeding. 2002. Available at: www.foodstandards. gov.uk/multimedia/pdfs/life02breastfeeding.pdf (accessed 12 December 2008).

Food Standards Agency (FSA) The eat well plate. 2007. Available at: www.eatwell.gov.uk/ healthydiet/ (accessed 12 December 2008).

Fox K. Obesity Resource Information Centre (ORIC) fact sheet: physical activity and obesity. Woodford Green: Association for the Study of Obesity; 2005. Available at: www.aso.org. uk/portal.aspx?mlmenuid=154&TargetPortal=36&ApplicationID=116&MID=&offset= (accessed 12 December 2008).

Franko D, Blais M, Becker A, *et al.* Pregnancy complications and neonatal outcomes in women with eating disorders. *Am J Psychiatry.* 2001; **158**(9): 1461–6.

Franko D, Spurrell E. Detection and management of eating disorders during pregnancy. *Obstet Gynecol.* 2000; **95**(6 Pt. 1): 942–6.

Galtier F, Raingeard I, Renard E, *et al.* Optimizing the outcome of pregnancy in obese women: from pregestational to long-term management. *Diabetes Metab.* 2008; **34**: 19–25.

Galtier-Dereure F, Boegner C, Bringer J. Obesity and pregnancy: complications and cost. *Am J Clin Nutr.* 2000; **71**(Suppl. 5): 1242s–8s.

Gate E, Ramsay J. Antenatal complications of maternal obesity: miscarriage, fetal abnormalities, maternal gestational diabetes and pre-eclampsia. In: Baker P, Balen A, Poston L, Sattar N, editors. *Obesity and Reproductive Health.* London: RCOG Press; 2007. pp. 127–44.

Gesink Law D, Maclehose R, Longnecker M. Obesity and time to pregnancy. *Hum Reprod.* 2007; **22**(2): 414–20.

Glazer N, Hendrickson A, Schellenbaurn G, *et al.* Weight change and the risk of gestational diabetes in obese women. *Epidemiology.* 2004; **15**: 733–7.

Hall L, Neubert A. Obesity and pregnancy. *Obstetric Gynecol Surv.* 2005; **60**: 253–60.

Hart R, Hickey M, Franks S. Definitions, prevalence and symptoms of polycystic ovaries and polycystic ovary syndrome. *Best Pract Res Clin Obstet Gynaecol.* 2004; **18**: 671–83.

Hendler I, Blackwell S, Bujold E, *et al.* The impact of maternal obesity on midtrimester sonographic visualization of fetal cardiac and craniospinal structures. *Int J Obes Relat Metab Disord.* 2004; **28**: 1607–11.

Heslehurst N, Lang R, Rankin J, *et al.* Obesity in pregnancy: a study of the impact of maternal obesity on NHS maternity services. *BJOG.* 2007; **114**(3): 334–42.

Hjern A, Lindberg L, Lindblad F. Outcome and prognostic factors for adolescent female in-patients with anorexia nervosa: 9–14-year old follow-up. *Br J Psychiatry.* 2006; **189**: 428–82.

Hoare J, Henderson L. *The National Diet, Nutrition Survey: adults aged 19 to 64 years: summary report.* (The National Diet, Nutrition Survey Volume 5). London: Stationery Office; 2004.

Irvine L, Shaw R. The impact of obesity on obstetric outcomes. *Curr Obstet Gynecol.* 2006; **16**(4): 242–6.

Izci B, Vennelle M, Liston W, *et al.* Sleeping-disordered breathing and upper airway size in pregnancy and post-partum. *Eur Respir J.* 2006; **27**: 321–7.

James D. Eating disorders, fertility and pregnancy: relationships and complications. *J Perinat Neonatal Nurs.* 2001; **15**(2): 36–48.

Juhasz G, Gyamfi C, Gyamfi P, *et al.* Effect of body mass index and excessive weight gain on success of vaginal birth after Caesarean delivery. *Obstet Gynecol.* 2005; **106**: 741–6.

Kaiser P, Kirby R. Obesity as a factor for Caesarean section in a low risk population. *Obstet Gynecol.* 2001; **97**(1): 39–43.

Kiel D, Dodson E, Artal R, *et al.* Gestation weight gain and pregnancy outcomes in obese women: how much is enough? *Obstet Gynecol.* 2007; **110**(4): 752–8.

Kiess W, Petzold S, Töpfer M, *et al.* Adiopocytes and adipose tissue. *Best Pract Res Clin Endocrinol Metab.* 2008; **22**(1): 135–53.

Kondo D, Sokol M. Eating disorders in primary care. *Post Med.* 2006; **119**(3): 59–65.

Kouba S, Hallstrom T, Lindholm C, *et al.* Pregnancy and neonatal outcomes in women with eating disorders. *Obstet Gynecol.* 2005; **105**: 255–60.

Kristensen J, Vestergaard M, Wisborg K, *et al.* Pre-pregnancy weight and the risk of stillbirth and neonatal death. *BJOG.* 2005; **112**: 403–8.

Kushner R, Foster G. Obesity and quality of life. *Nutrition.* 2000; **16**(10): 947–52.

Larrson G, Andersson-Ellstron A. Experience of pregnancy-related body shape changes and of breast-feeding in women with a history of eating disorders. *Eur Eat Disord Rev.* 2003; **11**: 116–24.

Lashen H, Fear K, Sturdee D. Obesity is associated with increased risk of first trimester and recurrent miscarriage: matched case-control study. *Hum Reprod.* 2004; **19**: 1644–6.

Lavender V. Body image: change, dissatisfaction and disturbance. In: Price S, editor. *Mental Health in Pregnancy and Childbirth.* Oxford: Churchill Livingstone; 2007. pp. 123–46.

Lean MEJ. *Clinical Handbook of Weight Management.* 2nd ed. London: Martin Dunitz; 2003.

Lewis G, editor. The Confidential Enquiry into Maternal and Child Health (CEMACH). *Saving Mothers' Lives: reviewing maternal deaths to make motherhood safer 2003–2005. The Seventh Report on Confidential Enquiries into Maternal Deaths in the UK.* London: CEMACH; 2007.

Little L, Lowkes E. Critical issues in the care of pregnant women with eating disorders and the impact on their children. *J Midwifery Womens Health.* 2000; **45**(4): 301–7.

Macdiarmid J, Blundell J. Assessing dietary intake: who, what and why of under-reporting. *Nutr Res Rev.* 1998; **11**: 231–53.

Mazzeo S, Slof-Op't Landt MC, Jones I, *et al.* Associations among postpartum depression, eating disorders, and perfectionism in a population-based sample of adult women. *Int J Eat Disord.* 2006; **39**(3): 202–11.

Mhyre J, Greenfield M, Polley L. Survey of obstetric providers' views on the anesthetic risks of maternal obesity. *Int J Obstet Anesth.* 2007; **16**(4): 316–22.

Micali N. Eating disorders and their effect on pregnancy. In: Baker P, Balen A, Poston L, *et al.*, editors. *Obesity and Reproductive Health.* London: RCOG Press; 2007. pp. 23–30.

Micali N, Simonoff E, Treasure J. Risk of major adverse perinatal outcomes in women with eating disorders. *Br J Psychiatry.* 2007; **190**: 255–9.

Mitchell A, Bulik C. Eating disorders and women's health: an update. *J Midwifery Womens Health.* 2006; **51**(3): 193–201.

Mond J, Hay P, Rodgers B, *et al.* Validity of the eating disorder examination questionnaire (EDE-Q) in screening for eating disorders in community samples. *Behav Res Ther.* 2004; **42**(5): 551–67.

Morgan J, Lacey J, Sedgwick P. Impact of pregnancy on bulimia nervosa. *Br J Psychiatry.* 1999; **174**: 35–140.

Morgan J, Lacey J, Chung E. Risk of postnatal depression, miscarriage and preterm birth in bulimia nervosa: retrospective controlled study. *Psychosom Med.* 2006; **68**: 487–92.

Morrill E, Nichols-Richardson H. Bulimia during pregnancy: a review. *J Am Diet Assoc.* 2001; **101**(4): 448–54.

National Institute for Health and Clinical Excellence (NICE). *Eating Disorders: core interventions in the treatment and management of anorexia nervosa, bulimia nervosa and related eating disorders: NICE guideline 9.* London: NICE; 2004. www.nice.org.uk/Guidance/CG9

National Institute for Health and Clinical Excellence (NICE). *Obesity: the prevention, identification, assessment and management of overweight and obesity in adults and children: NICE guideline 43.* London: NICE; 2006. www.nice.org.uk/Guidance/CG43

National Institute for Health and Clinical Excellence (NICE). *Antenatal Care: routine care for the healthy pregnant woman: NICE guideline 62.* London: NICE; 2008. www.nice.org.uk/Guidance/CG62

Nelson S, Fleming R. Obesity and reproduction: impact and interventions. *Curr Opin Obstet Gynecol.* 2007; **19**(4): 384–9.

Nohr E, Bech B, Vaeth M, *et al.* Obesity, gestational weight gain and preterm birth: a study within the Danish national birth cohort. *Paediatr Perinat Epidemiol.* 2007; **21**(1): 4–14.

Norman RJ, Noakes M, Wu R, *et al.* Improving reproductive performance in overweight/obese women with effective weight management. *Hum Reprod Update.* 2004; **10**(3): 267–80.

Obesity Resource Information Centre (ORIC). *Energy Balance.* Woodford Green: Association for the Study of Obesity; 2000. Available at: www.aso.org.uk/portal.aspx?mlmenuid=162&TargetPortal=36&ApplicationID=116&MID=&offset= (accessed 12 December 2008).

O'Brien T, Ray J, Chan W. Maternal body mass index and the risk of preeclampsia: a systematic review. *Epidemiology.* 2003; **14**: 368–74.

Ockenden J. Midwifery basics: diet matters (3). Obesity in pregnancy. *Pract Midwife.* 2007; **10**(11): 39–45.

Ogden J. *The Psychology of Eating: from healthy to disordered behaviour.* Oxford: Blackwell. 2003.

Ogston N. Obesity Resource Information Centre. *Understanding Obesity – Adipokines: signals derive.* Woodford Green: Association for the Study of Obesity; 2006. Available at: www.aso.org.uk/portal.aspx?mlmenuid=2036&TargetPortal=36&ApplicationID=116&MID=&offset= (accessed 12 December 2008).

Oken E, Gillman M. Fetal origins of obesity. *Obes Res.* 2003; **11**(4): 496–506.

Orbanic S. Understanding bulimia: signs, symptoms and the human experience. *Am J Nurs.* 2001; **10**(3): 35–42.

Pereira MA, Kartashov AI, Ebbeling CB, *et al.* Fast-food habits, weight gain, and insulin resistance (the CARDIA study): 15-year prospective analysis. *Lancet.* 2005; **365**: 36–42.

Perry M. *Eating Disorders for Pregnancy and the Primary Care Team.* Dinton: Mark Allen; 2002.

Powell K. Obesity: the two faces of fat. *Nature.* 2007; **447**(7144): 525–7.

Ramsay JE, Ferrell WR, Crawford L, *et al.* Maternal obesity is associated with dysregulation of metabolic, vascular and inflammatory pathways. *J Clin Endocrinol Metab.* 2002; **87**(9): 4231–7.

Rasmussen K, Kjolhede C. Prepregnant overweight and obesity diminish the prolactin response to suckling in the first week postpartum. *Pediatrics.* 2004; **111**: 465–71.

Ratnaike D. Eating disorders: shame and secrecy. *Midwives RCM.* 2007; **10**(4): 6.

Ravelli A, van der Meulen J, Michels R, *et al.* Glucose tolerance in adults after prenatal exposure to famine. *Lancet.* 1998; **351**: 173–7.

Reece A. Perspectives on obesity, pregnancy and birth outcomes in the United States: the scope of the problem. *Am J Obstet Gynecol.* 2008; **198**: 23–7.

Richens Y. Tackling maternal obesity: suggestions for midwives. *Br J Midwifery.* 2008a; **16**(1): 14–19.

Richens Y. Bring back the scales. *Br J Midwifery.* 2008b; **16**(8): 533–4.

Robinson S, Yu C. The epidemiology of obesity and pregnancy complications. In: Baker P, Balen A, Poston L, *et al.*, editors. *Obesity and Reproductive Health.* London: RCOG Press; 2007. pp. 113–26.

Rocco P, Orbitello B, Perinik L, *et al.* Effects of pregnancy on eating attitudes and disorders: a prospective study. *J Psychosom Res.* 2005; **59**: 175–9.

Roush S, Bell L. Obstructive sleep apnea in pregnancy. *J Am Board Fam Pract.* 2004; **17**: 292–4.

Russell G, Treasure J, Eisler I. Mothers with anorexia nervosa that underfeed their children: their recognition and management. *Psychol Med.* 1998; **28**: 93–108.

Salihu H, Dunlop A, Hedayatzadeh M, *et al.* Extreme obesity and risk of stillbirth among black and white gravidas. *Obstet Gynecol.* 2007; **110**(3): 552–7.

Saravanakumar K, Rao S, Cooper G. Obesity and obstetric anaesthesia. *Anaesthesia.* 2006; **61**: 36–48.

Sattar N. Obesity: age, ethnic and social variations. In: Baker P, Balen A, Poston L, *et al.*, editors. *Obesity and Reproductive Health.* London: RCOG Press; 2007. pp. 31–8.

Sattar N, Clark P, Holmes A, *et al.* Antenatal waist circumference and hypertension risk. *Obstet Gynecol.* 2001; **97**: 268–71.

Sebire N, Jolly M, Harris J, *et al.* Maternal obesity and pregnancy outcome: a study of 287,213 pregnancies in London. *Int J Obes.* 2001; **25**: 1175–82.

Serci I. Midwifery basics: diet matters (2). Maternal overweight in pregnancy. *Pract Midwife.* 2007; **10**(10): 36–42.

Serci I. Midwifery basics: diet matters (4). Weight gain in pregnancy. *Pract Midwife.* 2008; **11**(1): 29–33.

Shaw K, O'Rourke P, Del Mar C, *et al.* Psychological interventions for overweight and obesity. *Cochrane Database Syst Rev.* 2005; **2**: CD003818.

Sheiner E, Levy A, Menes T, *et al.* Maternal obesity as an independent risk factor of Caesarean delivery. *Paediatr Perinat Epidemiol.* 2004; **18**: 196–201.

Soens M, Birnbach D, Ranasinghe J, *et al.* Obstetric anesthesia for the obese and morbidly obese patient: an ounce of prevention is worth more than a pound of treatment. *Acta Anaesthesiolog Scand.* 2008; **52**(1): 6–19.

Steffan KJ, Mitchell JE, Roerig JL, *et al.* The eating disorders medicine cabinet revisited: a clinician's guide to ipecac and laxatives. *Int J Eat Disord.* 2007; **40**(4): 360–8.

Stein A, Woolley H, Cooper S, *et al.* An observational study of mothers with eating disorders and their infants. *J Child Psychol Psychiatr.* 1994; **35**: 733–48.

Stephansson O, Dickman P, Johansson A, *et al.* Maternal weight, pregnancy weight gain and the risk of antepartum stillbirth. *Am J Obstet Gynecol.* 2001; **184**: 463–9.

Stotland N. Obesity and pregnancy. *BMJ.* 2009; **338**: 107–10.

Thompson J. Eating disorders. *Community Pract.* 2000; **73**(5): 613–14.

Villamor E, Cnattingius S. Interpregnancy weight change and risk of adverse pregnancy outcomes: a population-based study. *Lancet.* 2006; **308**: 1164–70.

Waller D, Shaw G, Rasmussen S, *et al.* Prepregnancy obesity as a risk factor for structural birth defects. *Arch Pediatr Adolesc Med.* 2007; **61**(8): 745–50.

Walsh JM, Murphy DJ. Weight and pregnancy. *BMJ.* 2007; **335**: 169.

Ward V. Eating disorders in pregnancy. *BMJ.* 2008; **336**: 93–6.

Watkins M, Ramussen S, Honein M, *et al.* Maternal obesity and risk for birth defects. *Pediatrics.* 2003; **111**(5): 1152–8.

Werler M, Louik C, Shapiro S, *et al.* Prepregnant weight in relation to risk of neural tube defects. *J Am Med Assoc.* 1996; **275**: 1089–92.

Wilding J. Overview and prevalence of obesity in the UK. In: Baker P, Balen A, Poston L, *et al.*, editors. *Obesity and Reproductive Health.* London: RCOG Press; 2007. pp. 3–10.

Yu C, Teoh T, Robinson S. Obesity in pregnancy. *BJOG.* 2006; **113**: 1117–25.

Zaninotto P, Wardle H, Stamatakis E, *et al. Forecasting Obesity to 2010.* London: Department of Health; 2006.

Zerbe K. Eating disorders in the 21st century: identification, management, and prevention in obstetrics and gynecology. *Best Pract Res Clin Obstet Gynaecol.* 2007; **21**(2): 331–3.

Index